Hair Restoration

Editors

RAYMOND J. KONIOR
STEVEN P. GABEL

FACIAL PLASTIC SURGERY CLINICS OF NORTH AMERICA

www.facialplastic.theclinics.com

Consulting Editor
J. REGAN THOMAS

August 2013 • Volume 21 • Number 3

ELSEVIER

1600 John F. Kennedy Boulevard • Suite 1800 • Philadelphia, Pennsylvania, 19103-2899

http://www.theclinics.com

FACIAL PLASTIC SURGERY CLINICS OF NORTH AMERICA Volume 21, Number 3
August 2013 ISSN 1064-7406, ISBN-13: 978-0-323-18603-2

Editor: Joanne Husovski

Facial Plastic Surgery Clinics of North America (ISSN 1064-7406) is published quarterly by Elsevier Inc., 360 Park Avenue South, New York, NY 10010-1710. Months of issue are February, May, August, and November. Business and Editorial Offices: 1600 John F. Kennedy Blvd., Suite 1800, Philadelphia, PA 19103-2899. Periodicals postage paid at New York, NY, and additional mailing offices. Subscription prices are $373.00 per year (US individuals), $526.00 per year (US institutions), $425.00 per year (Canadian individuals), $628.00 per year (Canadian institutions), $509.00 per year (foreign individuals), $628.00 per year (foreign institutions), $153.00 per year (US students), and $245.00 per year (foreign students). Foreign air speed delivery is included in all *Clinics* subscription prices. All prices are subject to change without notice. POSTMASTER: Send address changes to *Facial Plastic Surgery Clinics*, Elsevier Health Sciences Division, Subscription Customer Service, 3251 Riverport Lane, Maryland Heights, MO 63043. **Customer service: 1-800-654-2452 (US and Canada); 1-314-447-8871 (outside US and Canada); Fax: 314-447-8029; E-mail:journalscustomerservice-usa@elsevier.com (for print support); journalsonline support-usa@elsevier.com (for online support).**

Reprints. For copies of 100 or more of articles in this publication, please contact the Commercial Reprints Department, Elsevier Inc., 360 Park Avenue South, New York, NY 10010-1710. Tel.: 212-633-3874; Fax: 212-633-3820; E-mail: reprints@elsevier.com.

Facial Plastic Surgery Clinics of North America is covered in *MEDLINE/PubMed* (*Index Medicus*).

Contributors

CONSULTING EDITOR

J. REGAN THOMAS, MD, FACS
Professor and Chairman, Department of
Otolaryngology, University of Illinois at
Chicago, Chicago, Illinois

EDITORS

RAYMOND J. KONIOR, MD, FACS
Clinical Professor, Department of
Otolaryngology – Head and Neck Surgery,
Loyola University Medical Center, Maywood,
Illinois; Chicago Hair Institute, Oakbrook
Terrace, Illinois

STEVEN P. GABEL, MD, FACS
Gabel Hair Restoration Center, Hillsboro,
Oregon

AUTHORS

MICHAEL L. BEEHNER, MD
Saratoga Hair Transplant Center, Saratoga
Springs, New York

KENNETH A. BUCHWACH, MD, FACS
Private Practice, Facial Plastic Surgery,
Kansas City, Missouri

JASON P. CHAMPAGNE, MD
Medical Director, The Champagne Center for
Facial Plastic Surgery and Hair Restoration,
Baton Rouge, Louisiana

JOHN P. COLE, MD
Private Practice, Alpharetta, Georgia

JERRY E. COOLEY, MD
Private Practice, Carolina Dermatology Hair
Center, Charlotte, North Carolina

JEAN DEVROYE, MD
International Society Hair Restoration Surgery
Member; Belgium Board of Medicine,
Etterbeek, Belgium

JEFFREY EPSTEIN, MD, FACS
Private Practice, Foundation for Hair
Restoration, Miami, Florida; Private Practice,

Foundation for Hair Restoration, New York
City, New York; Clinical Assistant Professor,
University of Miami, Florida

**BESSAM FARJO, MB, ChB, BAO, LRCPSI,
FICS**
Diplomate, American Board of Hair Restoration
Surgery; Fellow, International College of
Surgeons; Fellow and Medical Director,
Institute of Trichologists (UK); Hair Restoration
Surgeon and Director, Farjo Hair Institute,
Manchester, United Kingdom; Farjo Hair
Institute, London, United Kingdom

NILOFER FARJO, MB, ChB, BAO, LRCPSI
Diplomate, American Board of Hair Restoration
Surgery; Member, International Society of Hair
Restoration Surgery; Co-Editor, Hair
Transplant Forum International; Fellow,
Institute of Trichologists (UK); Hair Restoration
Surgeon and Director, Farjo Hair Institute,
Manchester, United Kingdom; Farjo Hair
Institute, London, United Kingdom

STEVEN P. GABEL, MD, FACS
Gabel Hair Restoration Center, Hillsboro,
Oregon

JAMES A. HARRIS, MD, FACS
Medical Director of the Hair Sciences Center of
Colorado, Greenwood Village, Colorado

CHRIS A. INGRAHAM, PhD
Aderans Research Institute, Marietta, Georgia

SHELDON S. KABAKER, MD, FACS
Private Practice, Oakland, California; Clinical
Professor, Department of Otolaryngology-
Head and Neck Surgery, University of
California, San Francisco, San Francisco,
California

JINO KIM, MD
Medical Director, New Hair Institute of Korea,
Yeoksam-dong, Korea

RAYMOND J. KONIOR, MD, FACS
Clinical Professor, Department of
Otolaryngology – Head and Neck Surgery,
Loyola University Medical Center, Maywood,
Illinois; Chicago Hair Institute, Oakbrook
Terrace, Illinois

E. ANTONIO MANGUBAT, MD
La Belle Vie Cosmetic Surgery and Hair
Restoration, Tukwila, Washington

BRYAN T. MARSHALL, PhD
Aderans Research Institute, Marietta, Georgia

ARON G. NUSBAUM, MD
Hair Transplant Institute of Miami, Coral
Gables, Florida

BERNARD P. NUSBAUM, MD
Hair Transplant Institute of Miami, Coral
Gables, Florida

JAE P. PAK, MD
Medical Director, New Hair Institute, A Medical
Group, Los Angeles, California

WILLIAM R. RASSMAN, MD
President, New Hair Institute, Los Angeles,
California

NICOLE ROGERS, MD, FAAD
Private Practice, Metairie, Louisiana; Assistant
Clinical Professor, Tulane University School of
Medicine, New Orleans, Louisiana

PAUL T. ROSE, MD
Hair Transplant Institute of Miami, Coral
Gables, Florida

PAUL SHAPIRO, MD
Private Practice, Shapiro Medical Group,
Minneapolis, Minnesota

RONALD SHAPIRO, MD
Adjunct Instructor, Department of
Dermatology, University of Minnesota; Private
Practice, Shapiro Medical Group, Minneapolis,
Minnesota

CAM SIMMONS, MD
Diplomate of the ABHRS; Seager Hair
Transplant Centre, Toronto, Ontario, Canada

SANUSI UMAR, MD
Dermatology Division, Department of
Medicine, University of California, Los Angeles,
Los Angeles; DermHair Clinic, Redondo
Beach, California

ROBIN H. UNGER, MD
Assistant Professor, Department of
Dermatology, Mount Sinai Hospital, New York
City, New York

KEN WASHENIK, MD, PhD
Aderans Research Institute, Marietta, Georgia;
Bosley, Beverly Hills, California

XUNWEI WU, PhD
Aderans Research Institute, Marietta, Georgia

Contents

Hairlines change shape with age, starting at birth. A good head of hair is frequently present some time after ages 3 to 5 years. The look of childhood has its corresponding hairline, and, as the child grows and develops into adulthood, facial morphology migrate changes from a childlike look to a more mature look. This article discusses the dynamics of hairline evolution and the phenotypic variations of the front and side hairlines in men and women. A modeling system is introduced that provides a common language to define the various anatomic points of the full range of hairlines.

It is crucial that hair restoration surgeons understand the basic clinical diagnosis and pathologic condition of other hair loss conditions that are not always amenable to successful hair transplantation. In this article nonscarring and scarring mimickers of androgenetic alopecia are discussed. Nonscarring conditions include alopecia areata, telogen effluvium, and tinea capitis. Some of the more common scarring alopecias include lichen planopilaris, frontal fibrosing alopecia, and central centrifugal cicatricial alopecia. Less common inflammatory conditions include pseudopelade of Brocq, discoid lupus erythematosus, and folliculitis decalvans.

This article is an update of the currently available options for medical therapies to treat androgenetic alopecia in men and women. Emerging novel therapeutic modalities with potential for treating these patients are discussed. Because androgenetic alopecia is progressive in nature, stabilization of the process using medical therapy is an important adjunct to any surgical hair-restoration plan.

Patient consultation, examination, and selection are crucial for successful outcomes in hair restoration surgery. The hair restoration surgeon must take a holistic approach in identifying those patients who are and who are not candidates for surgery. In this article, an overview of the consultation, pertinent physical examination features relating to patient candidacy, and several treatment paradigms are discussed. Additionally, those findings that may lead to poor results and conditions that are contraindications to hair restoration surgery are reviewed.

The authors' techniques for creating a natural frontal hairline are presented
in a video that accompanies this article

> Creating a natural hairline is one of the most important elements of a successful hair
> transplant. This article discusses the key skills needed to design a natural hairline.
> These are locating borders of the hairline as well as understanding and being able
> to mimic the visual characteristics of a hairline. Methods to locate the major borders
> and how to adjust them based on donor/recipient ratio are discussed. The visual
> characteristics of different hairline zones are described as well as techniques to
> recreate these characteristics using follicular unit grafting.

> The strip technique remains the most popular method of harvesting grafts. The chal-
> lenge in every patient is to maximize the number of grafts while minimizing the scar.
> Fortunately, there are many ways to ensure that the donor site will be inconspicuous.
> This article reviews the details of planning for follicle graft harvesting, including for-
> mulae for assessing scalp laxity and calculating strip dimensions. The procedure is
> discussed in detail, from preparation of the donor site and estimation of graft total
> through closure of the incision. The author presents his preferences for the tech-
> nique with rationale and surgical tips.

> The purpose of this article is to introduce the reader to the topic of follicular unit
> extraction (FUE) and to present an overview of the value of FUE to patients and phy-
> sicians. In addition to this, the various methods and instrumentation for performing
> this method of graft harvest are discussed as well as some of the technique's inher-
> ent advantages and disadvantages. Topics unique to FUE, including body hair graft-
> ing, plug/minigrafts repair, and donor area management are addressed as well.

> This article covers how to manage patients with extensive hair loss in whom com-
> plete, dense coverage is not possible. In addition to discussing planning a transplant
> pattern for already bald men, I discuss a conservative approach for recognizing and
> transplanting younger patients who have telltale warning signs that may evolve to
> extensive hair loss. For both groups, a variant of a frontal forelock-type pattern is
> usually the best course to follow.

> Treatment of alopecia of the crown possesses several unique challenges for hair res-
> toration physicians. In this article, the distinctive anatomic features and specific
> management paradigms related to the crown are discussed. This review also offers
> details on which surgical technique to implement for obtaining the most natural
> result possible that also yields the best possible apparent density.

> Female hair loss is a devastating issue for women that has only relatively recently
> been publicly acknowledged as a significant problem. Hair transplant surgery is
> extremely successful in correcting the most cosmetically problematic areas of alo-
> pecia. This article discusses the surgical technique of hair transplantation in women
> in detail, including pearls to reduce postoperative sequelae and planning strategies
> to ensure a high degree of patient satisfaction. A brief overview of some of the med-
> ical treatments found to be helpful in slowing or reversing female pattern hair loss is
> included, addressing the available hormonal and topical treatments.

> Surgical hair restoration allows male and female patients to achieve aesthetically
> natural results. The term megasession refers to transplanting greater then 3000 fol-
> licular unit grafts in a single procedure. By transplanting a large number of grafts,
> megasessions are capable of definitively treating a significant area of the scalp in
> 1 session. Patients must be carefully selected to determine whether they are appro-
> priate candidates for an extended procedure. An experienced and well-organized
> surgical team is mandatory to meet the demands of this technically challenging
> and lengthy procedure. This article reviews the indications, contraindications, and
> technical perspectives surrounding megasession hair transplantation.

> Dense packing is the philosophy of fitting more than 30 to 35 follicular unit grafts per
> square centimeter in one operation. The aim is to produce a more even, consistent,
> and natural looking flow of hair after just one procedure. Although desirable in prin-
> ciple, not all patients are suitable candidates nor is it possible to achieve in certain
> patients (eg, coarse or curly hair). Patients who have sufficient donor availability, rea-
> sonably stable hair loss, and high hair-to-skin color ratios are the ideal candidates.
> The authors highlight their philosophies and strategies for dense packing.

> Success in follicular unit extraction requires an understanding of forces, fluid dynam-
> ics, instrumentation, and individual patient variation. Sharp punches require a lower
> axial and tangential force to dissect follicular groups. The angle of hair emergence
> and the size of a punch influence the wound size and the depth of an incision. A pro-
> cedure must be individualized based on surface follicular group characteristics; hair
> splay; and strength of attachment between the outer root sheath, inner root sheath,
> and adipose with regard to hair follicles.

> Excellent surgical results and high patient satisfaction with hair transplantation
> depend on attaining optimal growth. Unfortunately, even experienced surgeons

acknowledge that graft survival often is not as high as is commonly stated. Hair transplant surgeons should be thoroughly familiar with the many variables that affect graft survival and refine their surgical techniques accordingly. This article provides a brief overview of the key factors that most significantly influence graft survival, including graft trauma, vascular/oxygenation factors, and biochemical injury.

Refinements in hair transplantation techniques allow the experienced surgeon to create natural-appearing facial hair transplants. Restoring eyebrows, beards/goatees, and sideburns have all become popular procedures, and the results can be outstanding. This article provides a comprehensive review of hair grafting techniques to achieve the best results in restoring various hair-bearing areas of the face, including the eyebrows, beard/goatee, and sideburns, and repairing the alopecic scarring from prior facial plastic surgery.

For many hair restoration patients with limited scalp donor hair it is possible to use nonhead hair sources to increase the potential follicle supply. Follicular unit extraction provides the hair restoration surgeon with a useful surgical means for accessing this valuable source of donor reserve. Nonhead hair can also be used to restore eyebrows, eyelashes, and moustaches. This article focuses on the use of body hair and beard in hair restoration. Discussed are the indications and effective techniques for performing hair transplants using non head hair donor sources, along with the pitfalls and risks of this surgical modality.

Hairline lowering or advancement, also known as forehead reduction, is a procedure that has been adapted and honed from scalp reduction and flap techniques. Although the high hairline can be found in both men and women of all races and ethnicities due to various diagnoses, hairline advancement is best suited for individuals, typically women, with a lifelong history of a high hairline and no familial or personal history of progressive hair loss. It is a procedure that is both effective and efficient in lowering the congenitally high hairline with very high patient satisfaction.

Repair of scalp defects is often challenging, because without careful planning, excision of the defect may leave unsatisfactory cosmesis. Contemporary techniques in hair restoration surgery allow creation of natural and undetectable results, but these techniques are often unsuitable for repairing large scarred areas of hair loss. However, by using older techniques of scalp reduction and tissue expansion, excision of many large scarring defects can be accomplished. Combining older methods with modern hair restoration surgery permits the satisfactory treatment of many previously untreatable conditions. This article focuses on tissue expansion as an adjunct to repairing large scalp defects.

FACIAL PLASTIC SURGERY CLINICS OF NORTH AMERICA

Advisory Board to Facial Plastic Surgery Clinics 2013

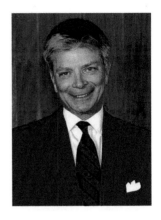
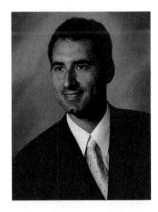
Facial Plastic Surgery Clinics is pleased to introduce the 2012-2013 **Advisory Board**.

Facial Plastic Surgery Clinics is widely available through the media of print, digital e-Reader, online via the Internet, and on iPad and smart phones.

Facial Plastic Surgery Clinics provides professionals access to pertinent point-of-care answers and current clinical information, along with comprehensive background information for deeper understanding.

Readers are welcome to contact the Clinics Editor or Board with comments.

BOARD MEMBERS 2013

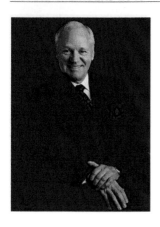

PETER A. ADAMSON, MD

Professor and Head
Division of Facial Plastic and Reconstructive Surgery
Department of Otolaryngology–Head and Neck Surgery
University of Toronto
Toronto, Ontario, Canada

Adamson Cosmetic Facial Surgery
Renaissance Plaza; 150 Bloor Street West; Suite M110
Toronto, Ontario M5S 2X9

416.323.3900
paa@dradamson.com
www.dradamson.com

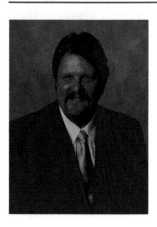

RICK DAVIS, MD

Voluntary Professor
The University of Miami Miller School of Medicine
Miami, Florida

The Center for Facial Restoration
1951 S.W. 172nd Ave; Suite 205
Miramar, Florida 33029

954.442.5191
drd@davisrhinoplasty.com
www.DavisRhinoplasty.com

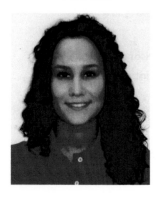

TATIANA DIXON, MD

University of Illinois at Chicago
Resident,
Department of Otolaryngology–Head and Neck Surgery

1855 W. Taylor
Chicago, IL 60612

312.996.6555
TFeuer1@UIC.EDU

STEVEN FAGIEN, MD, FACS

Aesthetic Eyelid Plastic Surgery
660 Glades Road; Suite 210
Boca Raton, Florida 33431

561.393.9898
sfagien@aol.com

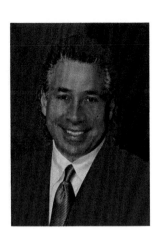

GREG KELLER, MD

Clinical Professor of Surgery, Head and Neck,
David Geffen School of Medicine,
University of California, Los Angeles;

Keller Facial Plastic Surgery
221 W. Pueblo St. Ste A
Santa Barbara, CA 93105

805.687.6408
faclft@aol.com
www.gregorykeller.com

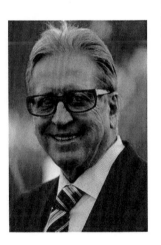

THEDA C. KONTIS, MD

Assistant Professor, Johns Hopkins Hospital
Facial Plastic Surgicenter, Ltd.
1838 Greene Tree Road, Suite 370
Baltimore, MD 21208

410.486.3400
tckontis@aol.com
www.facialplasticsurgerymd.com
www.facial-plasticsurgery.com

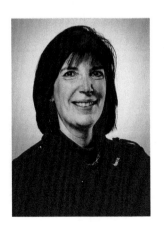

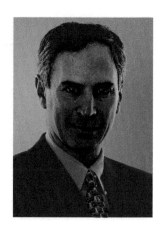

IRA D. PAPEL, MD

Facial Plastic Surgicenter
Associate Professor
The Johns Hopkins University
1838 Greene Tree Road, Suite 370
Baltimore, MD 21208

410.486.3400
idpmd@aol.com
www.facial-plasticsurgery.com

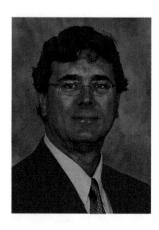

SHERARD A. TATUM, MD

Professor of Otolaryngology and
Pediatrics Cleft and Craniofacial Center
Division of Facial Plastic Surgery
Upstate Medical University
750 E. Adams St.
Syracuse, NY 13210

315.464.4636
TatumS@upstate.edu
www.upstate.edu

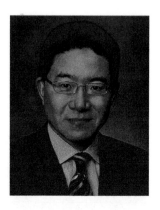

TOM D. WANG, MD

Professor
Facial Plastic and Reconstructive Surgery
Oregon Health & Science University
3181 Southwest Sam Jackson Park Road
Portland, OR 97239

503.494.5678
wangt@ohsu.edu
www.ohsu.edu/drtomwang

Preface
Hair Restoration: A Sophisticated Art Form

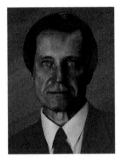
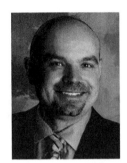

Raymond J. Konior, MD   Steven P. Gabel, MD
Editors

Hair restoration is truly an exciting and dynamic field that continues to fascinate and amaze. It has been nearly 20 years since *Facial Plastic Surgery Clinics of North America* published its first volume that was devoted exclusively to hair restoration. Numerous developments in medical and surgical treatment options at the time of that publication quickly advanced the specialty beyond the notorious "plug"-based restoration methods that predominated the hair restoration discipline for so many years beginning over a half century ago. The introduction of restoration protocols with the exclusive use of follicular unit grafts, which began around the time *Facial Plastic Surgery Clinics of North America* released "Hair Restoration Surgery" in 1994, initiated a period that produced consistent and predictable results of such naturalness as to be undetectable by even the most critical observer. The dramatic aesthetic leap forward at that time from the "plug" era gave one pause to believe that we reached the final frontier with respect to the evolution of hair restoration. However, the pause was very short lived and the specialty area of hair restoration has since continued to evolve at a breakneck speed.

An exclusive group of the world's premiere hair restoration experts has been assembled for this edition of the *Facial Plastic Surgery Clinics of North America* to provide the reader a thoroughly comprehensive, state-of-the-art review of hair restoration. This edition includes expert discussions on core topics relating to diagnostic pearls, medical therapy, hairline design, comprehensive surgical management schemes for male and female patients, and graft survival strategies. Several novel topics are also presented here that highlight the great strides that have most recently emerged in this specialty area. Innovative topics presented within include (1) a new and innovative ancillary treatment option—SMP (scalp micropigmentation), which offers great hope to patients with limited donor graft reserves; (2) new insights into the evolutionary progression of hairline maturation; (3) FUE (follicular unit extraction)—one of the most dynamic areas in hair restoration that has advanced surgical treatment options via the use of microscopic dissection to harvest individual follicular unit grafts from both scalp and body donor sites; and (4) the latest technological advancement in surgical

Facial Plast Surg Clin N Am 21 (2013) xv–xvi
http://dx.doi.org/10.1016/j.fsc.2013.08.003

management—robotic hair restoration. Finally, a cutting-edge discussion on follicular regeneration and neogenesis rounds out this compilation to highlight the future of things to come for this specialty area.

Surgical hair restoration has evolved into a sophisticated art form that consistently brings great joy to patients and treating physicians. The numerous dynamic changes in the field have been stimulating and thought-provoking and we feel extremely fortunate to have found a niche specialty that provides such extraordinary satisfaction. We extend our most sincere and heartfelt gratitude to the founding icons, who set the foundation for what has become an incredibly vibrant specialty area. Finally, we are extremely grateful to our distinguished authors for their time and expertise in creating this notably outstanding edition of *Facial Plastic Surgery Clinics of North America*.

Raymond J. Konior, MD
Chicago Hair Institute
1S280 Summit Suite C-4
Oakbrook Terrace, IL 60181, USA

Department of Otolaryngology Head and Neck Surgery
Loyola University Medical Center
2160 South First Avenue
Maywood, IL 60153, USA

Steven P. Gabel, MD
Gabel Hair Restoration Center
900 SE Oak Street, Suite 203
Hillsboro, OR 97123, USA

E-mail addresses:
drkonior@sbcglobal.net
http://www.chicagohairinstitute.com (R.J. Konior)
drgabel@gabelcenter.com
http://www.gabelcenter.com (S.P. Gabel)

Phenotype of Normal Hairline Maturation

William R. Rassman, MD[a],*, Jae P. Pak, MD[a], Jino Kim, MD[b]

KEYWORDS

• Phenotype • Hairline • Maturation • Facial morphology

KEY POINTS

- Hairlines have characteristic shapes in boys and girls and change predictably as children develop into adulthood.
- The hairline in male and female children is traditionally concave in shape in all races.
- The upward movement of the female hairline leaves a widow's peak in 81% of women.
- The concave shape of the male frontal hairline transitions to a convex shape between 18-29 years of age.
- The maturing recession of the temple mounds leaves a temple peak behind in boys and girls.
- Recession of the temple mound upwards and laterally in men leaves a balding corner.
- The leading edge of hair direction in the juvenile hairline is different than the hair direction in the mature hairline in adult men and some women.

INTRODUCTION

This article applies observational science to the process of how the hairline develops from childhood to adulthood in men and women. It also includes a summary of 1051 children from school yearbooks, aged 5 to 10 years and 15 to 18 years in boys and girls whose hairlines were not hidden by styling. It adds a missing link to the insights by Norwood and Shiell[1] and Hamilton[2] in their respective seminal articles on balding in men and women; however, this article's main focus is not about balding, but about the visual changes in the hairlines that are seen as humans age. What is seen in hairline changes results from environmental events (eg, traction alopecia), age, and hormones as they influence the genetics that code the various parts of the anatomic hairline. These genetics are evident in the phenotype of the hairline's evolution at each point in time. The available medical information on hairline evolution approaches hairline change as if it reflects a disease process or a genetic abnormality.

This article:

1. Provides physicians with a better understanding of how to educate the patient to better understand the changes seen in their hairlines
2. Will help decide whether the hairline changes are typical or not
3. Provides the physician with a more precise understanding of the genetic influences of the phenotype of hairline evolution from childhood to adulthood
4. Provides the hair restoration surgeon a foundation on which to design a hairline appropriate to meet each individual's needs, specific to their age and sex

People often ask or comment about their hairlines:

Is my hairline receding or getting thin? Am I seeing my hairline rise? Do changes in my hairline mean that I am balding like my father or mother? I don't like the shape or position of my hairline. Is there something I can do about it?

Disclosures: None.
[a] New Hair Institute, 5757 Wilshire Boulevard, Promenade #2, Los Angeles, CA 90036; [b] New Hair Institute, Gangnam Han-il B/D 7F, Yeoksam-dong 814-1, Korea
* Corresponding author.
E-mail address: wrassman@newhair.com

Facial Plast Surg Clin N Am 21 (2013) 317–324
http://dx.doi.org/10.1016/j.fsc.2013.04.001

With genetic balding already affecting up to 50% of the male and female population over their lifetimes, perceptions of what is abnormal are often preprogrammed by the genetic hair loss patterns of people's parents or grandparents. An uneven or eroding hairline creates a fuzzy, ill-defined border to the face, but a full leading hairline edge makes a statement that reflects a youthful, well-framed, and healthy image; an image that many people desire.

HAIRLINE ANALYSIS GROUP

We observed and analyzed the hairlines of 1051 adolescent and preadolescent boys and girls by analyzing school yearbooks. These measurement processes were limited by (1) hairline styles that often obscured the hairline, and (2) a single view of the subjects; these subjects were therefore omitted from the study. We supplemented these data by observing school athletic team photographs and swim teams photographs by performing Internet searches for schools all over the world, by observing children at school graduations and in recreation areas, and at social events (**Table 1**).

Widow's Peak and Temple Peak

It is apparent from the children studied in these yearbooks and from the multiple other observational and media sources (television, sports events, Olympic events from the 2012 Olympic Games) that male and female hairlines are similar in prepubertal children; all children start with a concave shaped hairline (ages 3–5 years). The leading central edge of the juvenile hairlines is always at the highest wrinkle of the furrowed brow. At the lateral temple borders, the forehead is narrowed in young children because of the presence of lateral temple mounds that help establish the concave shape. Widow's peaks are rare in

boys and girls between the ages of 5 and 10 years, whereas the incidence increases in teenage girls and boys. The widow's peak never extends below the highest crease of the furrowed brow (in children or adults) and, when it appears, it indicates a rising frontal hairline around it. The lateral temple mounds crowd the lateral borders of the forehead of young children, women, and some men, and there is rarely a temple peak in juvenile or female hairlines while the temple mounds are present. As the lateral temple mounds recede laterally and posteriorly, a temple peak often appears. Both the widow's peak and the temple peak are remnants of the midline juvenile hairlines and the lateral temple mound of the concave hairline.

Genetics, Hormones, Environment

Most prepubertal children have concave shaped hairlines. In most, there is little distinction between the hairlines of boys and girls until these children near puberty, when we believe hormone changes trigger genetic changes. These changes vary widely as children transition into adolescence and become young men and women. Although a great deal has been written about the importance of hair as a sign of health and vitality, subtle changes that show erosion of youthful hairlines greatly affect how people feel about themselves. The interplay between genetics, hormones, and possibly environmental factors (eg, traction on the hair from styling) can affect these changes.

There is little doubt that the hairlines we have studied can be influenced by traction brought on by pulling the hair back. Traction alopecia has been directly linked to hairline hair loss in African American children who have routinely worn tight braiding. This braiding has been known to produce a loss of some or all of the frontal and temple mound hair in a significant number of these children. What is unclear are the effects of the pony tail as a contributing factor affecting the evolution of what is seen in the hairlines of these girls. Considering that similar changes are seen in boys to a lesser degree, we think that styling adjuncts like the pony tail only rarely cause hairline alopecia. We were unable to distinguish the hairlines in the girls who did or did not routinely wear pony tails, and this reflects a limitation of the study and could affect the validity of some of our conclusions.

HAIRLINE MODEL SYSTEM

To develop language in order to define the various anatomic points of the hairline, the authors developed a modeled system, illustrated in **Fig. 1**, with the full range of hairlines. This model system can

Table 1				
Survey from school yearbooks in 1051 children				
Sex	Age (y)	# Subjects	WP (%)	TP (%)
Boys	5	38	0	0
Boys	5–10	170	6	0
Boys	15–17	374	36	14
Boys	18	51	14	16
Girls	5	28	8	0
Girls	6–10	56	11	0
Girls	15–17	281	31	19
Girls	18	53	11	25

Abbreviations: TP, temporal peak; WP, widow's peak.

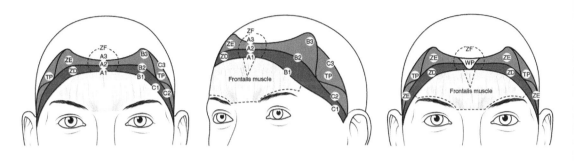

A1, B1, C1 = Juvenile Hairline   A2, B2, C2 = Intermediary Hairline   A3, B3, C3 = Adult Male Hairline

ZF = Forelock Zone   TP = Temporal Peak   WP = Widows Peak   ZD = Zone D (dark grey)   ZE = Zone E (light grey)

Fig. 1. Hairline locations.

be applied to men and women of all ages and of all races.

The border of the face is framed by the upper frontal hairline and lateral temple mounds. The anatomic location of the edges of these two structures need to be defined in order to understand the age-related standard, if there is a standard. We created a modeled system to be able to work out the changes in hairlines that we see. There are 3 critical areas that define a hairline:

1. A point where the central leading edge of the upper crease of the furrowed brow can easily be identified (point A)
2. Lateral leading edge of the upper temple hairline (point B)
3. Lateral temple mounds on the side of the forehead (point C)

The image of a face changes as a hairline recedes superiorly and laterally. As children, everyone has a hairline defined by points A1, B1, and C1 producing a hairline that is originally concave in shape (see **Fig. 1**).

RELEVANT HAIRLINE ANATOMY
Frontalis Muscle

A typical hairline cannot be understood without understanding the influence of the frontalis muscle, which lies under the forehead skin. The central, upper border of the muscle often has a small cleft in it and the skin of the forehead adheres to the muscle surface. Its edges attach to the eyebrows' deep fascia and the fascia of the upper nasal bone inferiorly. The muscle extends upward where it attaches to the galea aponeurosis, the dense fibrous tissue layer that extends across the upper part of the cranium. The superior border of the muscle is fixed and, when the muscle contracts, the eyebrows are raised. The

skin of the forehead adheres to the muscle so that, when the eyebrows are raised, the forehead develops transverse wrinkles. The lowest point of the hairline in the midline in children always touches the highest crease of the furrowed brow and this defines the medial inferior edge of a juvenile hairline.

The height of the frontalis muscle varies widely and is genetically determined. We think that there is a genetic relationship between the length of this muscle and the height of the hairline. If we are correct, people with a very short muscle will have a low hairline, whereas others with a very long muscle will have a high forehead and consequently a high hairline. Many adults with high hairlines tell me that they always had a high forehead when they present for a hairline lowering surgery. Point A1 in people with high hairlines is often located at the highest crease of the furrowed brow indicating that they always had a high hairline. On the side profile, there are lateral temple mounds that extend into the forehead, narrowing it considerably. The temple peaks, when they appear, reflect the loss of hair in Zones D and E (see **Fig. 1**).

Transition Zone

The leading edge of the frontal hairline begins with a transition zone made up of vellus hairs that are shorter (a few millimeters in height), and terminal hairs that are often lighter in color, finer, and single. The vellus hairs contribute to establishing a delicate marginal leading edge. These vellus hairs do not have a sebaceous gland associated with them, but they function during sweating, acting like the fins of a radiator for reducing body heat and promoting evaporation. The short vellus hairs decrease in numbers behind the leading edge where single, finer terminal hairs begin to appear. Posterior to the leading edge, the hair appears thicker because hairs grow in groups (follicular units) of between 2 and 5 terminal hairs each. The delicacy of the transition zone often makes it difficult to tell where the hairline starts. The wider the transition zone, the softer and more refined the hairline appears. Understanding this concept is critical for hair transplant surgeons because they must try to replicate the transition zone in all frontal hairlines.

Hairline Variations

There are wide variations in the presentation of the hairline in men and women related to age, sex, and genetic inheritance. The individual characteristics of the hair influence how it looks:

1. The color of the hair on the scalp
2. The degree of coarseness of the hair
3. Whether it is curly or straight
4. The density of the hair

However, these four characteristics are unrelated to the overall shape or the position of the hairline. The hairline shape, when combined with these four hair characteristics, profoundly affects a society's view of facial beauty, something that varies significantly in different cultures.

HAIRLINE MATURATION DYNAMICS

The male hairline has been well studied mainly because of the social impact of balding that starts in most men in their late teens or early 20s. This article does not address the balding patterns (behind points A3, B3, and C3) in men or women because they are discussed by Norwood and Shiell[1] and Hamilton.[2]

In his study of 360 women, Nausbaum and Fuentefria[3] recorded the high incidence of a widow's peak of 81% in this study group. The widow's peak is always located in zones D and E. Some balding men and women retain some or all of the hair in zones D and E, even if they are balding behind points A3, B3, and C3. This finding suggests that zones D and E have different genetic codes than the area behind these zones. The authors think that the genes in these zones may not be expressed when people bald. Genetic coding of the points anterior to A3, B3, and C3 may independently dictate a mix-and-match loss of hair in any individual. The statistical emergence of the widow's peak (8% in girls aged 5 years, 11% in girls aged 6 to 10 years, 31% in girls 15 to 17 years, and 81% of women average age 41 years) suggests that the hairlines of 81% of adult female hairlines recede posteriorly to A2 or A3 in most women as they age (see **Fig. 1**).

RECESSION PATH

Most Caucasian men, and some women, have a distinct upward and orderly recession path from their original juvenile hairline (points A1, B1, and C1) (see **Fig. 1**).

- For men, the leading edge of the central hairline recedes upward from the upper forehead crease (A1) to a distance of approximately 1.5 to 2 cm as the mature male hairline develops with the loss of hair in Zones D and E.
- The prominent temple mounds often recede laterally from point C1 in boys and young men.
- As the lateral wall of the side hairlines recedes, a temple peak often appears in both men and women, reflecting a remnant of hair in zones D and E.
- As the temple peaks become more distinct, the hair above these points often recede as well, creating a loss of hair to point B3.
- Point C1 can recede laterally to reveal a pointed temple peak at C2, which can remain into old age.

The genetic code of the temple peak is independent of the balding process common even in Norwood class 7 patterned balding men, as shown in **Fig. 2**. This is a Norwood class 7 pattern balding man (age 69 years) with a transplanted head of hair. Note that the temple peaks never receded. These temple peaks were never transplanted in this patient and they are often found in Norwood class 6 and 7 pattern patients. The temple peak is present (at some point in time) in most men and some women.

The hair above the lateral mounds (in zones D and E) in men becomes thinner and eventually becomes more transparent until the hair in the corners disappears to point B3. The disappearance of this hair may be rapid.

- When the hairline recedes to point B3, the convex shape of the typical mature male hairline pattern becomes evident.
- If the recession stops at points A2 and B2, a flat central hairline can remain.

In **Fig. 3**, Senator and vice presidential candidate Paul Ryan shows a widow's peak (a remnant of zone D) and a flat hairline showing a projection (dotted line) of where the authors think that Senator Ryan's juvenile hairline might have been. The classic mature hairlines in 90% of Caucasian men reflect a leading hairline location ranging from A2, B2, and C2 to A3, B3, and C3 in some combination. Points A, B, and C are not dependent

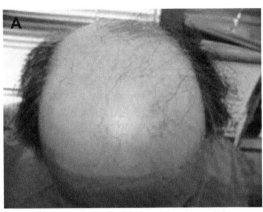

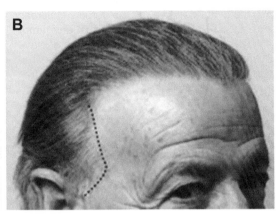

Fig. 2. (*A*) Preoperative view of 70-year-old man with a Norwood class 7 balding pattern. (*B*) Postoperative view with transplanted hairline. The temple peaks (*dotted line*) were not transplanted.

on one another, because one area can recede while another area may be fixed. These changes in men typically occur between the ages of 17 and 29 years and are stable providing that balding is not present. In many women, the corrugated patterns of the leading edges of their hairlines can be found in either zone D or zone E, or combinations of the two, and these remnants can make up the end-point appearance of the female hairline.

CENTRAL FORELOCK AND WIDOWS PEAK

In some men, a strong genetically inherited central forelock exists that commonly starts at the highest crease of the furrowed brow (A1), or at times at a higher point (A2 or A3), which is resistant to the changes of the hairline around it when balding

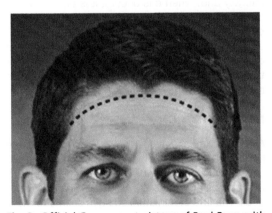

Fig. 3. Official Government picture of Paul Ryan with line showing where the author thinks his juvenile hairline probably was. The lowest point on the widow's peak rests on the highest crease of his furrowed brow.

patterns develop. These forelocks vary in width and height and may extend posteriorly and laterally a considerable distance from the midline (zone F). This forelock can persist well into adulthood, and often into older age. Television host David Letterman has a moderate sized forelock that frames the face and blocks visibility of the balding pattern behind it. In balding men, these forelocks can be seen in family inheritance patterns and, as such, are a heritable trait with a distinct phenotype. Likewise, a widow's peak may remain as a heritable remnant within zone D or even as an extension of the forelock. For women, according to Nausbaum and Fuentefria,[3] the widow's peak is present in 81% of mature women, and varies in size (from 0.8 cm to 1.8 cm). If a line is drawn from the lowest edge of the widow's peak to the lowest border of the temple mounds in women, the location of the child's hairline can be estimated (points A1, B1, and C1); a distinctly concave hairline shape is visible (**Fig. 4**).

Hormonal Influence on Hair Recession

Under the influence of hormones in the postadolescent male, the hairline starts a slow recession away from its youthful concave juvenile shape to a flat or convex shape, whereas the prepubertal female hairline may not change its shape to any significant degree in the same age groups. Most of the changes in male and female hairlines that occur with age do not reflect genetic balding, but rather a genetic heritable phenotypic pattern for the individual. When genetic balding does appear in men, the process does not usually start until the young men reach the age of ~17 years, and, when it appears in women, it may appear after menopause or even in women as early as their late teens and early 20s.

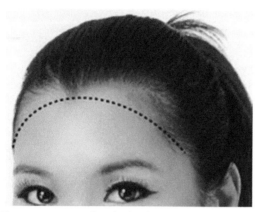

Fig. 4. A mature female hairline that shows some thinning in the temple mounds and where the hairline probably was located when she was very young (*dotted line*). The dotted line connects the tip of the widow's peak with the leading edge of the lateral mound. The suggested childhood hairline is concave.

Identifying Prepubertal Hairline

The lowest part of the hairline that hugs the wrinkled brow can identify the location of the prepubertal hairline when the eyebrow is lifted and the forehead wrinkles, regardless of the presence or absence of a balding pattern. Look at yourself in the mirror and test yourself by wrinkling your brow. Do you remember the day when your hairline was located there? As the hairline matures, parts of the juvenile hairline may remain. In a small group of Caucasian men, the juvenile hairline in zone D and zone E can be retained into adulthood, even if they bald in a typical class 7 Norwood balding pattern behind points A3, B3, and C3. This tendency suggests that the genetic code for zone D and zone E is phenotypically different than the hair behind it. The poorly named widow's peak is a genetically programmed remnant of the central portion of the original concave juvenile hairline that has not receded but has taken on a distinct, recognizable pattern in zones D and E. The leading edge of the widow's peak never extends lower than the highest wrinkle of the furrowed brow.

Some men retain their juvenile hairline well into adulthood. The best example of this is former President Bill Clinton (**Fig. 5**). President Clinton's hairline is concave in shape and the authors think that this is the same hairline (less the mild erosion lateral to the midpoint) he had since childhood, suggesting that even our former President is showing some minimal signs of an aging hairline. As in all juvenile hairlines, his forehead is crowded from the sides with prominent lateral temple mounds. He has no temple peaks because he has strong temple mounds covering the area where the temple peaks

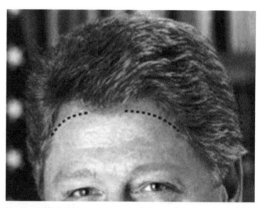

Fig. 5. Official Government picture of former President Bill Clinton with line showing where the author thinks his juvenile hairline probably was. A full concave hairline with strong temple mounds can be seen. In this picture, President Clinton has early recession of his frontal hairline to the sides of the midline.

would be. Other photographs of Clinton (search Google Images) show emotional moments. His forehead creases at point A1 as shown in the dotted hairline in **Fig. 5**.

HAIR DIRECTION

The hair direction of the juvenile hairline hair found in zones D and E is different than the hair direction posterior to points A3 and B3. Moving laterally from the midpoint of zone D, the hair direction, which frequently points forward and parallel to the ground in the midline (above A3), gradually points more downward toward the ears. When a centrally located widow's peak remains, it may point forward or laterally depending on what direction it took in its prepubertal location in zones D and E. It is common for this widow's peak to point laterally and, when this occurs, it is often referred to as a lick. In many women whose hairline recedes to A3 and B2, remnants of hair in zones D and E can take on a minicorrugated pattern. This corrugated appearance is an important feature that should be created in a transplanted hairline if it is to look natural.

MINIATURIZATION

As frontal and side hairlines erode and recede, the nonpermanent hair often undergoes miniaturization (thinning of the individual hair shafts) and, if this process is rapid, the hair may quickly disappear. The fate of miniaturized hairs seems to manifest itself clinically in 3 ways:

1. Slow progressive miniaturization, with or without moderate prolonged hair cycling (anagen/telogen cycle)

2. Hairs that remain miniaturized and do not appear to grow or cycle
3. Hairs that reach the end of their genetically determined number of growth cycles, and do not return after a given cycle (where apoptosis is the cause of the hair loss)

Miniaturization in the upper lateral corners of zone E to point B3 in women often presents with a prolonged period of miniaturization that could extend for years and, when this process occurs in men, the disappearance of the corners is usually more rapid. Miniaturized hairs in these corners appeared in many of the female athletes in the 2012 summer Olympics, possibly the result of hormone influences in athletes or traction from the pony tails worn to keep their hair away from their faces. When women lose their corners to point B3, there is a distinctly male shape to the hairline (**Fig. 6**).

As points B1 and C1 recede, the concave shape of the child's hairline disappears. The V shape is characteristic of the mature male hairline and is the most common presentation in Caucasian men as the hair in the corners disappears. When this occurs in women, it may affect their feminine image. African and Asian men (Indian, Chinese, Korean, and Japanese) maintain the A2, B2, and C2 points more commonly than Caucasian men.

In the mature male hairline at A3, the hairs point forward and parallel to the ground, not downward to the sides, where it may have pointed had the hairs been measured at points A1 and A2 in zone D (in childhood). The distance between point A1 and point A3 is 1.5 to 2 cm. As men see the development of a mature hairline with loss of hair in zones D and E, many ask, "Is this a sign of balding?" and, "When will this recession stop?" The mature hairline in men often appears between

the ages of 17 and 29 years. The changes within zone D and zone E are genetically controlled and they are probably heavily influenced by testosterone. We do not classify miniaturization changes in zones D and E as balding, although men often look at these changes as the beginning of the balding process, particularly if there is balding in the family line.

The female hairline often remains stable for many years past puberty and well into adulthood. Significant changes in the location and shape of the temple mounds may appear with age, even before or just after puberty. The shape of the female hairline most often remains concave into adulthood. When there is lateral recession of the temple mounds, it often leaves a temple peak similar to men (point C2 and C3). In these women, the corners of the hairline in zone E to point B3 may remain full, with healthy terminal hairs. Movement of the central hairline to point A2 or A3 creates a high hairline and many women still retain points B2 and C2, even if the central hairline rises to A3. The shape of the rounded concave hairline and the crowded forehead from prominent temple mounds can be an attractive female look. If the forehead is long and significantly above the highest wrinkle of the furrowed brow, even young girls become concerned that they are losing their feminine look, or that they may be balding. Some girls have high hairlines, even before puberty, but they rarely become concerned until they are in their midteens. Hairline lowering procedures or transplants into zones D and E are good approaches to the high female hairline.

As women age, there are changes in the hairline that start to appear as early as preadolescence. These hairlines may develop slowly in the age range of 18 to 50 years. The corners (zone E to

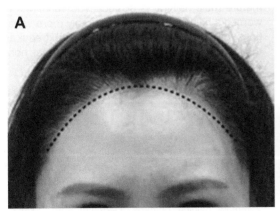 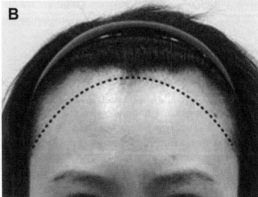

Fig. 6. Female corner hairline correction. (*A*) Before. (*B*) After transplants were done. Remnants of the lateral temple mounds (temple peaks) were barely visible before surgery. The lateral temple wall was restored in this patient, incorporating remnants of the lateral temple peaks within the repair.

point B3) may start to undergo miniaturization, producing thinning in the corners, and this is a common problem for many women of all races. The terminal hair in this area can become miniaturized, changing the overall shape of the hairline from a female concave shape toward a typical male flat or convex shape as the bare corners, normally not visible in the concave hairlines with normal terminal hairs, become thin. The corner hairs may become thinner and the normal hair growth cycle may change in zone E from B2 to B3. The upper corner hair of zone E may even stop growing, which may produce a wider forehead and an upward receded frontal leading edge. These changes may reflect a variance of a mature female hairline, but I do not think that this is a normal maturing process and many women are not happy with these changes. The hairs in the corners that originally pointed downward and to the sides are the hairs that become miniaturized, which produces a flat or convex shape more typical of the male hairline. Sometimes, the central hairlines rise and the corners become miniaturized. The shape of the female hairline may follow ethnic patterns. People from India often have prominent crowding of the forehead, with strong and dominant, persistent lateral temple mounds and a low hairline. The authors assume that a low frontal hairline reflects a short frontalis muscle and a narrow forehead, which is also found in Indian men. We believe that there is no cause and effect between the low hairline and a short frontalis muscle.

The discussions on normal female hairline shapes reflect normal healthy Caucasian women who do not have the genetic effects of balding. Changes in hairline shape, the disappearance of the corner hairs secondary to miniaturization, and a recession of the frontal hairline are seen in most Caucasian women as they age. In those who have undergone facial plastic surgery, these changes are probably induced by the trauma of the cosmetic procedures.

HAIRLINE PATTERNS: OBSERVATIONS BY THE AUTHORS

To assess the patterns described in this article, thousands of observations were made of individuals who participated in school teams (through the Internet) and viewed by observations with photographs in school yearbooks. The hairline patterns that were recognized led to the hairline schema presented in this article. We have had the opportunity to study it further, viewing the hairlines of female athletes from the 2012 Olympic shown on television, and children at weddings, birthday parties, athletic events, and school graduations over the past 6 months. Mature women were included in our study, as well. We continued analyzing the hairlines of all women at shopping centers, airports, and conventions. It was a worthy exercise; to validate the schema presented here, which shows the wide variety of hairlines of children, men, and women of all ages. We challenged our model of female hairline evolution in thousands of individuals. The phenotype that has emerged was observed over and over again. We think that the hairline evolution model presented here will be validated by further scrutiny.

We realized that the patterns in female hairline evolution that we observed were orderly and logically reflective of what we observed clinically. Once we realized that all human hairlines developed from a common concave shape, the patterns we studied in men and women of all ages could be categorized. Combined with our extensive clinical experience, we suspected that we had discovered a process that previously was not well defined in the medical literature. The phenotype we observed can only be explained by genetic coding within the anatomic hairline outlined in **Fig. 1**. With this model, we think that we are better equipped to explain the hairline changes seen in men and women and their relationships with age. These insights will be invaluable for modern hair restoration surgeons.

SUMMARY

This article presents phenotypic variations of the front and side hairlines found in men and women of all ages. There is a migration of the hairlines as people age, because most children start with a common concave hairline that migrates to some variant as shown in **Table 1**. The Caucasian, mature male hairline is distinct. The variations in women's hairlines show considerably more variations, at times resulting in changes as extreme as those found in the mature hairlines of normal, nonbalding men.

REFERENCES

1. Norwood OT, Shiell RC. Hair transplantation surgery. 2nd edition. Springfield (IL): Charles C Thomas; 1984. p. 5–10.
2. Hamilton JB. Patterned loss of hair in man: types and incidence. Ann N Y Acad Sci 1951;53:708–27.
3. Nausbaum BP, Fuentefria S. Naturally occurring female hairline patterns. Dermatol Surg 2009;35: 907–13.

Imposters of Androgenetic Alopecia
Diagnostic Pearls for the Hair Restoration Surgeon

Nicole Rogers, MD

KEYWORDS

- Hair loss • Alopecia areata • Cicatricial alopecia • Lichen planopilaris • Frontal fibrosing alopecia
- Folliculitis decalvans • Hair transplantation

KEY POINTS

- Hair restoration surgeons should understand the basic clinical diagnosis and pathologic condition of hair loss conditions that are not always amenable to successful hair transplantation.
- There are several nonscarring and scarring mimickers of androgenetic alopecia that may fool even the most experienced hair transplant surgeon.
- When these conditions are transplanted, they either may not grow at all or may grow in the short term but fall out in the long term.
- Perifollicular erythema, shiny alopecia with loss of follicular ostia, yellow dots, unexplained pruritis and burning, and exclamation mark hairs are important clinical clues to identify androgenetic alopecia imposters.
- A scalp biopsy may help to definitively rule out imposters of androgenetic alopecia.

INTRODUCTION

The most frequent cause of hair loss in both men and women is androgenetic alopecia (AGA), affecting up to 50% of both genders. It is also known as male or female pattern hair loss. This male or female pattern hair loss is usually inherited and can progress over time. Fortunately, it is amenable to medical and surgical therapy, such as minoxidil, finasteride, and hair transplantation. However, other forms of hair loss are not always amenable to hair transplant surgery. It may be technically possible to transplant these conditions, but their underlying cause may be related to an inflammatory or cicatricial (scarring) nature. These conditions may fool even the most experienced hair transplant surgeons by appearing consistent with androgenetic alopecia, but when they are transplanted, they either may not grow at all or may grow in the short term but fall out in the long term.

Although it is not always possible to recognize these conditions early on, this article is important to provide as many clues as possible for recognizing such imposters of AGA. In this article a variety of the clinical, dermatoscopic, and symptomatic criteria are covered that help distinguish these conditions from male and female pattern hair loss. Hair surgeons who have training in dermatology may already be able to recognize some of these criteria. Others who do not may consider referral to a dermatologist or at least performing a scalp biopsy before hair transplantation

Disclosure: No conflicts of interest to report.
Private Practice, 701 Metairie Road, Suite 2A205, Metairie, LA 70005, USA
E-mail address: nicolerogers11@yahoo.com

Facial Plast Surg Clin N Am 21 (2013) 325–334
http://dx.doi.org/10.1016/j.fsc.2013.04.002

to rule out any inflammatory or cicatricial condition. It is also highly valuable to cultivate a good relationship with your local dermatopathologist to help interpret these results. In many cases, a team approach is necessary and can offer the most accurate and helpful plan for patients.

Nature of the Problem

Patients presenting for hair transplantation have sometimes done extensive research on the Internet and have already made their diagnosis and treatment plan before even seeing a hair surgeon. It may be tempting for the hair surgeon to agree to transplant before understanding the true nature of the problem. They may assume the patient has no contraindications to surgery. However every hair surgeon must inspect the scalp and surrounding skin extremely carefully before proceeding with surgery. If there are any clues to suggest inflammation or scarring, they should stop and either perform a biopsy or refer to a dermatologist before agreeing to transplant.

In some cases of cicatricial alopecia the area may be transplanted, but it should only be done after 2 to 5 years' time, at the point when the condition has become completely "burned out." This stable period occurs when there is no further evidence of active inflammation on biopsy. Such inflammation could consume the transplanted grafts and result in their loss. However even then there is no guarantee of good or permanent growth. Some cases may grow well in the short run, only to flare years later with the loss of the transplanted grafts. Others may have only 20% to 50% of the hair growth even 12 months after surgery, which can be devastating to patients and disappointing to physicians. It is imperative that both parties have extensive discussion and management of expectations before hair transplant surgery.

NONSCARRING ALOPECIAS
Alopecia Areata

Alopecia areata (AA) represents an autoimmune form of hair loss in which the body's inflammatory T cells mistakenly attack the hair follicle. The mechanism is highly complicated, but seems to have both a genetic and an environmental cause. It is unclear whether this is a result of attack against the hair bulb or just the pigmented portion of the hair bulb. It usually presents as smooth round or oval patches of hair loss anywhere on the scalp, beard area, or body. Poliosis (whitening of the affected hairs) may occur with regrowth. Different terms are used to classify the body area affected. AA refers to one or more localized patches of hair loss; alopecia totalis refers to loss of all the hair on the head, and alopecia universalis refers to loss of all the hair on the body. A symmetric, single patch of hair loss in the vertex could certainly be confused with AGA (**Fig. 1**).

Diffuse AA /alopecia incognito

A less common form of AA (but more concerning mimicker of AGA) is diffuse alopecia areata, or alopecia incognito. This form of hair loss results in massive widespread and diffuse hair loss. In the short run, it may be confused with telogen effluvium, and in the long run, it may be confused with AGA. Practitioners should be on the lookout even for overlapping conditions such as a diffuse alopecia areata in the setting of male pattern hair loss. Clinical history can be valuable in sorting out the exact diagnosis.

Although the scalp biopsy is the gold standard, dermoscopy can be helpful in diagnosing this condition. There are unique features seen on microscopic examination of these patients. The most sensitive is yellow dots, which represent dilated infundibula filled with keratin debris. In diffuse alopecia areata, these yellow dots appear in and among normal (unaffected) follicles (**Fig. 2**). The most specific dermoscopic feature in AA is exclamation point hairs. These are short broken hairs that are tapered proximally. Both yellow dots and exclamation point hairs are shown in **Fig. 3**.

Patients may complain of a slight tingling or itching just before the affected area loses hair. On histology this may be related to the "swarm of bees" described as numerous T cells surrounding a hair bulb and attacking, resulting in sudden hair loss. The good news is that these patients frequently regrow their hair either with topical or with intralesional steroids or no treatment at all.

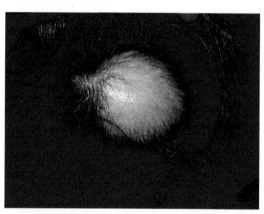

Fig. 1. Alopecia areata: large round patch of nonscarring hair loss in the vertex could mimic AGA.

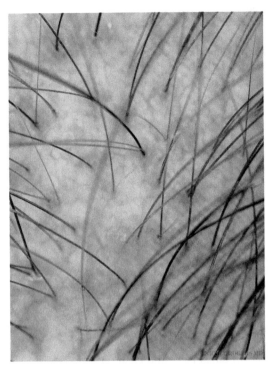

Fig. 2. Alopecia areata: yellow dots seen in dermoscopy represent dilated infundibula.

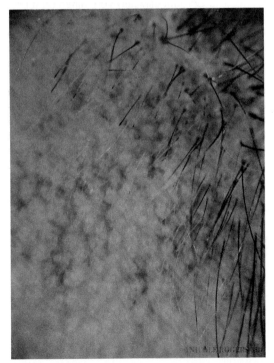

Fig. 3. Alopecia areata: yellow dots and exclamation point hairs are characteristic.

Treatment options for diffuse alopecia areata include the following:

- High potency topical steroids under occlusion
- Systemic corticosteroids
- Topical sensitizers, such as squaric acid, diphenylcyclopropenone, or anthralin
- In longstanding cases of alopecia, the author has successfully used immunosuppressive agents, such as methotrexate and mycophenolate mofetil.
- Light-based therapies, such a psoralen + ultraviolet-A phototherapy (PUVA), narrowband ultraviolet B therapy (UVB), and low-level light therapy,[1] also seem to have some role in down-regulating the inflammation associated with AA.

Hair transplantation for AA

The results of hair transplantation for AA can be uncertain. In long-standing cases there can be fibrosis with dissolution of the underlying follicles. In these cases little inflammation may remain to attack the transplanted follicles. However AA is a chronic condition that can recur at any time. Thus, patients must understand and be comfortable with the possibility of a flare at any time point. The flare may affect either transplanted hairs, hairs near the donor area, or totally unrelated hairs. A few reports of successful hair transplantation into AA exist, in which the transplanted area was quiescent with good growth at 11.5 months.[2,3] Nonetheless each case should be approached cautiously and the patients should be thoroughly consented to understand all possible outcomes of proceeding with surgery.

Telogen Effluvium

Patients undergoing major physiologic stress may report rapid and diffuse hair loss 3 to 6 months later. It can occur when a large number of hair follicles enter the resting phase at once. Major causes include general anesthesia, crash dieting, childbirth, high fever, or prolonged illness. Certain medications such as isotretinoin or high-dose vitamin A may also contribute. No treatment is generally necessary.

Tinea Capitis

Another unusual presentation of diffuse hair loss may be cutaneous fungal infection (**Fig. 4**). Diagnosis should be made with either scalp biopsy or a scraping of the affected scalp area and subsequent staining with potassium hydroxide. Cases of tinea and AGA may coexist. The author transplanted one woman with longstanding AGA only after treatment with griseofulvin for biopsy-proven tinea capitis.

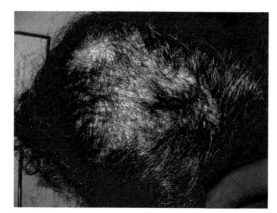

Fig. 4. Tinea capitis: young female patient presenting with diffuse and rapid hair loss.

SCARRING ALOPECIAS

Cicatricial alopecias may also be mistaken for AGA. These conditions can result in permanent hair loss and can cause deep emotional distress to affected patients. Successful transplantation of these conditions is tenuous due to the waxing and waning nature of the inflammatory infiltrate. Transplanted follicles may grow in the short run but be lost with a recurrent flare of the condition months or years later.

Cicatricial alopecias are traditionally classified by their inflammatory infiltrate (lymphocytic, neutrophilic, mixed). These and other less common forms of hair loss are summarized in **Table 1**. For the purposes of this article these conditions are addressed according to their prevalence and clinical relevance.

Table 1
Imposters of androgenetic alopecia and their corresponding infiltrate

Form of Inflammation	Condition
Lymphocyte-associated	Alopecia areata Lichen planopilaris (LPP) Frontal fibrosing alopecia (FFA) Discoid lupus erythematosus (DLE) Pseudopelade of Brocq Central centrifugal cicatricial alopecia (CCCA)
Neutrophilic infiltrate	Folliculitis decalvans Dissecting cellulitis
Mixed infiltrate	Folliculitis (acne) keloidalis Erosive pustular dermatosis

Lichen Planopilaris

Lichen planopilaris (LPP) is a relatively uncommon form of hair loss resulting in permanent destruction of the pilosebaceous unit. It results in a shiny alopecia of the midscalp, vertex, or parietal areas (**Fig. 5**). Patients in the early stage may complain of itching, burning, and diffuse hair loss. Close inspection during the acute stage may reveal a bright red perifollicular erythema with slight scaling (**Fig. 6**). In more longstanding cases the erythema may subside or exist only along the periphery of affected patches (**Fig. 7**). Centrally affected areas may be completely white (as in Caucasians) and have total loss of follicular openings.

Treatment of LPP involves combating the inflammation as soon as possible to minimize ongoing destruction of follicles. Topical and intralesional corticosteroids are a first-line therapy but may not be enough. Systemic anti-inflammatory medications can also be required. Prednisone, doxycycline, hydroxychloroquine, and mycophenolate mofetil have all shown promise in halting the inflammation. Pioglitazone (a PPAR-γ agonist) has been shown effective in one case report based on the loss of PPAR-γ functionality in mouse models of scarring alopecia.[4,5]

Frontal Fibrosing Alopecia

Frontal fibrosing alopecia (FFA) is histologically identical to LPP but clinically very different. It presents with a recession of the hairline along the sideburns and central scalp, leaving behind a zone of atrophic, ivory-colored skin (**Fig. 8**). This atrophic, ivory-colored skin contrasts with the sun-damaged skin of the forehead and can indicate the location of the original hairline. Often there is also partial or total loss of the eyebrows. Dermoscopy reveals follicular hyperkeratosis with a very mild erythema (**Fig. 9**). Some patients develop a cobblestoning of the skin on the cheeks and chin

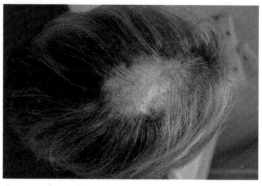

Fig. 5. Lichen planopilaris: middle-aged woman with shiny alopecia in vertex.

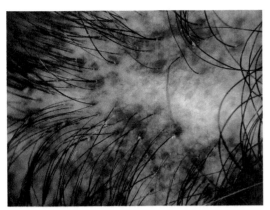

Fig. 6. Acute lichen planopilaris: bright red markings are seen around follicles.

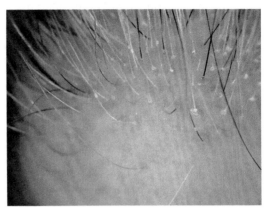

Fig. 9. Frontal fibrosing alopecia: mild erythema with follicular hyperkeratosis.

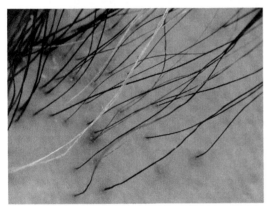

Fig. 7. Chronic lichen planopilaris: mild erythema with white scar tissue.

(**Fig. 10**). This cobblestoning has been suggested to represent involvement of the facial vellus hairs as well.[6]

The condition was originally described by Kossard in 1994 in postmenopausal women. However, it has since been reported in premenopausal women as well as men. In the author's experience,

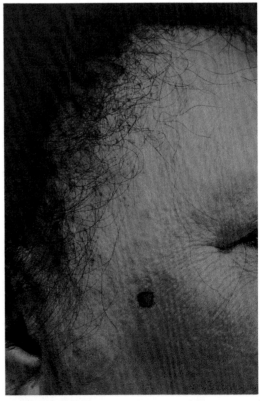

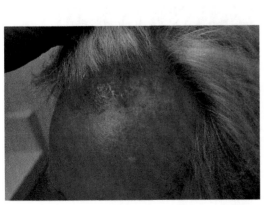

Fig. 8. Frontal fibrosing alopecia: recession of frontal hairline with atrophic, ivory-colored zone of hair loss.

Fig. 10. Frontal fibrosing alopecia: cobblestoning of the cheeks and chin.

it frequently coexists with other autoimmune-related conditions, such as thyroid disease, lupus, diabetes, and Sjogren syndrome.[7] For unknown reasons, the condition seems to be increasing in prevalence.[8]

The treatment of FFA also involves the use of topical, intralesional, and systemic anti-inflammatory treatments. Unfortunately, the condition can wax and wane over a lifetime. Patients can undergo surgery and may have good growth in the short run; however, the long-term growth of transplanted follicles cannot be guaranteed.[9] See Case 3 for further discussion.

Pseudopelade of Brocque

It is unclear whether this form of hair loss is a distinct entity or whether it represents a burned-out, late stage of cicatricial alopecia, in which all the inflammation has resolved. It may appear clinically similar with AA, with flesh-colored, smooth "footprints in the snow" (**Fig. 11**). For this reason the word pseudopelade is the French term for "false alopecia areata." It has been reported to either spontaneously resolve or improve with systemic medications such as hydroxychloroquine. However, the hair seldom regrows.[10]

Folliculitis Decalvans

Folliculitis decalvans is a form of scarring alopecia that can present in the vertex area and usually affects men (**Fig. 12**). Dermatoscopic examination of the scalp will usually reveal white pustules, a golden crust, and tufting of hair follicles (where surrounding scar tissue compresses 2 or more follicular units together) (**Fig. 13**). The condition is in most cases idiopathic; however, there is a case report of a patient developing the condition 20 years after hair transplant surgery.[11]

Histologically, there is a neutrophilic infiltrate in and among hair follicles. These pustules can be

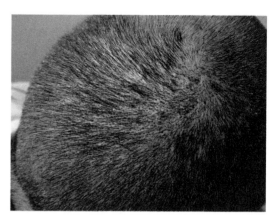

Fig. 12. Folliculitis decalvans: male patient with vertex involvement.

sterile but are frequently colonized with *Staphylococcus aureus*. Treatment involves topical and oral antibiotics (doxycycline, clindamycin, trimethoprim-sulfamethoxazole) as well as the antineutrophilic agent dapsone.

Central Centrifugal Cicatricial Alopecia

Central centrifugal cicatricial alopecia (CCCA) occurs primarily in African American women (**Fig. 14**).[12] It has long been thought a result of lye-based chemical relaxers, tight braids, or other damaging grooming techniques. More recent reports suggest a genetic role. The author has identified a positive family history in many affected patients. The condition generally begins with itching and tenderness in the vertex of the scalp. Subsequent hair loss occurs in a symmetric and centrifugal distribution. In areas of active disease, dermatoscopic examination may reveal a perifollicular erythema. In areas of longstanding disease, follicular ostia are replaced by tiny white dots of fibrosis (**Fig. 15**).

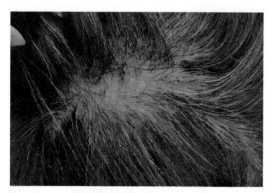

Fig. 11. Pseudopelade of Brocq: scarring alopecia with no evidence of erythema.

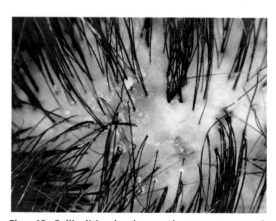

Fig. 13. Folliculitis decalvans: dermoscopy reveals golden crusts with tufting of follicles.

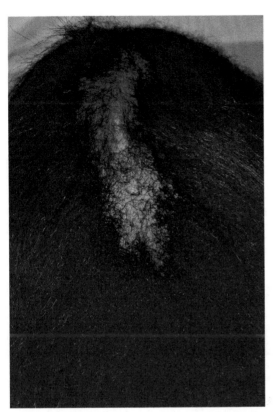

Fig. 14. CCCA: young woman with loss of follicular ostia in vertex of scalp.

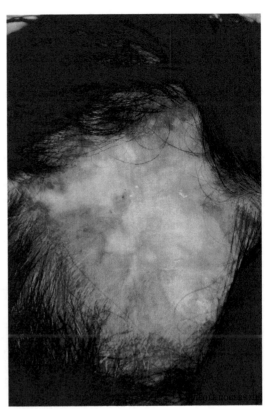

Fig. 16. Discoid lupus: young woman with large depigmented alopecic patch.

Discoid Lupus Erythematosus

Discoid lupus (also called chronic cutaneous lupus erythematosus) is limited to the skin and is seen in African Americans slightly more frequently than Caucasians. In the scalp, it appears as shiny permanent alopecia with frequent loss of pigmentation centrally (**Fig. 16**). On dermoscopy, atrophy with follicular plugging may be present (**Fig. 17**). First-line treatment options include topical and

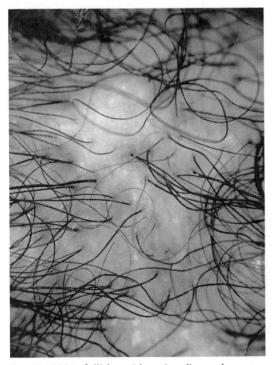

Fig. 15. CCCA: follicles with active disease have erythema; white dots indicate fully fibrosed follicles.

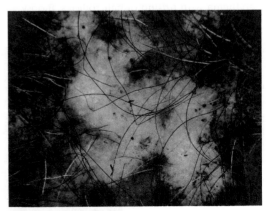

Fig. 17. Discoid lupus: dermoscopy reveals follicular plugging and loss of pigmentation.

intralesional steroids, hydroxychloroquine, and sun protection.

Overlapping Conditions

Occasionally, primary scarring alopecias are seen in addition to other scalp conditions. It is not uncommon to diagnose AA or lichen planopilaris in the presence of male or female pattern hair loss. Sometimes a longstanding diagnosis of LPP is only identified after transplanted hairs do not grow. African Americans can also develop overlapping conditions such as CCCA in the presence of discoid lupus.

CASE STUDIES

Case 1:

A 46-year-old man presented for a refill of his prescription finasteride. He has been taking the medicine for 5 years under the care of his primary doctor. He denied any symptoms of scalp itching or burning. On physical examination he had diffuse thinning on the frontal scalp. However, on close inspection, there were areas of shiny alopecia with irregular distances between the hairs (**Fig. 18**).On dermoscopy, there was bright red erythema around follicles (**Fig. 19**). The area was biopsied and found to be consistent with lichen planopilaris. He was placed on doxycycline in addition to renewing the finasteride but has failed to follow-up for further treatment.

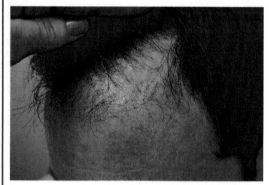

Fig. 18. Case of LPP believed to be AGA by patient and previous MD.

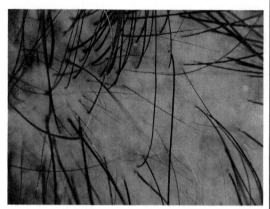

Fig. 19. LPP: dermoscopy reveals erythema and irregular space between follicles.

Case 2:

A 33-year-old man with hair loss in the vertex presented for treatment options (**Fig. 20**). He had not been evaluated by other doctors and complained of no symptoms. However, on close examination, he had erythema with tufting of hair follicles. Biopsy was consistent with folliculitis decalvans. The condition improved with doxycycline.

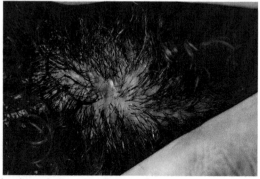

Fig. 20. Case of folliculitis decalvans believed to be AGA by patient.

Case 3:

A 65-year-old woman with a diagnosis of frontal fibrosing alopecia was seen for hair transplantation (**Fig. 21**). Her condition had been stable for 5 years following extensive medical treatment at the Cleveland Clinic. Biopsy showed no inflammation. After extensive discussion about the limitations of hair transplant surgery, the patient elected to proceed. Eight hundred grafts were placed along the frontal hairline. Follow-up at 1 year demonstrated very poor growth (**Fig. 22**).

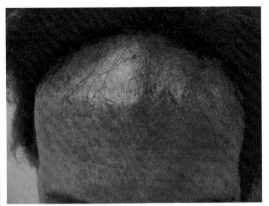

Fig. 21. Case of FFA prior to hair transplantation.

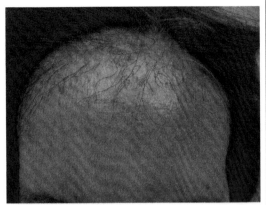

Fig. 22. Case of FFA 1 year after hair transplantation with poor growth.

Case 4:

A 61-year-old woman presented with 10-year history of hair thinning over the crown of her scalp (**Fig. 23**). She denied any symptoms of itching or burning. She was interested in medical and/or surgical options for AGA. Close examination revealed shiny, increased space between follicles with slight erythema around the follicles. Biopsy revealed late-stage lichen planopilaris.

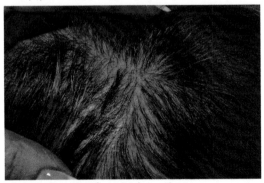

Fig. 23. Longstanding case of LPP believed to be AGA by patient.

SUMMARY

Hair transplant surgeons are expected to be experts of all things concerning hair. In this vein, it is essential to recognize certain warning signs before proceeding with surgery. Perifollicular erythema, shiny alopecia with loss of follicular ostia, yellow dots, unexplained pruritis and burning, and exclamation mark hairs are important clinical clues to identify AGA imposters. The use of polarized light with magnification can ease the recognition of these signs. Physicians who are not comfortable looking for these features may consider routinely performing a scalp biopsy to rule out such imposters of androgenetic alopecia definitively.

REFERENCES

1. Wikramanayake TC, Rodriguez R, Choudhary S, et al. Effects of the Lexington Lasercomb on hair regrowth in the C3H/HeJ mouse model of alopecia areata. Lasers Med Sci 2012;27:431–6.
2. Unger R, Dawoud T, Albaqami R. Successful hair transplantation of recalcitrant alopecia areata of the scalp. Dermatol Surg 2008;34:1589–94.
3. Barankin B, Taher M, Wasel N. Successful hair transplant of eyebrow alopecia areata. J Cutan Med Surg 2005;9:162–4.
4. Karnik P, Tekeste Z, McCormick TS, et al. Hair follicle stem-cell specific PPAR gamma deletion causes scarring alopecia. J Invest Dermatol 2009;129:1243–57.
5. Mirmirani P, Karnik P. Lichen planopilaris treated with peroxisome proliferator-actived receptor gamma agonist. Arch Dermatol 2009;145:1363–6.
6. Donati A, Molina L, Doche I, et al. Facial papules in frontal fibrosing alopecia: evidence of vellus follicle involvement. Arch Dermatol 2011;147:1424–7.
7. Cevasco NC, Bergfeld WF, Remzi BK, et al. A case-series of 29 patients with lichen planopilaris: the Cleveland Clinic Foundation experience on evaluation, diagnosis, and treatment. J Am Acad Dermatol 2007;57:47–53.
8. MacDonald A, Clark C, Holmes S. Frontal fibrosing alopecia: a review of 60 cases. J Am Acad Dermatol 2012;67(5):955–61.
9. Nusbaum BP, Nusbaum AG. Frontal fibrosing alopecia in a man: results of follicular unit test grafting. Dermatol Surg 2010;36:959–62.
10. Harries MJ, Sinclair RD, MacDonald-Hull S, et al. Management of primary cicatricial alopecias: options for treatment. Br J Dermatol 2008;159:1–22.
11. Otberg N, Wu WY, Kang H, et al. Folliculitis decalvans developing 20 years after hair restoration surgery in punch grafts: case report. Dermatol Surg 2009;35:1852–6.
12. Gathers RC, Lim HW. Central centrifugal cicatricial alopecia: past, present, and future. J Am Acad Dermatol 2008;60:660–8.

Nonsurgical Therapy for Hair Loss

Aron G. Nusbaum, MD, Paul T. Rose, MD,
Bernard P. Nusbaum, MD*

KEYWORDS

- Androgenetic alopecia • Medical therapy for pattern hair loss • Minoxidil • Finasteride • Dutasteride
- Low-level laser therapy for hair loss

KEY POINTS

- Topically applied minoxidil results in increased hair weight with a less dramatic increase in hair counts, suggesting that its therapeutic effect is primarily due to increasing the diameter of existing hairs.
- Finasteride is a type II 5α-reductase inhibitor that decreases serum and scalp levels of dihydrotestosterone. Administered orally at a dose of 1 mg daily, it is by far the most effective FDA-approved treatment of male pattern hair loss.
- Although a small number of men claim that they have suffered permanent sexual dysfunction despite discontinuation of finasteride, most large, double-blind, placebo-controlled studies do not confirm the claims of persistent sexual dysfunction. In a subset of men, however, prolonged sexual side effects lasting weeks to months have been reported and patients should be advised to report promptly any side effects.
- The optimal frequency, power, and duration of low-level light therapy for treating pattern hair loss have yet to be determined. Current treatment protocols are determined on an empiric basis. Theoretically, it is possible that too high a dose could result in a reversal of therapeutic benefit.

INTRODUCTION

The introduction of minoxidil in the late 1970s and systemic 5α-reductase inhibitor therapy in the late 1990s each provided, for the first time, an effective means for halting the progression of male pattern baldness and, in some cases, achieving regrowth.[1] Medical therapy is most effective when started in the early phases of pattern hair loss and patients may elect to be treated solely with nonsurgical modalities. Undoubtedly, as long as surgical hair restoration is limited by a finite donor supply, medical therapy will play a central role as an adjunct to surgical treatment by preventing loss of surrounding native hair and thus enhancing the overall aesthetic result.

MINOXIDIL

Minoxidil was originally developed as an antihypertensive agent that attracted interest as a potential hair loss therapy when patients receiving this drug via the oral route were noted to develop generalized hypertrichosis.[2] This observation led to its topical formulation, which has become a first-line treatment of pattern hair loss in men and women.[3] Topically applied minoxidil is currently available as an over-the-counter preparation in either a 2% or 5% solution, or as a 5% foam.

Mechanism of Action of Minoxidil

Minoxidil's mechanism of action was originally thought to be secondary to vasodilation but,

Hair Transplant Institute of Miami, Coral Gables, FL, USA
* Corresponding author. 4425 Ponce De Leon Boulevard #230, Coral Gables, FL 33146.
E-mail address: drnusbaum@miamihair.com

Facial Plast Surg Clin N Am 21 (2013) 335–342
http://dx.doi.org/10.1016/j.fsc.2013.04.003

recently, it has been linked to the opening of potassium channels.[4] In the stump-tail macaque, minoxidil was shown to increase follicle size in histologic sections as well as the percentage of anagen follicles.[5] These findings have been confirmed in clinical studies of male-pattern hair loss (MPHL).[6] Topically applied minoxidil increases hair weight with a less dramatic increase in hair counts, suggesting that its therapeutic effect is primarily due to increasing the diameter of existing hairs.[7] In MPHL, the 5% concentration is superior in efficacy to 2%, with 45% more hair growth after 48 weeks of treatment.[8] It should be noted that, although the package label states that minoxidil is indicated for treatment of the vertex, in the authors' experience it is effective for treating the top scalp and frontal areas.

Side Effects of Minoxidil

The most commonly observed side effect is allergic or irritant contact dermatitis. This is predominately in reaction to propylene glycol, which is used to enhance minoxidil solubility in the liquid vehicle. It should be noted that, although less frequent, true allergic reactions to minoxidil also occur. Irritant contact dermatitis occurs less frequently with the 2% compared with the 5% solution. Patients exhibiting this type of reaction can be switched to the 5% foam vehicle, which is formulated without propylene glycol.[9] If reactions persist, contact allergy to minoxidil is likely and, therefore, all minoxidil preparations should be discontinued. In the absence of contact reactions, compliance issues may arise either from the cosmetic appearance of the hair following application (which may influence the choice of foam or liquid) or from the need for twice daily use. Compounding tretinoin into a minoxidil solution may increase its efficacy and improve compliance because once daily application of 5% minoxidil with 0.01% tretinoin was shown to be equal in efficacy to twice-daily 5% minoxidil alone.[10]

Minoxidil Use in Females

For women, minoxidil is marketed only as a 2% solution because the 5% solution is associated with a greater incidence of hypertrichosis.[11] In a study of 1333 women with female-pattern hair loss (FPHL), 4% developed hypertrichosis outside the area of application. This was more frequent with the 5% solution than the 2% solution and generally resolved 1 to 3 months after discontinuation.[11] A more recent study showed equal efficacy in women who applied the 2% solution twice daily compared with a single daily application of the 5% foam, with the latter resulting in less pruritus and flaking.[12] There is increasing evidence that FPHL is associated with a significant inflammatory component and a formulation of 5% minoxidil with 0.025% retinoic acid and 0.05% betamethasone dipropionate has been shown to be effective in treating women with FPHL (**Fig. 1**).[13] It should be noted that minoxidil might be harmful in women who are pregnant or breastfeeding.

FINASTERIDE

Finasteride is a type II 5α-reductase inhibitor that decreases serum and scalp levels of dihydrotestosterone (DHT).[1] It is administered orally at a dose of 1 mg daily and is by far the most effective FDA-approved treatment of MPHL. It acts predominantly by increasing hair diameter and growth rate, although increased hair counts are also observed to a lesser degree.[1] In 1553 men, daily treatment with 1 mg finasteride resulted in stabilization of pattern hair loss in 51% and regrowth in 48% of subjects.[14] The first signs of efficacy are usually seen at 3 months when men who complain

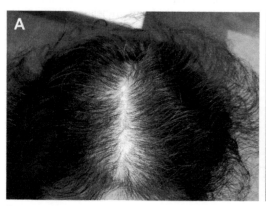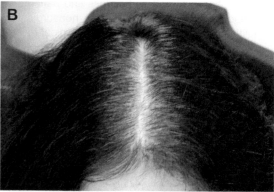

Fig. 1. A 39-year-old woman with FPHL. (*A*) Before and (*B*) after 10 months of treatment with once daily applications of a minoxidil 2%, retinoic acid 0.025%, betamethasone dipropionate 0.05% solution.

of increased hair shedding during their hair loss process begin to notice improvement in this parameter. To assess fully stabilization and/or regrowth, 12 months of therapy are required.

Side Effects of Finasteride

Finasteride was evaluated for safety in a large clinical trial of subjects with MPHL. The most common drug-related side effects were decreased libido (1.9%), erectile dysfunction (1.4%), and decreased ejaculate volume (1.0%).[14] Resolution of these side effects occurred in those men who discontinued the drug and in many of those who continued therapy. In the authors practice, we have observed resolution of side effects in some patients simply by prescribing every-other-day dosing. In a dose-ranging study of men ages 18 to 36 years, 0.2, 1, and 5 mg daily were shown to be effective compared with placebo. Doses of 1 and 5 mg daily had similar efficacy, whereas 0.2 mg daily showed 70% to 90% of the effect seen with 1 mg, depending on the parameter being measured.[15] The effectiveness of lower doses may serve as a rationale for decreasing daily dosage or frequency of administration in patients who develop side effects. Postmarketing side effects reported include breast tenderness and/or enlargement, breast nodules, depression, allergic reactions, testicular pain, and rare cases of male breast cancer. Although a small number of men claim that they have suffered permanent sexual dysfunction despite discontinuation of the drug,[16] most large, double-blind, placebo-controlled studies do not confirm the claims of persistent sexual dysfunction.[14,15] In a subset of men, however, prolonged sexual side effects lasting weeks to months have been reported[17] and patients should be advised to report promptly any side effects.

Men older than age 45 should be advised that finasteride affects the results of prostate-specific antigen testing and, therefore, should report the use of this medication to their physician. In the 7-year prostate cancer prevention trial, men older than age 55 taking finasteride 5 mg daily (5 times the daily dose of Propecia) had an overall decrease in the incidence of prostate cancer, but those who did develop prostate cancer had a higher proportion of histologically high-grade tumors.[18] It has not been clearly established whether this effect was due to histologic grading artifacts that have been observed with androgen deprivation therapy[18] or to increased sampling density bias from reducing prostate volume,[19] or if 5α-reductase inhibitors may increase the risk of developing high-grade prostate cancer. Additional validation is necessary to draw firm conclusions. Women

should not handle crushed or broken finasteride tabs when they are pregnant or trying to become pregnant because of the possibility of percutaneous absorption and subsequent risk to the male fetus.

Finasteride Use in Females

Finasteride therapy for FPHL was first evaluated in a large well-controlled study of postmenopausal women in which a 1 mg daily dose was shown to have no effect.[20] Although a handful of case reports have demonstrated stabilization of hair loss with some regrowth using higher doses than what is used in men (2.5–5 mg daily), the limited clinical studies available show varying results. Thirty-seven premenopausal women with no evidence of hyperandrogenism were treated with 2.5 mg of finasteride orally plus an oral contraceptive agent containing ethinyl estradiol and drospirenone for 12 months.[21] Scalp photography showed improvement in 62% of the subjects, of which half were slightly improved and half were moderately to greatly improved. Thirty-five percent of the study subjects had stabilization of their hair loss. In addition, there was a statistically significant increase in the hair density score in 12 subjects. No adverse reactions to the drug were reported. In a separate study of 87 normoandrogenic premenopausal and postmenopausal women, 5 mg of finasteride daily for 12 months showed a statistically significant improvement in hair density and hair thickness on phototrichogram.[22] In addition, 81.4% improved on global photographic assessment. Although finasteride would be expected to be particularly effective in women with hyperandrogenism, a study of 48 premenopausal women with documented hyperandrogenism showed that finasteride 5 mg daily did not result in a statistically significant improvement as measured by Ludwig score and subjective assessment of clinical improvement.[23] Finasteride is not approved by the FDA for the treatment of FPHL and, therefore, is prescribed off label. Pregnancy must be ruled out before instituting therapy and women should be maintained on strict birth contraception during treatment.

Other Antiandrogens for Female Hair Loss

Other antiandrogens for systemic use in FPHL include spironolactone and cyproterone acetate (the latter not available in the United States). Spironolactone requires 6 to 12 months to exhibit a therapeutic effect and treatment is generally initiated with a low dose of 25 to 50 mg daily, which is then gradually increased to a maintenance dose of 100 to 200 mg daily, which is the dose required to attain a therapeutic benefit. In a study of 80 FPHL subjects, 200 mg daily of spironolactone was equivalent to 100 mg daily of cyproterone acetate, resulting in 44% of subjects experiencing regrowth, 44% with stabilization, and 12% with further hair loss.[24] It should be noted that spironolactone may elevate serum potassium levels and regular monitoring is necessary. In addition, patients should be advised to adhere to strict, effective birth contraception while taking antiandrogens because they pose a risk to the fetus.

DUTASTERIDE

Dutasteride inhibits both type I and type II 5α-reductase and was approved by the FDA in 2002 for the treatment of benign prostatic hyperplasia at a dose of 0.5 mg per day.[1] Since then, dutasteride has been used off label for the treatment of MPHL and FPHL. Compared to finasteride, dutasteride is 3 times more potent for inhibiting type II 5α-reductase and 100 times more potent for inhibiting the type I enzyme in vitro.[25] In a study of 416 men ages 21 to 45 years, various doses of dutasteride were compared with finasteride 5 mg or placebo for 24 weeks of treatment.[26] Finasteride 1 mg was not available at the time of the study and previous data showed that 1 and 5 mg of finasteride were equal in efficacy for treatment of MPHL. All dutasteride doses tested (0.05, 0.1, 0.5, 2.5 mg) and finasteride 5 mg were significantly better than placebo at 12 and 24 weeks, but only dutasteride at a 2.5 mg daily dose was statistically superior to finasteride with respect to hair counts. There was no significant difference in adverse events, but it is noteworthy that 9 of 71 subjects treated with dutasteride 2.5 mg daily developed decreased libido, whereas only 1 of 68 subjects treated with dutasteride 0.5 mg complained of this side effect. Because scalp DHT suppression most likely correlates with clinical efficacy, we might speculate that a dutasteride 0.5 mg daily dose should be superior to finasteride as reflected by the 51% scalp DHT reduction observed with dutasteride 0.5 mg compared with the 32% suppression of finasteride.[26] Although dutasteride 2.5 mg showed a 79% reduction, the frequency of sexual side effects cited above suggests that, from a risk benefit ratio, 0.5 mg daily may be the optimal dose. In fact, this dose was evaluated in a phase III 6 month trial of 153 men ages 18 to 49 years that showed a statistically significant improvement compared with placebo with regard to hair counts, self-assessment scores, and photographic assessment.[27]

Side Effects of Dutasteride

Sexual dysfunction was reported in 4.1% of the subjects in the treatment group compared with 2.7% of those receiving placebo. Unfortunately, the study did not evaluate sperm parameters; concern in this regard has been raised by a study that showed decreased sperm counts after 26 weeks of treatment with dutasteride 0.5 mg daily in 27 subjects, with 2 subjects developing greater than 90% reduction in sperm count that, after 24 weeks of discontinuing therapy, improved by only 20%.[28] This brings to light concern with dutasteride side effects because the half-life of the drug is 4 to 5 weeks compared with the half-life of finasteride, which is only 6 to 8 hours.[26] Therefore, any side effects that occur secondary to dutasteride may take much longer to resolve than with finasteride. Additionally, this drug should be used with caution in men with MPHL due to concerns of infertility. The authors suggest that dutasteride should be reserved for cases of MPHL that are refractory to finasteride therapy. We have observed stabilization of hair loss in such patients with a 0.5 mg daily dose (**Fig. 2**). Of the first three such patients treated, all in their early twenties, two developed profoundly decreased sperm counts that gradually returned to normal after discontinuing the drug. A case report describes a patient who was experiencing decreased response to finasteride after 4 years of therapy and experienced an increase in hair density 3 months after the addition of dutasteride at 0.5 mg weekly.[29] The extended half-life of dutasteride serves as a rationale for intermittent dosing even though the optimal frequency interval has not been determined.

LOW-LEVEL LIGHT OR LASER THERAPY

Light was first reported to stimulate hair growth in 1967 in a mouse model.[30] More recent reports of paradoxic hair growth in subjects receiving laser therapy for hair removal serve as a basis for evaluating this modality in treating patients with pattern hair loss.[31]

Mechanism of Action of Light and Laser Therapy for Hair Loss

It is presumed that the mechanism of action for hair stimulation is mediated by absorption of photons by cytochrome oxidase in the mitochondrial respiratory chain, resulting in increased oxygen consumption and ATP production.[32] Gene regulation resulting in decreased apoptosis is presumed to occur as a result.

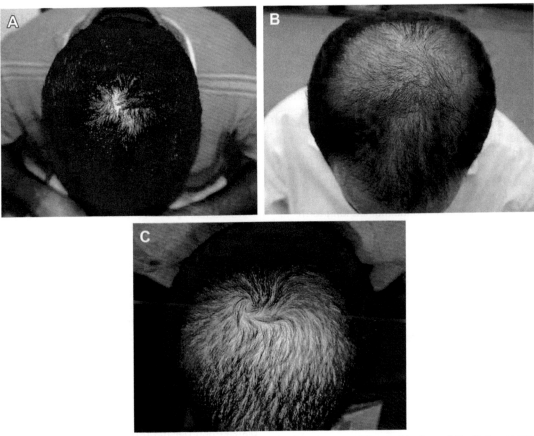

Fig. 2. A 24-year-old man with FPHL. (*A*) Pretreatment. (*B*) After 4 years of finasteride 1 mg daily. Note progression of MPHL. (*C*) Discontinuing finasteride and starting dutasteride 0.5 mg daily for 9 months resulted in stabilization.

Laser and Light Devices for Hair Loss

Several devices are available that emit wavelengths of 630 to 680 nm. In a study of 123 men with MPHL, treatment with the HairMax Laser-Comb (Lexington International [Boca Raton, FL, USA]) resulted in a statistically significant increase in hair counts compared with a sham device.[33] The HairMax received 510(k) clearance from the FDA in 2005 and is recommended for use 3 times per week for 10 to 15 minutes with results expected after approximately 4 months of treatment. The handheld, home-use devices, such as the Hair-Max, Sunetics Laser Hair Brush (Sunetics International, Las Vegas, NV, USA), and X5 Hair Laser (Spencer Forrest, Inc [Los Angeles, CA, USA]), must be sequentially moved over the affected area by the patient during the treatment period, which may affect compliance. In-office systems such as the Sunetics Model G and MEP90 system (Midwest RF, LLC [Hartland, WI, USA]), the latter cleared by the FDA, resemble hair salon dryer hoods and deliver higher total doses than the handheld devices. However, compliance may be limited because of the frequent office visits required (2 to 3 times per week), especially in the initial treatment period. A home-use system, LaserCap (Transdermal Cap, Inc [Cleveland, OH, USA]), with more power than most in-office systems is available (**Fig. 3**). It contains 224 5 mW

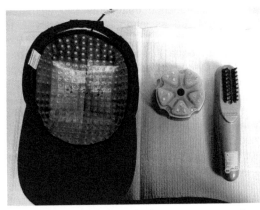

Fig. 3. Low-level laser devices for home use. Left to right: LaserCap, X5 Hair Laser, HairMax LaserComb.

laser diodes in a helmet-type configuration that fits under a hat or cap. Powered by a rechargeable battery, it is portable and treatment can be administered while on the go. LaserCap is currently available for purchase only through physicians.

The optimal frequency, power, and duration for treating pattern hair loss with low-level light therapy has yet to be determined and current treatment protocols are determined on an empiric basis. Theoretically, it is possible that too high a dose could result in a reversal of therapeutic benefit[32] and more well-controlled studies are needed to determine optimal wavelength, power, treatment frequency, and duration, as well as whether benefits can be maintained long term.

ADDITIONAL THERAPIES FOR HAIR LOSS
Prostaglandin Analogues

The FDA approval of topical bimatoprost for eyelash hypotrichosis has spurred interest in the use of prostaglandin (PG) analogues for the treatment of pattern hair loss. The PG pathway is intimately related to hair growth because PGE_2 and $PGF_2\alpha$ promote hair growth, whereas PGD_2 inhibits hair growth in both mice and human follicles.[34] Latanoprost (a $PGF_2\alpha$ analogue) applied as a 0.1% solution resulted in a statistically significant increase in hair density in 16 men with MPHL compared with placebo.[35] Allergan (Irvine, CA, USA) is currently conducting a multicenter study evaluating the safety and efficacy of bimatoprost for the treatment of pattern hair loss.

Mesotherapy

Mesotherapy consists of superficial scalp injections of pharmaceuticals and vitamin compounds that have been previously used to treat hair loss via the topical or systemic routes of administration. Injections are often administered initially at weekly intervals and subsequently with longer intervals so that maintenance treatments can ultimately be administered as infrequently as every 2 to 3 months. Multiple, small-volume injections (0.02–0.05 ml) are equally spaced approximately 5 mm apart to cover the affected area (Fig. 4). Although there are no established treatment protocols, the rationale is to deliver active compounds directly to the follicle, avoiding systemic administration with its possible side effects. In addition, the treatment schedules used are designed to enhance compliance compared with topical agents that require once or twice daily topical applications. Compounds used include minoxidil, finasteride, dutasteride, biotin, tretinoin, pantothenic acid, pyridoxine, procaine, and other vitamins and minerals. In a study of 126 subjects with FPHL injected with a

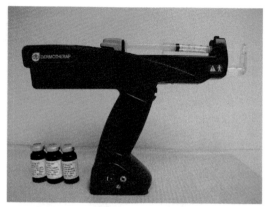

Fig. 4. Power injector to enhance ergonomics of mesotherapy. These devices provide depth control as well as metered injections.

combination of dutasteride, biotin, pyridoxine, and D-panthenol, photographic improvement was seen in 63% compared with 17.5% with saline placebo.[36] Minimal side effects were reported. Further studies are necessary to determine which compounds are active and at what concentrations so that optimal efficacy can be achieved via this route.

Platelet-Rich Plasma

The finding that platelets are a rich reservoir for cytokines and growth factors has led to the use of platelet-rich plasma (PRP) in dentistry, maxillofacial surgery, orthopedics, and treatment of chronic wounds. Its use for hair loss stems from reports of enhanced growth of transplanted follicular units.[37–39] PRP therapy consists of injecting concentrated autologous platelets into the scalp that, when activated, release growth factors such as platelet-derived growth factor, transforming growth factor, vascular endothelial growth factor, insulin-like growth factor, epidermal growth factor, and interleukin-1.[40] Some claim that this treatment delivers stem cells, which is a fallacy because there are no stem cells present. Although small studies have demonstrated the effectiveness of PRP in accelerating healing in hair transplant surgery,[41] data to support direct stimulation of hair growth is limited. PRP applied to dermal papilla cells in vitro stimulates their proliferation and upregulates components of the Wnt pathway, which is intimately related to hair growth.[40] Injection of mice with PRP induced a faster telogen to anagen transition[40] and, in a clinical trial of 26 men and women with pattern hair loss, PRP showed an increase in target hair counts compared with control.[42] When PRP was administered with dalteparin and protamine microparticles as carriers for controlled release of growth factors, the effect on hair counts was similar, yet the combination was superior to

PRP alone with respect to increasing hair shaft diameter.[42] A drawback to this study was that target sites for baseline and posttreatment measurements were localized by measuring landmarks rather than tattooing. Various PRP products are available that differ in their method of preparation, platelet concentration, and type of platelet activator used. Well-controlled studies are needed to evaluate PRP as a hair loss therapy.

SUMMARY

The treatments described in this article can be used alone as monotherapy or in various combinations. Therapeutic modalities that act by different mechanisms may be additive in their effects or, in some cases, synergistic. Pattern hair loss gradually progresses in severity if left untreated and medical therapy is most effective in the early stages. Patients must understand that current treatments for hair loss are not curative and, therefore, must be continued indefinitely. As research in hair basic science continues to unravel the molecular signals that regulate the hair cycle, it is expected that novel therapeutic agents will be developed to directly arrest follicular miniaturization and revert affected follicles into robust, cosmetically pleasing terminal hairs.

REFERENCES

1. Schweiger ES, Boychenko O, Bernstein RM. Update on the pathogenesis, genetics and medical treatment of patterned hair loss. J Drugs Dermatol 2010;9(11):1412–9.
2. Rogers NE, Avram MR. Medical treatments for male and female pattern hair loss. J Am Acad Dermatol 2008;59(4):547–66 [quiz: 567–8].
3. Tsuboi R, Itami S, Inui S, et al. Guidelines for the management of androgenetic alopecia (2010). J Dermatol 2012;39(2):113–20.
4. Shorter K, Farjo NP, Picksley SM, et al. Human hair follicles contain two forms of ATP-sensitive potassium channels, only one of which is sensitive to minoxidil. FASEB J 2008;22(6):1725–36.
5. Brigham PA, Cappas A, Uno H. The stumptailed macaque as a model for androgenetic alopecia: effects of topical minoxidil analyzed by use of the folliculogram. Clin Dermatol 1988;6(4):177–87.
6. Abell E. Histologic response to topically applied minoxidil in male-pattern alopecia. Clin Dermatol 1988;6(4):191–4.
7. Price VH, Menefee E, Strauss PC. Changes in hair weight and hair count in men with androgenetic alopecia, after application of 5% and 2% topical minoxidil, placebo, or no treatment. J Am Acad Dermatol 1999;41(5 Pt 1):717–21.
8. Olsen EA, Dunlap FE, Funicella T, et al. A randomized clinical trial of 5% topical minoxidil versus 2% topical minoxidil and placebo in the treatment of androgenetic alopecia in men. J Am Acad Dermatol 2002;47(3):377–85.
9. Friedman ES, Friedman PM, Cohen DE, et al. Allergic contact dermatitis to topical minoxidil solution: etiology and treatment. J Am Acad Dermatol 2002;46(2):309–12.
10. Shin HS, Won CH, Lee SH, et al. Efficacy of 5% minoxidil versus combined 5% minoxidil and 0.01% tretinoin for male pattern hair loss: a randomized, double-blind, comparative clinical trial. Am J Clin Dermatol 2007;8(5):285–90.
11. Dawber RP, Rundegren J. Hypertrichosis in females applying minoxidil topical solution and in normal controls. J Eur Acad Dermatol Venereol 2003; 17(3):271–5.
12. Blume-Peytavi U, Hillmann K, Dietz E, et al. A randomized, single-blind trial of 5% minoxidil foam once daily versus 2% minoxidil solution twice daily in the treatment of androgenetic alopecia in women. J Am Acad Dermatol 2011;65(6):1126–1134.e2.
13. Magro CM, Rossi A, Poe J, et al. The role of inflammation and immunity in the pathogenesis of androgenetic alopecia. J Drugs Dermatol 2011;10(12): 1404–11.
14. Kaufman KD, Olsen EA, Whiting D, et al. Finasteride in the treatment of men with androgenetic alopecia. Finasteride Male Pattern Hair Loss Study Group. J Am Acad Dermatol 1998;39(4 Pt 1):578–89.
15. Roberts JL, Fiedler V, Imperato-McGinley J, et al. Clinical dose ranging studies with finasteride, a type 2 5alpha-reductase inhibitor, in men with male pattern hair loss. J Am Acad Dermatol 1999;41(4): 555–63.
16. Irwig MS, Kolukula S. Persistent sexual side effects of finasteride for male pattern hair loss. J Sex Med 2011;8(6):1747–53.
17. Traish AM, Hassani J, Guay AT, et al. Adverse side effects of 5alpha-reductase inhibitors therapy: persistent diminished libido and erectile dysfunction and depression in a subset of patients. J Sex Med 2011;8(3):872–84.
18. Lucia MS, Epstein JI, Goodman PJ, et al. Finasteride and high-grade prostate cancer in the Prostate Cancer Prevention Trial. J Natl Cancer Inst 2007;99(18): 1375–83.
19. Cohen YC, Liu KS, Heyden NL, et al. Detection bias due to the effect of finasteride on prostate volume: a modeling approach for analysis of the Prostate Cancer Prevention Trial. J Natl Cancer Inst 2007;99(18): 1366–74.
20. Price VH, Roberts JL, Hordinsky M, et al. Lack of efficacy of finasteride in postmenopausal women with androgenetic alopecia. J Am Acad Dermatol 2000; 43(5 Pt 1):768–76.

21. Iorizzo M, Vincenzi C, Voudouris S, et al. Finasteride treatment of female pattern hair loss. Arch Dermatol 2006;142(3):298–302.

22. Yeon JH, Jung JY, Choi JW, et al. 5 mg/day finasteride treatment for normoandrogenic Asian women with female pattern hair loss. J Eur Acad Dermatol Venereol 2011;25(2):211–4.

23. Carmina E, Lobo RA. Treatment of hyperandrogenic alopecia in women. Fertil Steril 2003;79(1):91–5.

24. Sinclair R, Wewerinke M, Jolley D. Treatment of female pattern hair loss with oral antiandrogens. Br J Dermatol 2005;152(3):466–73.

25. Clark RV, Hermann DJ, Cunningham GR, et al. Marked suppression of dihydrotestosterone in men with benign prostatic hyperplasia by dutasteride, a dual 5alpha-reductase inhibitor. J Clin Endocrinol Metab 2004;89(5):2179–84.

26. Olsen EA, Hordinsky M, Whiting D, et al. The importance of dual 5alpha-reductase inhibition in the treatment of male pattern hair loss: results of a randomized placebo-controlled study of dutasteride versus finasteride. J Am Acad Dermatol 2006; 55(6):1014–23.

27. Eun HC, Kwon OS, Yeon JH, et al. Efficacy, safety, and tolerability of dutasteride 0.5 mg once daily in male patients with male pattern hair loss: a randomized, double-blind, placebo-controlled, phase III study. J Am Acad Dermatol 2010;63(2):252–8.

28. Amory JK, Wang C, Swerdloff RS, et al. The effect of 5alpha-reductase inhibition with dutasteride and finasteride on semen parameters and serum hormones in healthy men. J Clin Endocrinol Metab 2007;92(5):1659–65.

29. Boyapati A, Sinclair R. Combination therapy with finasteride and low-dose dutasteride in the treatment of androgenetic alopecia. Australas J Dermatol 2013;54(1):49–51.

30. Hamblin MR, Demidova TN. Mechanisms of low level light therapy. Proc SPIE 2006;6140:1–12.

31. Bernstein EF. Hair growth induced by diode laser treatment. Dermatol Surg 2005;31(5):584–6.

32. Farjo N. An interview with Professor Michael Hamblin. Hair Transplant Forum Int'l 2010;20(3):83.

33. Leavitt M, Charles G, Heyman E, et al. HairMax LaserComb laser phototherapy device in the treatment of male androgenetic alopecia: a randomized, double-blind, sham device-controlled, multicentre trial. Clin Drug Investig 2009;29(5):283–92.

34. Garza LA, Liu Y, Yang Z, et al. Prostaglandin D2 inhibits hair growth and is elevated in bald scalp of men with androgenetic alopecia. Sci Transl Med 2012;4(126):126ra134.

35. Blume-Peytavi U, Lonnfors S, Hillmann K, et al. A randomized double-blind placebo-controlled pilot study to assess the efficacy of a 24-week topical treatment by latanoprost 0.1% on hair growth and pigmentation in healthy volunteers with androgenetic alopecia. J Am Acad Dermatol 2012;66(5): 794–800.

36. Moftah N, Abd-Elaziz G, Ahmed N, et al. Mesotherapy using dutasteride-containing preparation in treatment of female pattern hair loss: photographic, morphometric and ultrustructural evaluation. J Eur Acad Dermatol Venereol 2012;27(6): 686–93.

37. Rinaldi F. Improving the revascularization of transplanted hair follicles through up-regulation of angiogenic growth factors. Hair Transplant Forum Int'l 2005;17(4):117–26.

38. Greco J, Brandt R. Preliminary experience and extended applications for the use of autologous platelet-rich plasma in hair transplantation surgery. Hair Transplant Forum Int'l 2007;17(4):131–2.

39. Uebel CO, da Silva JB, Cantarelli D, et al. The role of platelet plasma growth factors in male pattern baldness surgery. Plast Reconstr Surg 2006;118(6): 1458–66 [discussion: 1467].

40. Li ZJ, Choi HI, Choi DK, et al. Autologous platelet-rich plasma: a potential therapeutic tool for promoting hair growth. Dermatol Surg 2012;38(7 Pt 1): 1040–6.

41. Reese R. A single-blinded, randomized controlled study of the use of autologous platelet rich plasma (PRP) as a medium to reduce scalp hair transplant adverse effects. Hair Transplant Forum Int'l 2008; 18(2):51–2.

42. Takikawa M, Nakamura S, Ishirara M, et al. Enhanced effect of platelet-rich plasma containing a new carrier on hair growth. Dermatol Surg 2011; 37(12):1721–9.

Patient Selection, Candidacy, and Treatment Planning for Hair Restoration Surgery

Raymond J. Konior, MD[a,b,*],
Cam Simmons, MD, Diplomate of the ABHRS[c]

KEYWORDS

- Patient selection • Candidacy • Treatment planning • Hair restoration surgery • Hair transplant
- Hair transplant philosophy

KEY POINTS

- Hair restoration physicians must determine which patients are appropriate candidates for successful hair transplantation and understand the physical characteristics that may lead to less than optimal results.
- Hair restoration physicians must be cautious in selecting a young patient to transplant because these patients often desire aggressive restoration patterns in the setting of an unpredictable future of hair loss.
- Hair loss is progressive and can be unpredictable at any age.
- A thorough preoperative evaluation is essential to exclude those patients with conditions that are contraindications to hair restoration surgery and may require referral to a dermatologist.
- A detailed, long-term treatment plan must be prepared to ensure the patient's goals coincide with the anticipated outcomes outlined by the physician.

INTRODUCTION

Male-pattern baldness (MPB), also known as androgenetic alopecia (AGA), is the most common cause of hair loss. In affected areas, genetically sensitive hair follicles exposed to normal levels of dihydrotestosterone (DHT) go through progressively shorter anagen (growth) phases. New generations of terminal hairs miniaturize, becoming shorter, finer, and lighter in color, and they conceal the scalp less. In its final phase, the terminal hairs transition into vellus hairs. Miniaturization may be gradual or can come in waves, and the course and extent of AGA are unpredictable. There is polygenic inheritance and variable penetrance, so family history alone is not predictive.

Hair transplantation involves relocating unaffected donor hair follicles to a recipient area of thinning or balding with the expectation that the transplanted follicles will continue to produce unaffected terminal hairs. Experts once believed that the donor area was separated from the recipient area by a well-demarcated line. That definition of MPB stated that a man established a pattern, balding occurred within the pattern, and the pattern did not change significantly after midlife. The inference was that the surgeon could predict the patient's final pattern or the lowest line of

Disclosures: None.
[a] Department of Otolaryngology, Head and Neck Surgery, Loyola University Medical Center, 2160 South First Avenue, Maywood, IL 60153, USA; [b] Chicago Hair Institute, 1S280 Summit, Suite C-4, Oakbrook Terrace, IL 60181, USA; [c] Seager Hair Transplant Centre, Suite 418, The Court at Centenary, 2863 Ellesmere Road, Toronto, Ontario M1E 5E9, Canada
* Corresponding author. Chicago Hair Institute, 1S280 Summit, Suite C-4, Oakbrook Terrace, IL 60181.
E-mail address: drkonior@sbcglobal.net

Facial Plast Surg Clin N Am 21 (2013) 343–350
http://dx.doi.org/10.1016/j.fsc.2013.04.004
1064-7406/13/$ – see front matter © 2013 Elsevier Inc. All rights reserved.

facialplastic.theclinics.com

demarcation when a man reached an age somewhere between 30 and 45. Unfortunately, we now know that terminal hair has the potential to progress to vellus hair decades beyond the initiation of the balding process. The clear line that once was presumed to be permanent is actually an indistinct line that can advance inferiorly in many more cases, and often at much later ages, than we once thought possible.

PATIENT SELECTION

With regard to devising a surgical protocol, MPB must be defined as an event that proceeds into the ages of 50s, 60s, and beyond.[1] If MPB was a static process, the surgeon could easily choose a surgical procedure that would suit the patient for life. However, MPB is a dynamic process that can alter a patient's eligibility for any given procedure depending on the stage of baldness (**Fig. 1**). If, at age 30 years, the patient's baldness is defined as class IV, the physician must consider the risk of the baldness progressing to class V, VI, or VII in later years. The physician must factor in the variable of progression and select an appropriate treatment based on the patient's final pattern. If the surgeon would not perform a particular procedure on a 55-year-old man with class VI or VII baldness, he should not perform that same procedure on a 30-year-old man with class IV baldness because he may be the same patient 25 years later.

Patient Consultation

An in-depth consultation allows the patient to communicate their goals and desires for the hair restoration procedure.[2] The surgeon must take into account the patient's age, medical history, family history of alopecia, facial features, and hair characteristics (caliber, texture, color) that may have an effect on the final outcome. Young patients usually request a full head of hair even though future balding can make them poor surgical candidates for the procedures that are recommended. The surgeon must counsel young patients about their denial of how bald they will become and about any unrealistic fantasy of regaining a full head of hair. The fact is that hair transplantation does not create new hair; it only rearranges existing hair. The patient must understand his condition and the limitations of surgical restoration so that the surgeon can create an honest and logical treatment plan. Wherever possible, it is best to demonstrate before and after photographs of patients who faced similar limitations to show surgical candidates what results they can realistically expect.

Clinical Examination

Simple procedures can be used to uncover subtle signs and improve diagnosis.[3,4] Some physicians advocate wetting the hair to determine the line of demarcation between permanent terminal hair and thinning vellus hair. Wetting the hair can help identify currently thinning hair but does not predict future thinning. What appears to be terminal hair on the wet head of a 30-year-old man is not guaranteed to be terminal hair when he is 40 or 50 years old. However, wetting the head is useful for communicating a treatment plan to the patient and helping the patient appreciate the significance of his future pattern.

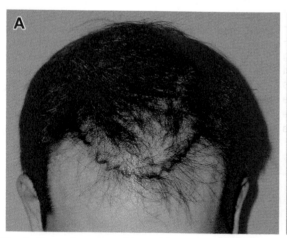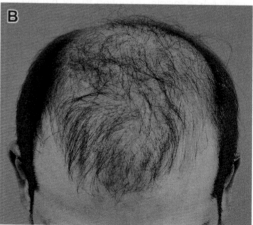

Fig. 1. Dynamic nature of MPB. (*A*) The planned hairline (*purple line*) for a 21-year-old who underwent frontal and midscalp hair transplantation. (*B*) Same patient only 6 years later demonstrates a dramatic and unexpected progression of AGA throughout the grafted area and surrounding scalp. Persistent miniaturization along his superior temporal fringe suggests that the balding process has yet to stabilize.

Parting the hair in various areas may demonstrate differences in density or miniaturization. Because hair hangs down, parting is essential to assess the quality and density of donor hair. High-power magnification with a hand-held microscope camera, densitometer, or even loupe makes miniaturization, scarring, or hair abnormalities easier to see.[5] Trimming hairs first can show miniaturized hairs that are normally hidden by longer terminal hairs. A pull test can be used to check for effluvium. Typically, a cluster of 30 to 40 hairs is grasped at the base then pulled slowly. If five or more telogen hairs are pulled out, it is considered a positive test, and surgery should be postponed until the cause of the hair loss is discovered. Simple mechanical devices are also available to measure hair volume to help detect subtle volume changes that develop before miniaturization may be noticed. Finally, a full-depth scalp biopsy can be submitted for histopathological diagnosis to help identify the cause of any suspected inflammatory or scarring hair loss condition.

TRANSPLANTATION CANDIDACY

Although most patients with hair loss are good candidates for hair replacement surgery (HRS), some are not. To identify noncandidates and nonideal candidates, the hair replacement surgeon must examine every prospective patient carefully and actively look for warnings or red flags (**Table 1**).[6]

The extent to which hair can be replaced on a given individual's head depends on the following law of MPB: the balder a man is, the more grafts he will need to restore the bald area. The more grafts he needs, the fewer grafts he will have because of the inverse reciprocal relationship between the donor and recipient areas. Almost every man is a candidate for hair transplantation provided he accepts the limitations of surgery and understands the final hair loss pattern that will result. Even a patient with advanced class VII baldness can be a candidate if the donor supply is sufficient to meet his individual expectations.

Good Candidates

Good HRS candidates have realistic goals, stable and high-quality donor hair, and a recipient area that will support growth of the transplanted hair. They should have enough donor hair available in their lifetime to cover enough of the eventual balding or thinning pattern to maintain a natural hair (loss) pattern and to fulfill individual recipient-site density expectations.

Noncandidates

Unrealistic expectations
After the initial greeting, it is best to ask an open-ended question such as "What are your goals for your hair?" This simple question can help determine whether the patient has reasonable expectations related to the limitations of surgical restoration, the progressive nature of hair loss, and the finite nature of donor supply. Transplanted hairlines do not recede, but patients' faces age. It is both impossible and undesirable to restore a patient's hairline, density, and coverage to teenager levels. Young patients are particularly prone to excessive expectations because they compare

---

Table 1
Possible exclusionary criteria for HRS and some associated conditions

Red Flags	Some Associated Factors or Conditions
Unrealistic expectations	Generally younger patients
Mental illness	Body dysmorphic disorder, depression, anxiety, obsessive-compulsive disorder, psychosis
Donor miniaturization	Diffuse unpatterned alopecia
Unusual hair loss pattern	Trichotillomania, traction alopecia, scarring alopecia (eg, lichen planopilaris), nonscarring alopecia (eg, alopecia areata)
Many broken hairs	Trichotillomania, hair shaft disorders, styling trauma
Excessive shedding	Telogen effluvium, anagen effluvium
Scalp inflammation	Scarring alopecia, psoriasis, tinea capitis, folliculitis, discoid lupus erythematosus
Unexplained scarring	Scarring alopecia, lichen planopilaris, frontal fibrosing alopecia, Brocq pseudopelade
Pain, burning, alopecia zone pruritus	Scarring and inflammatory conditions

themselves to their recent past and to their peers. Ironically, they need a more conservative plan than do older patients with a similar pattern of loss. Younger patients have a higher risk of extensive loss because they have more years of hair loss ahead and may have faster hair loss. Many young patients, but not all, do not have the maturity or foresight to temper their short-term expectations to achieve their best long-term goals.

Patients with depression, obsessive-compulsive disorder, or body dysmorphic disorder may be psychologically unable to be satisfied with any HRS results.[7] Mental illness may also make the recovery period difficult to bear.

Donor hair issues

Some patients do not have a stable supply of donor hair. For example, diffuse unpatterned alopecia is an uncommon variation of AGA in which hair follicles in the traditional donor area are also sensitive to DHT and will miniaturize (**Fig. 2**). Transplanting DHT-sensitive donor hairs can result in poor growth or later loss of transplanted hair. Donor scars can also become visible with

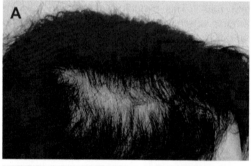

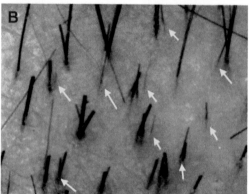

Fig. 2. Diffuse unpatterned alopecia. (*A*) Hair combed upward reveals extensive donor site thinning. (*B*) Microscopic evaluation shows diffuse miniaturization throughout the donor area (*arrows*). Graft harvesting is contraindicated because the remaining normal follicles are at risk for future miniaturization and because removing grafts from this zone will further diminish the already low density.

progressive thinning in the donor area. Other examples of unstable donor hair include active alopecia areata, primary scarring alopecia, and active effluvium (see **Table 1**).

Recipient issues

Some recipient area conditions can cause poor survival or later destruction of the transplanted hair. If the examination reveals patchy or unpatterned hair loss, a cause other than AGA should be considered and a scalp biopsy or referral to a dermatologist may be warranted. For example, patients with a primary scarring alopecia such as lichen planopilaris can have inflammation and scarring that destroys both native and transplanted hair. Trichotillomania and traction alopecia are self-inflicted conditions that can destroy transplanted hair. Active alopecia areata can cause temporary or permanent loss of grafts. Anagen or telogen effluvium can adversely affect both donor and recipient site hair.

Nonideal Candidates

Nonideal candidates represent a distinct group who may benefit from hair restoration, but these patients generally should have lower expectations than good candidates do because of varying intrinsic factors that can limit their aesthetic outcome (**Table 2**). The surgeon must identify those factors that can adversely affect the result so that appropriate expectations can be set before scheduling surgery. Negative factors include unfavorable hair characteristics, potential for advanced hair loss, and limited donor hair (**Fig. 3**). Nonideal candidates are best treated conservatively and by experienced surgeons.

PLANNING

It is important to appreciate that a man's concern about baldness generally changes with age. Unacceptable baldness to a 25-year-old man is baldness anywhere on the head: front, top, or back. Most 60-year-old men, on the other hand, consider unacceptable baldness as no hair in the front. Posterior baldness diminishes in importance to most men as they age because most of their counterparts also have developed a thin or bald spot on their heads. A 60-year-old patient also tends to understand and accept the limitations of surgical hair restoration more readily than does a 25-year-old patient.

The outcome of surgical hair restoration varies depending on the patient's final pattern. The single-most important factor to consider is how bald the patient will become over time with regard to the final width, shape, and density of the fringe.

Table 2
Nonideal candidates

Hair Characteristics	Fine hair
	Low density grafts (few hairs per graft)
	High hair–scalp color contrast
Large (potential) Recipient Area	Skull size and shape
	Extensive family history
	Young age of onset
	Rapid progression
	Low residual hairline
	Miniaturization in superior fringe region
	Temporal thinning and/or recession
Limited Donor Hair Supply	Tight scalp (strip harvesting)
	Low donor density
	Narrow donor fringe
	Retrograde alopecia (Fig. 3)
	Previous surgical or traumatic scarring

If the fringe will remain high, the surgeon can connect the hairline to the fringe and may be able to reestablish a frontal density that mimics the fringe hair. However, if there are any doubts about how extensive the hair loss will be in time, one may have to opt for a more conservative restoration scheme. The plan for the nonideal patient may require a strategic modification, such as

1. Starting with a higher, more receded hairline
2. Reducing the transplanted density to cover a larger area more lightly
3. Increasing the density to cover a key area better
4. Accepting incomplete coverage and designing a pattern that mimics less severe natural hair loss.

Most conservative treatment plans limit or avoid grafting the posterior scalp region and focus on framing the frontal hairline zone with a lower density restoration plan. These are graft-sparing strategies intended to maintain donor reserves for the future. The question of the best way to transplant the area posterior to the frontal zone can be answered later when the final pattern is demarcated more fully. Graft preservation is also important if future balding could separate the superior fringe hair from the transplant zone (Fig. 4). Progressive hair loss of this type creates a bald alley between the graft zone and the inferiorly receded temporal fringe, which will look unnatural if the two zones cannot be reconnected.

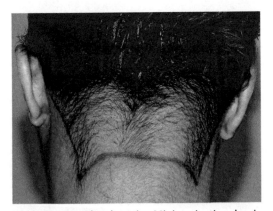

Fig. 3. Retrograde alopecia. Miniaturization begins inferiorly at the nape of the neck and extends superiorly. The blue line marks the inferior limit of his once thick donor region. This process can dramatically reduce the size of a donor area well beyond that which is seen with the inferior migration of the superior fringe that characterizes AGA.

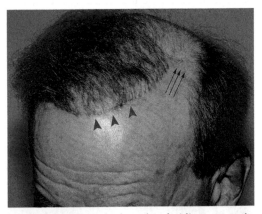

Fig. 4. This patient had a plug hairline restoration 25 years earlier. He noted a very subtle disconnect between his plugs and the adjacent temporal hairline about 10 years after that procedure. Progressive balding over the ensuing 15 years resulted in exposure of the frontal plugs (*red arrowheads*) and the creation of a wide bald alley (*black arrows*) that resides between the lateral graft margin and the residual temporal fringe.

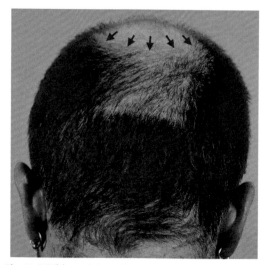

Fig. 5. Visible recipient site scar (*inferior arrows*) that resulted from a strip harvest 8 years earlier in an unstable donor location. The patient experienced unexpected, progressive miniaturization between his once thick superior donor fringe (*superior arrows*) and the now exposed scar.

Although most patients can be managed in a variety of ways, the most important criterion for an aesthetically correct treatment plan is undetectability. Therefore, the surgeon should prioritize recreating a head of hair that looks as natural as one that exists in men who have not undergone HRS. Many patients will see the advantages of a modified conservative plan after education by the physician. If patients are shown realistic expectations but would not be satisfied with those results, it is better to defer HRS than to perform it and have an unhappy patient.

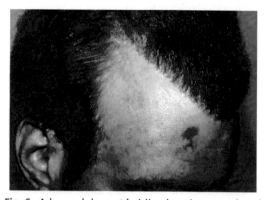

Fig. 6. A low, adolescent hairline location was placed on this patient when he was 21 years old. Unanticipated progression of MPB over 10 years resulted in significant temporal hairline recession. The result of failing to anticipate the dynamic nature of the balding process is a very low, strangely shaped hairline.

Donor Site Considerations

If a safe donor site is not chosen in the face of progressive MPB, donor site scars, grafted hair loss, and recipient site scars will occur years after transplants are performed (**Fig. 5**). There are no reliable guidelines for determining a safe donor area, especially in younger patients. The older the patient is, the more secure the physician can be in choosing a safe donor area. However, a physician must accept his or her inability to accurately predict the extent of future hair loss for a young

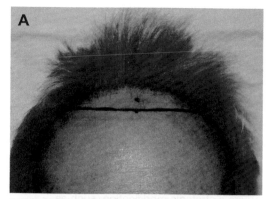

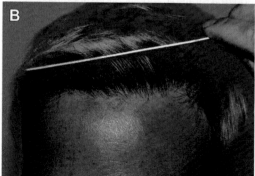

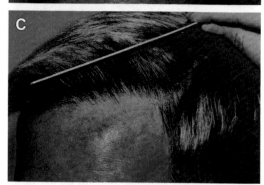

Fig. 7. High-density transplant. This strategy densely packs grafts with minimal spacing to recreate a final density that compares to nonbalding scalp. (*A*) Preoperative isolated frontal hairline recession. (*B, C*) Postoperative dense-pack graft placement results in a high-density hairline.

patient and therefore be cautious and conservative about estimating the supply of safe donor hair. The consequences of counting on a larger donor area than may be available in the future result in permanent disfigurement for the patient.

A lack of density in the patient's fringe is not necessarily a contraindication for transplanting. The goal of transplanting the front of the patient's head is to achieve a hair density that best mimics density in the fringe. Patients with diminished donor hair density have to understand and accept that their transplanted hair will be as thin, or thinner, on top than it is in the sides and back. Although most people can comfortably lose 40% to 60% of their donor hair and maintain a normal appearance, excessive graft harvesting via strip or follicular unit extraction can lead to clinically apparent donor site thinning and scarring.

Recipient Site Considerations

The area that is circumscribed for graft distribution to create a hairline must be appropriate to the patient's face, age, and donor area.[8] One can have a

transplanted area that looks undetectable, but the quality of the transplant is ruined if the shape of the transplanted area is incorrect (too low, too wide, or unnatural curves). Hairline design on an older patient who has experienced most of his baldness is usually easy because such a patient rarely objects to conservative hairline placement. The most difficult consultation is the young patient who desires his adolescent hairline be restored. Replacing that adolescent hairline (too low or too wide) not only depletes the finite donor supply, it can cause the patient to look odd with age and future balding (**Fig. 6**). The guideline for hairline design on a young person is to err in making the hairline too high, knowing that it can always be lowered in the future if enough donor hair remains. It is very difficult to raise a hairline that was made too low, too wide, or both.

Transplant Philosophy

There are two ways to conceptualize planning the recipient site: high-density (dense-pack) transplanting and lower density transplanting (any

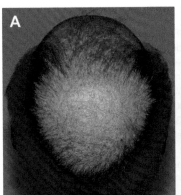
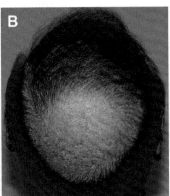
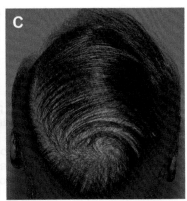

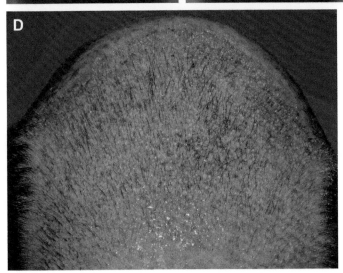

Fig. 8. Lower density transplant. This strategy intentionally leaves spaces between the grafts with the goal of producing a natural, thinning appearance. (*A*) Preoperative class 6 MPB. (*B*) Session 1: frontal-midscalp restoration. (*C*) Session 2: crown restoration. (*D*) Immediate postoperative graft placement demonstrates a 20% to 25% density restoration.

degree of density that is less than maximum dense-pack). It is the surgeon's intent with high-density transplanting to cover the bald area with tightly packed grafts so that the completed transplant area attains a visual density comparable to the surrounding fringe (**Fig. 7**).

When performing lower density HRS, it is the surgeon's deliberate intent to leave spaces between the transplanted grafts. A lower density transplant attempts to create an illusion of higher density despite the spaces that are present between the grafts. A natural thin look is possible with widely or moderately spaced follicular units because the result replicates the appearance of naturally thinning hair (**Fig. 8**). Although most mature men readily accept a thinning look, younger patients may not.

One can transplant the front, top, and back of a patient with advanced baldness using widely spaced follicular unit grafts if the patient accepts having diffusely thin hair all over his head and understands that all of the hair placed posteriorly could have been used in the front to make a denser frontal hairline. In general, a patient can have any distribution of hair he desires as long as it looks natural and he is aware of the final density that will be achieved with the proposed graft distribution plan.

SUMMARY

It is critical for the hair restoration surgeon is to know when to and when not to perform HRS. Consultation with the patient to determine their goals followed by a discussion on realistic, age-appropriate results are imperative for a successful outcome. It is important to identify factors that can negatively affect results before performing HRS. A long-term treatment plan is imperative so patients can have realistic expectations and the HR surgeon can plan appropriately. A methodical approach to patient evaluation and consultation may reduce the risk of missing a warning symptom or sign.

REFERENCES

1. Marritt E, Konior RJ. Patient selection, candidacy, and treatment for hair replacement surgery. Facial Plast Surg Clin North Am 1994;2(2):111–34.
2. Stough D. The consultation. In: Stough D, editor. Hair transplantation. Philadelphia: Elsevier; 2006. p. 43–8.
3. Price V, Mirmirani P. Clinical assessment of the patient. In: Price V, Mirmirani P, editors. Cicatricial alopecia. New York: Springer; 2011. p. 7–13.
4. Olsen EA. Clinical tools for assessing hair loss. In: Olsen EA, editor. Disorders of hair growth: diagnosis and treatment. 2nd edition. New York: McGraw-Hill; 2003. p. 75–86.
5. Bernstein RM, Rassman WR. Densitometry and video-microscopy. Hair Transplant Forum Int'l 2007; 17(2):41.
6. Ruston A. "Red flags" in hair restoration surgery. In: Unger WP, Shapiro R, editors. Hair transplantation. 5th edition. London: Informa Health Care; 2011. p. 76–81.
7. Diagnostic and statistical manual of mental disorders. 4th edition. Washington, DC: American Psychiatric Association; 2000. http://dx.doi.org/10.1176/appi.books.9780890423349.
8. Unger W, Beehner M. Planning and organization of the recipient area. In: Unger WP, Shapiro R, editors. Hair transplantation. 4th edition. New York: Dekker; 2004. p. 92–106.

Hairline Design and Frontal Hairline Restoration

Ronald Shapiro, MD[a,b,*], Paul Shapiro, MD[b]

KEYWORDS

- Hairline • Naturalness • Transition zone • Lateral hump • Frontal tuft • Frontal-temporal angle
- Lateral epicanthi line • Temporal point

KEY POINTS

- Do not make the hairline too low.
- Do not flatten or totally fill in the frontal temporal angle.
- The frontal temporal angle lies and remains on the lateral epicanthal line as hair loss progresses.
- Take future hair loss into consideration when planning the hairline.
- The frontal hairline consists of micro-irregularity and macro-irregularity.

 The authors' techniques for creating a natural frontal hairline are presented in a video that accompanies this article at http://www.facialplastic.theclinics.com

INTRODUCTION

Creating a natural hairline is one of the most important elements of a successful hair transplant and many excellent reviews have been written on the subject.[1–6] Patients expect and deserve undetectable hairlines. We are better equipped now to create hairlines that meet this high expectation (**Fig. 1**A, B). In part, this is a result of the exclusive use of follicular unit (FU) grafts in the hairline region. FU grafts have given us a finer paintbrush with which to create a hairline. Equally important has been a better understanding and recognition of the visual characteristics that make up a normal hairline. Simply using FU grafts without a deliberate attempt to reproduce these characteristics does not guarantee naturalness (**Fig. 2**A, B).

In other words, to create the most natural looking hairline, we cannot simply *use* a finer paintbrush; we must also know *how to paint*. There are 2 major skills needed to paint a natural hairline:

1. The ability to locate the appropriate borders of a hairline and adjust these boarders based on donor/recipient ratio.

2. The ability to mimic the visual characteristics of a natural hairline at these boarders.

The authors techniques for creating a natural frontal hairline are presented in the (Video 1).

MAJOR COMPONENTS OF THE HAIRLINE

The hairline consists of more than its most anterior frontal border. It is an extended area that consists of a number of borders and zones that work together to frame the face and create the final aesthetic look. These components are briefly described as follows and are illustrated in **Fig. 3**A, B. They are discussed in greater detail throughout the article.

- Frontal hairline: Frames the front of the face and runs horizontally from temple to temple.
  - Mid-frontal point (MFP): The most anterior point of the frontal hairline in the midline.
  - Mid-pupillary point (MPP): Point lateral to the MFP where the hairline begins to bend posteriorly on a line drawn vertically from the pupil.

[a] Department of Dermatology, University of Minnesota, 516 Delaware Street SE, MMC98, Minneapolis, MN 55455, USA; [b] Shapiro Medical Group, 5270 West 84th Street, #500, Minneapolis, MN 55437, USA
* Corresponding author.
E-mail address: Rshapiromd@shapiromedical.com

Facial Plast Surg Clin N Am 21 (2013) 351–362
http://dx.doi.org/10.1016/j.fsc.2013.06.001
1064-7406/13/$ – see front matter Published by Elsevier Inc.

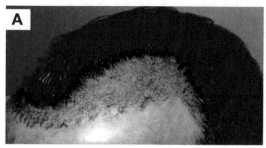
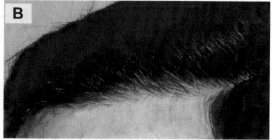

Fig. 1. Natural transplanted hairline. (A) Naturally transplanted hairline immediate postoperative pattern. (B) Naturally transplanted hairline 1 year postoperative.

- o Transition zone (TZ): The most anterior zone of the frontal hairline. It should appear soft and irregular containing both micro and macro irregularity.
- o Defined zone (DZ): Located directly behind the TZ and the point where the frontal hair line begins to appear denser and less see through.
- o Frontal tuft (FT): An oval zone overlying the central (midline) portion of the DZ. This is an aesthetically critical area for the appearance of density.
- Frontal temporal angle (FTA): The point where the frontal hairline meets the temporal hairline. It typically lies on a line drawn vertically from the lateral epicanthi of the eye.
- Temporal hairline: Frames the side of the face running from the FTA to the sideburn.
- The lateral hump (LH) or lateral fringe: The strip of hair located on the side of the head in the temporal-parietal region that connects the permanent donor hair below to the mid scalp above. Its anterior border is the temporal hairline.
- Temporal points (TP): A triangular-shaped protrusion located on the lower aspect of the temporal hairline.

NATURAL CHARACTERISTICS THE HAIRLINE

The frontal hairline is an area approximately 2 to 3 cm deep that bridges the bald forehead to the hair-bearing scalp. It can be visualized as an extended area that consists of 3 zones: the anterior portion or TZ; the posterior portion or DZ; and an oval-shaped area in the center of the DZ called the FT (see **Fig. 3**A, B; **Fig. 4**).[1] All 3 zones make their own unique contribution to the overall appearance of the hairline.

Transition Zone

The TZ consists of the first 0.5 to 1.0 cm of the hairline (see **Figs. 3**A and **4**). It should initially appear irregular and ill-defined, but gradually takes on more definition and substance as it reaches the DZ. Close observation of normal TZs reveals a number of specific elements that work together to create this overall effect. They are described in the following sections.

Single hair grafts
One-hair grafts should be used only in the anterior portion of the TZ with a shift toward 2-hair grafts in the posterior portion. This helps ensure a natural, softer look.

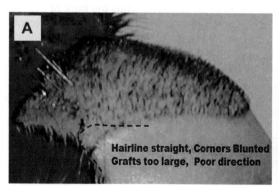
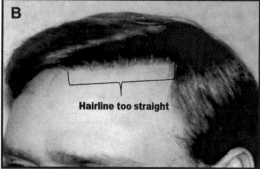

Fig. 2. Unnatural transplanted hairline. (A) Hairline is too straight, grafts are misdirected, and the FTA has been abnormally filled in. (B) Hairline is too straight with no irregularity, even though only 1-hair FU grafts were used.

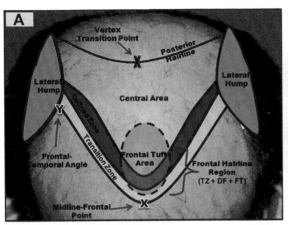
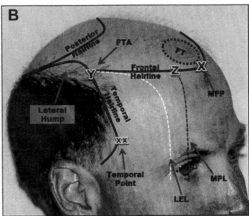

Fig. 3. Major borders, landmarks, and zones of the hairline. The hairline consists of many components that work together to obtain the final aesthetic look. (*A*) Top view. (*B*) Side view.

Sentinel hairs

A few isolated, very fine single hairs called *sentinel hairs* can be found scattered randomly in front of the TZ. Sentinel hairs contribute to softness and irregularity.

Micro-irregularity

Close examination of the TZ reveals small, intermittent clusters of hairs along its border (see **Fig. 4**). These clusters vary in shape and depth but often resemble ill-defined triangles of various sizes. Their existence creates variable and intermittent density along the TZ. This form of irregularity is referred to as *micro-irregularity* because it is more noticeable viewed close-up than from a distance. Parsley called these areas *clusters* and the area between them *gaps*.[7,8] There is a natural mistaken urge to fill in the gaps between these clusters when working on the TZ. This impulse must be overcome to prevent the creation of a straight or solid-appearing hairline.

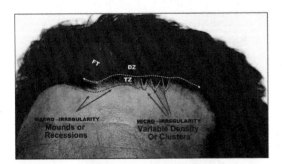

Fig. 4. Micro and macro irregularity. A normal non-transplanted hairline. The *white dotted line* separates the TZ from the DZ. The *black dotted line* follows the macro-irregular undulating anterior border. Notice the micro-irregularity within the TZ. FT is the frontal tuft.

Macro-irregularity

If one stands back and looks at a normal hairline from a distance, the path of the anterior border is seen to be more serpentine or curvaceous than linear. This form of irregularity is referred to as *macro-irregularity* because it is more obvious when one stands back and observes the hairline from a distance (see **Fig. 4**). Martinick used the term "snail-tracking" to describe this appearance.[9] Parsley[8] attributed this macro-irregularity to existence of 1 to 3 "mounds" or "protrusions" along the path of the hairline. Both micro-irregularity and macro-irregularity are needed in the TZ to create a natural-looking hairline.

Defined Zone

The DZ sits directly behind the TZ (see **Figs. 3**A and 4). In this area, the hairline should develop a higher degree of definition and density. Increasing density in the DZ creates a fuller looking hairline by limiting the distance seeable through the TZ.[1,10] As a benefit, it creates this effect without placing hair directly in the TZ, limiting the chance of creating an unnatural straight or solid appearance (**Fig. 5**A, B). Increasing density in the DZ is a safe and effective way to make the hairline appear thicker.

FT Area

The FT is a small but aesthetically significant oval-shaped area that overlies the central portion of the DZ (see **Figs. 3**A, B and 4). The density in this area should be higher than the rest of the DZ. James Arnold impressed on me the aesthetic importance of density in the FT with the following example.[11] He would say, "Consider a patient who is totally bald except for a fairly full residual FT area. Imagine he is standing in an elevator facing the door

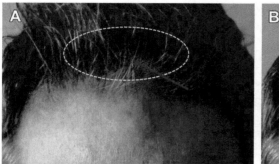
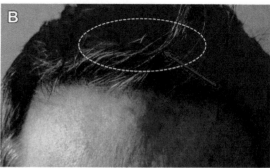

Fig. 5. The importance of density in the DZ. (A) The DZ is thinning and the hairline appears to be see through. (B) The hairline looks much fuller but no hairs were added to the TZ. Hair was only manually compressed in the DZ, making it less see through. This indirectly made the TZ look fuller.

with you facing him on the other side. When the door opens your first impression, looking at him face on, would be of a person with a fairly full head of hair. It would only be when you walked by him that you noticed he was bald everywhere else." Creating fullness in this area has a tremendous influence on the overall appearance of fullness (**Fig. 6**A, B).

FTA Area

Slight temporal recession or weakness of the FTA is normal in the white male hairline. Therefore, flattening or densely filling in this recession is a mistake and would make the hairline look artificial

(see **Fig. 2**). Like the TZ, the anterior border of the FTA should not appear solid but instead soft and ill-defined.

In certain ethnic groups (black, Middle Eastern, Asian, and Hispanic), it is more common to see broader, flatter hairlines with less recession. In these groups, if the donor/recipient ratio is good, a more aggressively filled in FTA may occasionally be acceptable. However, even if a flatter hairline is more common in certain ethnic groups, if the donor/recipient ratio is poor, some temporal recession still needs to be created. Female hairlines are the only true exception. With women, the FTA is more medial, rounded, and filled in.

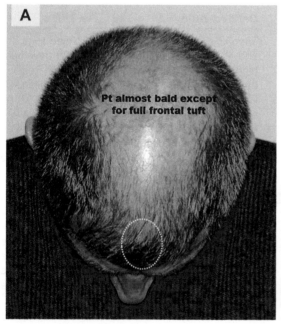
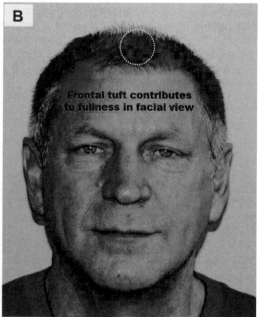

Fig. 6. The importance of the FT. (A) From the top view, he looks bald. (B) From a frontal view, the patient appears to have a fairly full head of hair thanks solely to this tuft.

Proper Angle and Direction

Angle and direction are distinct entities. Angle refers to the degree of elevation that hair has as it exits the scalp. Direction refers to the way hair points (right or left) when leaving the scalp. It is important to pay attention to changes in *both* angle and direction as one transplants different parts of the hairline (**Fig. 7**A, B). Often there are residual miniaturized hairs that act as a road map for the physician to follow.

- In the mid scalp, hair usually exits at 30° to 45° and points forward toward the nose.
- As one reaches the frontal hairline, the angle becomes more acute at 15° to 20°, and the direction usually remains pointing forward. On occasion, hair in this area may bend slightly to the left or right.
- As one moves laterally along the hairline, the direction remains forward until nearing the FTA.
- As one reaches and sweeps around the FTA toward the temporal hairline, there is a gradual change in direction from forward to inferior lateral. Simultaneously, a gradual change in angle occurs from approximately 15° in the frontal hairline to almost flat (5°–10°) in the temporal hairline.

From a side view, the incisions resemble a fan pointing forward and changing from a medial to lateral direction at the level of the FTA (see **Fig. 7**A).

- As one continues down the temporal hairline toward the TP, the direction can change to more posteriorly and the angle should be as flat as possible. Coronal incisions should be used in the temporal hairline to ensure a more acute angle.

Selective Distribution of Grafts

Selective distribution is an important tool that helps us mimic the density gradient found in normal hairlines (**Fig. 8**). It is a safer and more powerful tool than increasing incisional density. For example, at identical incisional densities of 30/cm^2, 3-hair grafts create 3 times the hair volume as 1-hair grafts. To accomplish the same increase in hair volume *entirely* with incisions would require an increase in incisional density from 30/cm^2 to an unrealistic 90/cm^2. In general, we use the following selective distribution of grafts.

- The TZ contains only 1-hair grafts with a shift to 2-hair grafts toward the posterior aspect of this zone. One-hair grafts can vary in thickness. The finer 1-hair grafts should be used for sentinel hairs and in the most anterior portion of this zone.
- The DZ contains predominantly 2-hair grafts.
- The FT area contains a greater concentration of 3-hair grafts. *Follicular pairing* is a useful tool to use in the FT area if not enough 3-hair grafts are found naturally. With follicular pairing, a 1-hair graft and a 2-hair graft are combined to make an artificial 3-hair graft.[11]

Graft Numbers and Incisional Density

Physicians learning hair transplantation often ask "How many grafts do I need?" or "What incisional density should I use?" There is no single correct answer. In our experience, incisional densities ranging from 25 to 35 FU/cm^2 are most commonly used. Higher densities are possible, but more controversial with respect to survival, and typically not needed for good results.[12] The frontal hairline measures about 20 to 30 cm^2 if all 3 zones (TZ +

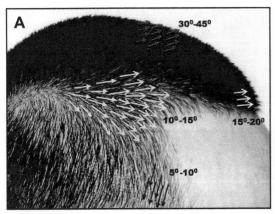
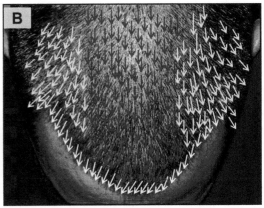

Fig. 7. Changes in angle and direction. Exit angles are different in the mid scalp (30°–45°), frontal hairline (15°–20°), FTA (10°–15°), and temporal hairline (5°–10°). Notice the gradual fan-shaped change in direction from medial to inferior/lateral around the FTA. (*A*) Lateral view. (*B*) Top view.

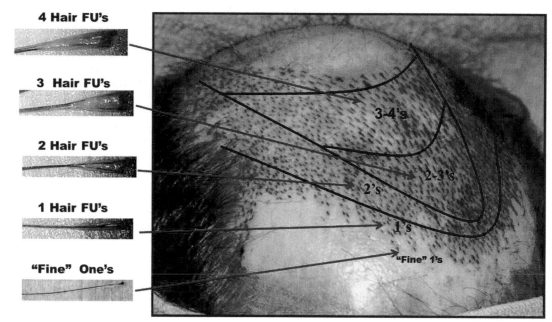

4 Hair FU's

3 Hair FU's

2 Hair FU's

1 Hair FU's

"Fine" One's

3-4's

2-3's

2's

1's

"Fine" 1's

Fig. 8. Selective distribution of grafts: a powerful tool for controlling density. One-hair FUs are used in the TZ, 2-hair FUs in the DZ, and 3-hair FUs in the FT zone.

DZ + FT) are included. If you do the math, a range of 500 to 1050 FU grafts may be needed. Of these, approximately 200 to 400 are 1-hair grafts placed in the TZ and the rest are 2-hair to 3-hair grafts placed in the DZ and FT area.

Minor changes in incisional density can be used to influence the appearance of fullness. However, incisional density does not change dramatically, typically remaining somewhere near 25 to 35 FU/cm^2. Caution should be urged against trying to use very high incisional densities in the FT area, where a more fragile blood supply combined with dense packing could lead to necrosis or poor growth.[12]

Cowlicks

Cowlicks often present a challenge when creating hairlines. They occur more often in women. If a patient has a residual cowlick that is very weak and looks like it will be gone within a couple of years, we usually ignore it. However if a cowlick is strong, we may attempt to use the presence of existing hairs to follow its direction. We usually re-create a cowlick by starting at its periphery, where the direction of hair is obvious, and slowly work inward toward the point of swirl.

LOCATING THE BORDERS OF THE HAIRLINE

The borders of the hairline consist of a frontal hairline and a temporal hairline that meet at the FTA. When hair loss begins, there is simultaneous recession of both the frontal and temporal hairline, causing the FTA to move posteriorly and widen. As this process progresses, the FTA moves farther posteriorly and temporal recession deepens. An important observation is that the FTA remains on a line drawn perpendicular from the lateral epicanthi of the eye as hair loss worsens (**Fig. 9**).[1,2]

A primary decision that physicians need to make is how aggressive to be when recreating the

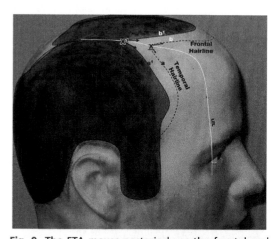

Frontal Hairline

Temporal Hairline

LEL

Fig. 9. The FTA moves posteriorly as the frontal and temporal hairlines recede. The FTA remains on the LEL as temporal recession deepens. x and x^1 = original and receded FTA; a and a^1 = original and receded temporal hairline; b and b^1 = original and receded frontal hairline.

hairline. By aggressive, we mean how far forward the frontal hairline, temporal hairline, and FTA can be restored with respect to their original position. This is strongly influenced by the relationship between a patient's age, current hair loss, potential future hair loss, and donor supply. Future hair loss is particularly important in younger patients, in whom there is more time for progression to occur. If future loss is not considered, unnatural patterns may be revealed as hair recedes from transplanted areas. With a depleted donor supply this may be difficult to fix.

In general, the younger the patient, the more severe the hair loss, and the poorer the donor supply, the more conservative the hairline should be. It is a matter of supply and demand (ie, donor/recipient ratio). If we had unlimited donor supply we could create aggressive hairlines on everyone. Unfortunately, this is not the case.

If there is any concern, it is better to err on the side of conservatism and follow the basic tenant, "do not place the hairline too low." Following this advice is often difficult, as many patients request hairlines that are lower than prudent.

Locating the MFP

Locating the MFP is one of the first steps in hairline recreation. The MFP is located in the midline and is the most anterior point of the frontal hairline. A number of guidelines can aid in the proper location of the MFP; however, 2 guidelines that should not be used are the "4 Finger Breaths Rule" and Leonardo da Vinci's "Rule of Thirds." The 4 Finger Breaths Rule states that the MFP should be located 4 finger breaths above the glabella. This is unreliable, as fingers vary in size from person

to person. Leonardo da Vinci's "Rule of Thirds" states the perfect face should be divided into equal thirds with the distance between the chin to the nose, nose to the glabella, and glabella to the hairline all being the same.[1,6] However, a hairline located with this rule is meant for a young patient with no hair loss. It is not the reconstructed hairline typically achievable in an alopecic adult with the constraints of a limited donor supply. It would be too aggressive for most patients. More appropriate guidelines for locating the MFP include the following (**Fig. 10**):

- 7-cm to 10-cm Rule: The MFP lies on point drawn somewhere between 7 and 10 cm above the glabella.
- Curve of the Forehead Rule: The forehead takes on a gentle curve as it transitions from the vertical plane of the face to meet the horizontal plane of the scalp. The MFP usually lies somewhere within this curve. A good starting point is a line drawn to this curve from the intersection of these 2 planes. This places the MFP somewhere in the middle of the curve.[1,2]

These rules are only guidelines and should be adjusted based the patient's age, severity of hair loss, and donor supply. In patients with more severe hair loss, raising the MFP by 1 to 2 cm may be appropriate; however, it should not be placed so high that it falls on the horizontal plane of the scalp where it loses the aesthetic effect of framing the face. In patients with good donor/recipient ratios, the MFP can be placed lower, but caution needs to be exercised. It should never be placed on the vertical plane of the face, as this seldom will look natural in a restored hairline.

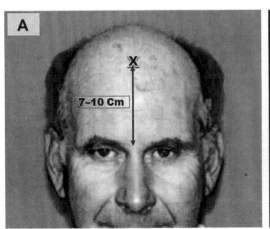
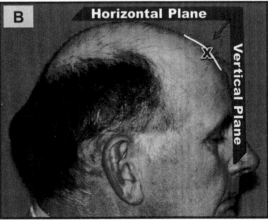

Fig. 10. Finding the MFP. (*A*) Seven to 10 cm above the glabella. (*B*) The middle of the curve that occurs as the vertical plane of the face meets the horizontal plane of the scalp. Adjust the MFP up or down based on severity of hair loss.

A specific situation worth mentioning is the patient who has a very low persistent FT. In this patient, the physician should ignore the hair in the preexisting tuft and place the MFP at a higher, more appropriate point.

Locating the FTA

As stated previously, all mature male hairlines have an FTA formed by the junction of the frontal and temporal hairlines. The superior arm of the FTA is the frontal hairline and the inferior arm of the FTA is the temporal hairline. The apex of the FTA is where they meet. The FTA moves increasingly posterior as hair loss progresses. In our opinion, locating and deciding how far forward the FTA should be restored when reconstructing a hairline is one of the more important and difficult tasks in hairline design. The following guidelines are useful for locating the FTA.

- The Lateral Epicanthus Line Rule: This rule states the FTA lies on a line drawn vertically from the lateral epicanthus of the eye called the lateral epicanthi line (LEL). An important observation is that the FTA remains on this line as it moves increasingly posterior with worsening temporal recession. The FTA is located at the point where the LEL intersects the temporal hairline (see **Fig. 9**; **Fig. 11**).
- Up-Sloping Line Rule: A line drawn from the MFP to the FTA should always slope slightly upward when viewed from the side. It should never slope downward.

In mild degrees of hair loss (ie, types 3 and 4), in which patients have very little recession of the temporal hair line, these guidelines work well. The *existing* temporal hair usually becomes the inferior

border of the FTA, whereas the *future* frontal hairline will become the superior border of the FTA.

In moderate to severe degrees of hair loss (ie, types 5, 6, and 7), in which the temporal hair has receded, finding the FTA using only the LEL rule is not sufficient. With severe hair loss, the temporal hairline and lateral fringe may have dropped below a point where the LEL can intersect. There is no temporal hairline for the LEL to meet. In more moderate degrees of hair loss, the LEL can still intersect the temporal hairline, but the point of intersection may be farther back than optimally desired. In either case, the following additional guidelines are useful.

- Visualizing and re-creating the LH: The LH is an upside-down C-shaped area located superior to the ear that connects the permanent donor hair below to the mid scalp above. It is the last part of the lateral fringe to recede. If you look at normal lateral profiles you can see that one can be very bald and still retain a residual LH. Visualizing and re-creating an LH gives the LEL a target to intersect to find the FTA. The down-sloping frontal border of the LH, just anterior to this intersection, becomes the superior portion of the temporal hairline. The degree to which the LH travels forward before sloping down and intersecting the LEL will determine the location of the reconstructed temporal hairline (**Fig. 12A, B**).
- Using lines parallel to the sideburns: From a side view, multiple lines can be visualized running parallel to the sideburn and intersecting the LEL. The point where these lines intersect the LEL helps approximate the location of the FTA in different degrees of hair loss. If a patient has severe hair loss or is destined to become a type 6 to 7, We use a line located behind the sideburn. Of interest is that this is similar to the anterior position of the FTA in Beehner frontal forelock design for severe hair loss.[12] If a patient has moderate hair loss, we use a line starting somewhere in the middle of the sideburn. For minimal hair loss with low risk of progression, we can be more aggressive and use a line located just in front of the sideburn (**Fig. 13**). Anything more anterior is potentially too aggressive.

Determining the Shape and Contour of the Frontal Hairline

Once the locations of the MFP and FTA have been determined, the frontal hairline is created by drawing a gently curving line that connects the MFP to both FTAs. The MPP is an additional landmark that assists in the drawing of this line. The MPP sits on

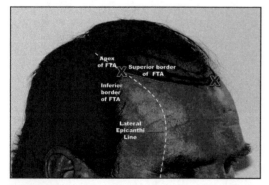

Fig. 11. Finding the FTA/LEL. The FTA lies on a line drawn vertical to the lateral epicanthi. The point where the LEL meets the temporal hairline is the FTA. The temporal hairline becomes the inferior arm of the FTA.

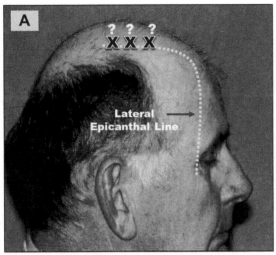
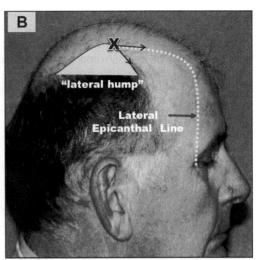

Fig. 12. Finding the FTA/LH. (*A*) As hair loss advances, the temporal hairline recedes and the lateral fringe drops, making it more difficult to know how far back to place the FTA on the LEL. (*B*) Visualizing the LH gives the LEL a target it can intersect. The anterior border of the LH becomes the temporal hairline.

a line drawn vertically from the midpoint of the pupil and is the point where the frontal hairline begins to curve more acutely posterior toward the FTA (see **Fig. 3B**).

The contour of the frontal hairline can range from round, to oval, to bell shaped. The more conservative a hairline needs to be, the more its shape moves from a rounder shape toward an oval or bell-shaped

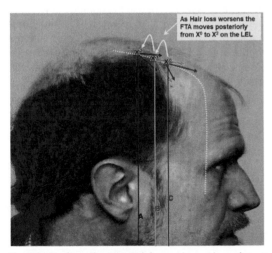

Fig. 13. Finding the FTA/Sideburn Lines. Lines drawn parallel to the sideburn at different distances from the ear help approximate how far forward to place the FTA on the LEL (*yellow dotted line*) in different degrees of hair loss. Severe hair loss = line behind the sideburn (*black line* A). Moderate hair loss = line through the middle of the sideburn (*green line* B). Mild hair loss = line parallel to the anterior border of the sideburn (*red line* C).

design. The increasing lateral concave suppression that occurs as one moves from round to bell shape corresponds to the increasing temporal recession that occurs in more severe hair loss.[6] Beehner[12] visualized creating this concavity by taking his index finger and gently pushing in the lateral border of the hairline. An alternative way that we create this concavity is by making the lateral border of the hairline weaker and more see through. We create this weakness by using more 1-hair grafts at a lower density as we approach the FTA. This basically mimics the process that occurs in nature.

Adjusting the Hairline Downward

As alluded to earlier, patients often want a lower hairline than recommended. It is not uncommon for them to look at the hairline drawn during a consult and plead for it to be lower. It is imperative for physicians to learn to say "no" to patients in whom the request is inappropriate. However, in some cases there may be some room to adjust the hairline downward. The following are 2 methods we use to accomplish this goal in the safest way possible.

- If the patient wants the midpoint of the hairline to be lower, creating a small widow's peak is a relatively safe and graft-economical way to do this. Sometimes just a tiny protrusion can be enough to satisfy the patient.
- Other patients are more concerned with temporal recessions and request filling in the FTA by lowering the lateral aspect of their frontal hairline. This would flatten the FTA and look abnormal. If there is enough room, a safer

way of lowering the FTA is to visualize its current location and imagine sliding it slightly forward. This moves both the temporal and frontal arms of the FTA and maintains the presence of an angle.

Temporal Points

Recession of the TP contributes a great deal to the appearance of baldness by making the forehead look larger. Before the use of FU grafts, the TP could not be transplanted naturally. Now, with the use of FU grafts, it can be done. However, this is an extremely visible area that is unforgiving to mistakes. It requires a high level of skill and should not be undertaken lightly by novices. Mayers' classification of temporal hair loss is[13]:

- Normal (N): The there is no hair loss or recession.
- Thinning (T): The TP is present but thin and beginning to recede. Transplanting at this stage is not typically necessary.
- Parallel (P): The TP is gone and the temporal hairline from the FTA to the sideburn appears straight and flat.
- Reverse (R): The TP has receded to the point that it has a concave border along the sideburn.

In general, the TP does not need to be transplanted until it reaches the very late T or early P stage.

A common rule for finding the TP is the intersection of the following 2 lines:

- Line 1 is drawn from the tip of the nose, over the center of the pupil.
- Line 2 is drawn from the tip of the earlobe to the proposed MFP.

This rule should be used only as a starting point, as it finds the location of the TP that existed before any hair loss occurred and can be fairly aggressive. Surgeons should use their artistic judgment to finalize the design. We generally prefer to create a more conservative TP with an anterior point closer to the temporal hairline. Haber suggested raising the distal aspect of Line 2 slightly above the MFP to bring the point closer (**Fig. 14**).[14] Two other useful observations are that the bottom border of the TP is often parallel to the lateral aspect of the eyebrow and the top border should slope gently backward toward the temporal hairline. Often there are miniaturized hairs from the preexisting TP that act as a road map for the location and direction of hair.

The angle of hair in the TP should be flat or as close to 0° as possible. To accomplish this, coronal incisions should be used. The direction of hair points downward and posterior toward the ear.

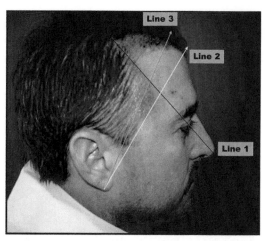

Fig. 14. Finding the TP. Common rule for finding the TP is intersection of a line drawn from tip of nose through the pupil (*red line*) and a line drawn from tip of ear lobe to the MFP (*yellow line*). For a more conservative TP, a line slightly superior to the *yellow line* is used (*green line*).

STEP-BY-STEP APPROACH FOR CREATING A NATURAL HAIRLINE

The following is a step-by-step approach we have found useful when creating our hairlines. It is not meant to be dogmatic. Other methods exist that also work well. With this approach, an initial framework is built that is then repeatedly fine-tuned. We prefer this approach as opposed to completing our design in one pass. We use the analogy of writing a paper. Each time we put it away, when we come back to it we find improvements that can be made. The following step-by-step approach is also illustrated in the video that accompanies this article.

1. Draw the initial hairline design with a marking pen using the guidelines discussed earlier.
   ○ Find the MFP, MPP, and FTA using the guidelines described earlier in this article.
   ○ Connect the MFP to the MPP and then the FTA with a gently curved line to create the anterior border of the TZ.
   ○ After the anterior border of the TZ has been drawn, sketch in the rest of the zones.
2. Check the symmetry of your design.

Symmetry can be checked multiple ways. Looking at the hairline in a mirror or through a camera lens reveals asymmetry. From a frontal view, holding a pencil horizontally at the level of the MFP also reveals asymmetry. One can measure the distance of both FTAs from the midline to see if they are equal. Asking your assistants for their opinions can be helpful. Pathomvanich and Ng[15] recently

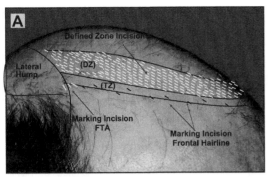
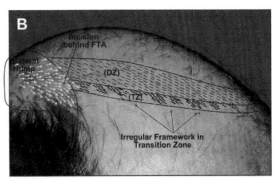

Fig. 15. (A) Early steps when creating a hairline: Marking incisions (*blue*) along anterior border of the TZ; marking incision (*yellow*) around the FTA. Incisions (*white*) in the DZ are done before working on the TZ. (B) Later steps when creating a hairline: Incisions (*blue*) are made in front of the DZ and into the TZ in an irregular wavy pattern of varying depth. Incisions (*yellow*) are also made behind the FTA changing in direction from medial to inferior lateral around the FTA.

described the use of a laser light leveling device. Unique aides that have been specifically created to check for hairline symmetry are Pathomvanich and Ng's laser leveling device and Cole's "aid to hairline design" measuring device.[15,16]

3. Make initial marking incisions along the anterior border of the TZ and in the FTA.

Marking incisions preserve the location of the hairline design even if the lines drawn with the marking pen are washed off. Placing these initial marking incisions at various distances from the DZ begin the process of creating irregularity (**Fig. 15A**).

4. Make incisions in the DZ first.

Making incisions in the DZ first and then moving anteriorly into the TZ gives me more control over the shape and irregularity of our TZ. We make the analogy to painting a wall. We do the easy central part first and then move to the more delicate fine trim last. Incisions in the DZ are placed in a staggered pattern (see **Fig. 15A**).

5. Move to the TZ and create the initial framework of irregularity.

Incisions are now made in front of the DZ and into the TZ in an irregular wavy pattern of varying depth.

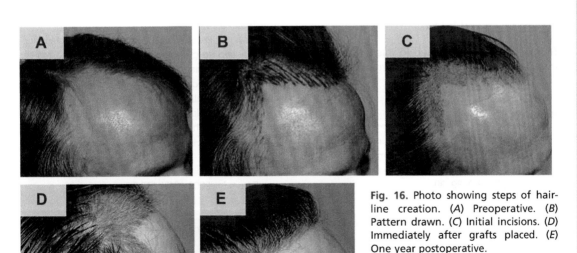

Fig. 16. Photo showing steps of hairline creation. (A) Preoperative. (B) Pattern drawn. (C) Initial incisions. (D) Immediately after grafts placed. (E) One year postoperative.

Some physicians freehand this pattern. Others will start by connecting the DZ to the irregularly spaced initial marking incisions created earlier. Either technique is meant to begin an initial framework of irregularity that will be refined with further passes (see **Fig. 15B**).

6. Make multiple passes in both the DZ and TZ.

Multiple passes and artistic skills are used to increase density in the DZ and fine-tune the irregularity of the TZ.

7. Final fine-tuning with the "stick-and-place" technique.

About 100 to 300 grafts are usually saved for the end of the procedure, to further fine-tune the hairline. The physician can get an aesthetic preview of the way the hairline will look and what is needed because the hairs have been left 2 to 4 mm long.

SUMMARY

The principles and techniques outlined in this article will help the physician create hairlines with the high degree of naturalness and substance expected by today's discerning patients (**Fig. 16**). It is not enough to "just use FU grafts." Finding the appropriate borders and then mimicking the natural characteristics of a hairline at these borders are the skills needed for success. My approach is to create an initial framework based on the principles of hairline design and then use artistic ability and experience to fine-tune this framework.

SUPPLEMENTARY DATA

Supplementary data related to this article can be found online at http://dx.doi.org/10.1016/j.fsc.2013.06.001.

REFERENCES

1. Shapiro R. Creating a natural hairline in one session using a systemic approach and modern principles of hairline design. Int J Cosm Surg Aesthetic Dermatology 2001;3(2):89–99.

2. Unger W. Hairline zone. In: Unger W, Shapiro R, editors. Hair transplantation. 5th edition. Informa; 2011. p. 133–40 Chapter 6A.

3. Shapiro R. How to use follicular unit transplantation in the hairline and other appropriate areas. In: Unger WP, Shapiro R, editors. Hair transplantation. 4th edition. New York: Marcel Dekker; 2004. p. 454–69.

4. Stough D, Khan S. Determination of hairline placement. In: Stough D, Haber R, editors. Hair replacement: surgical and medical. Mosby-Year Book; 1996. p. 425–9.

5. Rose PT, Parsley WM. The science of hairline design. In: Haber RS, Stough DB, editors. Procedures in cosmetic dermatology. Hair transplantation. Philadelphia: Elsevier Saunders; 2006. p. 55–72.

6. Lam S. Hairline design. In: Hair transplant 360. Jaypee Brothers Medical Pub; 2011. Chapter 50.

7. McAndrews P. Hairlines based on natural patterns of hair loss. In: Unger W, Shapiro R, editors. Hair transplantation. 5th edition. Informa; 2011. p. 152–62 Chapter 6B1.

8. Parsley WM. Natural hair patterns. Facial Plast Surg Clin North Am 2004;12:167–80.

9. Martinick J. 2005 ISHRS Annual Meeting, Australia Live Surgery Workshop. Sydney, August 27, 2005.

10. Unger W. Hairline zone and "egg." In: Unger W, Shapiro R, editors. Hair transplantation. 5th edition. Informa; 2011. p. 372–4 Chapter 12f1.

11. Mayer and Keene's study comparing Fu growth with different planting densities. Presented at the 2003 annual meeting of the International Society of Hair Restoration Surgeons.

12. Beehner ML. A frontal forelock/central density framework for hair transplantation. Dermatol Surg 1997;23:807–15.

13. Mayer M, Perez-Meza D. Temporal points: classification and surgical techniques for aesthetic results. ESHRS Journal 2003;3(2):6–7.

14. Haber B. Lecture on Hairline Design. 2nd Annual Hair Restoration Surgery Cadaver Workshop. St Louis, MO, November, 2009.

15. Pathomvanich D, Ng B. Laser assisted hairline placement. Hair Transplant Forum Int 2008;18(5):169.

16. Cole J. Aid to hairline design (AHD). Hair Transplant Forum Int 2008;18(5):173.32.

Graft Harvesting and Management of the Donor Site

Kenneth A. Buchwach, MD*

KEYWORDS

- Donor site • Donor scar • Harvesting grafts • Strip technique • Tricophytic closure

KEY POINTS

- Remove only enough donor width that will close without tension.
- Remove donor strip in portions to accurately judge graft yield and laxity in different areas and to avoid a large open wound.
- The lateral donor areas have less laxity, afford less camouflage, and yield fewer grafts.
- The deep stitch is critical in a good closure.
- Use a single incision when doing multiple sessions.

INTRODUCTION

The donor strip technique has been the predominant method of harvesting grafts for decades.[1–8] Like every aspect of hair transplantation, it has undergone numerous refinements. These changes became necessary as patients began wearing their hair shorter and requesting larger graft sessions. Patients having more than one procedure expect to have just one incisional scar, not a series of stripes. It is no longer acceptable to have an excellent result at the recipient site and a telltale wide scar at the donor site. The following discussion highlights how we can accomplish the goal of harvesting adequate grafts via the strip technique with a resultant inconspicuous scar.

PREOPERATIVE PLANNING
Safe Donor Area

Grafts should be harvested only from areas with terminal hairs that will grow forever. This safe donor area (**Fig. 1**) is different for every patient, but a few guidelines are helpful. The superior boundary should be at least 2 cm below where

crown thinning is predicted to occur. In class V-VII patients, this is easy to determine, but in patients who are still losing more hair it may be slightly challenging. The inferior boundary should be about 2 cm above the nape of the neck. Patients will often thin naturally in the lower occipital area so one does not want to harvest donor hair in this area. Laterally, one can harvest from the supra-auricular area, but it is important to keep in mind that the density here is less, the skin is tighter, and there is less superior hair for covering the incision.

Scalp Laxity

As we strive to harvest more grafts for accommodating large sessions, scalp laxity has become a very important issue. The parameters that influence the dimensions of strip size in the donor area are length and width. Length is more finite, as one can only go from one supra-auricular area to the other. The maximum length usually ranges from 24 to 30 cm depending on the size of the patient's head. Width is much more variable and depends on local soft tissue laxity. Less width

Disclosures: None.
Private Practice, Facial Plastic Surgery, Kansas City, MO, USA
* 11550 Granada Lane, Leawood, KS 66211.
E-mail address: doc2708@aol.com

Facial Plast Surg Clin N Am 21 (2013) 363–374
http://dx.doi.org/10.1016/j.fsc.2013.05.001

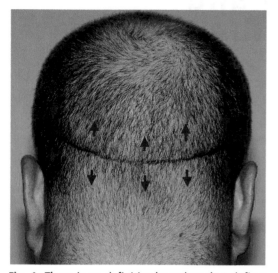

Fig. 1. There is no definitive boundary that defines the safe donor area. In general, the safest donor zone is found in the center (*blue line*) of the horseshoe-shaped, hair-bearing region that typifies a later-stage balding pattern. Removing follicles from above or below this central location increases the risk that harvested follicles will thin or bald later in life. Any evidence of donor site miniaturization (area above and below *arrow* points) should caution the surgeon from entering these zones for a follicular harvest.

can usually be excised laterally and more in the occipital area. Depending on the baseline donor laxity, a safe strip width will generally vary from 10 to 25 mm. The upper limit of a safe strip width depends on being able to close the incision without tension, and this is primarily determined by scalp laxity.

Over the years, there have been many methods to predict donor site laxity. Laxity estimation can be accomplished most simply by squeezing the scalp between your fingers. This technique is, of course, very subjective and relies on experience, but for an experienced surgeon it often proves quite reliable. Alternatively, an experienced surgeon can determine the donor laxity parameter by measuring superior and inferior soft tissue excursion at the center of the planned strip excision site (**Fig. 2**).

Scalp elasticity formula

Mayer and Pauls[3] developed a formula for determining scalp elasticity. With their method, a 50-mm line is first marked on the occipital donor area, and then the borders are squeezed together along the horizontal axis. Their formula is:

Scalp elasticity = (50 mm − x) (100%)/50 mm where x is the length of the compressed skin segment.

They found that scalp elasticity in 400 patients ranged between 10% and 45%, with the average being 24%. They concluded that 10% elasticity represents a tight scalp and 45% elasticity represents a very elastic scalp. From a practical consideration, these data suggest that a tight scalp (10% elasticity) may yield a 5-mm strip, an average scalp (24% elasticity) may yield a 12-mm strip, and a very loose scalp (45% elasticity) may yield a 22.5-mm strip.

Preoperative scalp massage is recommended to increase laxity. The results are variable, but it is quite simple and the potential benefits justify encouraging patients to use this exercise. They are instructed to vigorously massage the donor area in a vertical fashion for 3 to 5 minutes frequently during the day and to continue this regimen for 2 to 4 weeks before surgery.

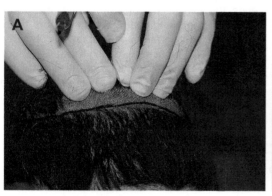
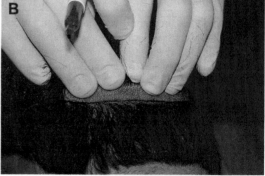

Fig. 2. Scalp laxity can be assessed by determining the limits of superior movement (*A*) and inferior movement (*B*) at the proposed harvest site.

Calculating Strip Dimensions

Predicting how many follicular unit grafts (FUs) can be harvested from the donor area is essential in every case. Most hair restoration surgeons calculate strip dimensions and donor graft harvest capabilities based on local follicular unit density and regional donor elasticity. First, the surgeon approximates regional follicular unit density with a device such as a densitometer (**Fig. 3**). This magnification device allows the surgeon to quickly count the number of follicular units in one square centimeter, so as to allow for an overall appraisal of the donor site density. Next, the donor site elasticity is evaluated to determine the maximum safe width for the strip that will be removed (**Fig. 4**). The donor density and the strip width calculations are then used to determine the necessary strip length for the required graft session size (**Fig. 5**). These parameters will also allow the surgeon to calculate the maximum graft yield possible for any given individual.

For example, if one estimates that a maximum donor width of 1 cm can be removed and that the average density throughout the strip measures 60 FUs/cm^2, harvesting a 25-cm-long strip should yield approximately 1500 grafts. However, sufficient laxity for the safe removal of 2 cm from the donor would now require only a 12.5-cm-long strip to obtain 1500 grafts. Alternatively, assuming sufficient laxity, a 2-cm width could double the graft yield to 3000 FUs for the same 25-cm-long strip.

It is common to witness variable FU densities within different zones of the donor area. The temple region often demonstrates a significantly lower density than the central occipital scalp. It is prudent to evaluate donor density in a minimum of 2 different zones. Adjustments can be made for varying regional densities to ensure avoiding miscalculation of the graft harvest.

Hair Color

The presence or absence of color of the hair follicles is important. Patients with white hair often have follicles that are literally translucent. This makes it hard to see the follicles when excising the strip and equally difficult to see the follicles when preparing the grafts under the microscope. There is no ideal remedy for this. We have found it helpful to dye the donor area with a hair coloring solution to facilitate visualization of the hair shafts, but variable uptake of the dye onto the hair can limit its usefulness.

Preexisting Donor Scars

The goal is to have only one incision regardless of the number of sessions, so precise planning is necessary when a scar exists from a previous procedure. A scar will affect the donor site in numerous ways. A scar affects how wide the subsequent donor strip can be. Usually the removal of a preexisting scar along with a new donor strip will result in a much wider incision than one would expect. For example, if the previous scar measures 3 mm in width and the donor width to be removed measures 1 cm, one might expect the resultant wound to be 1.3 cm wide. However, this is usually not the case, and the wound width has the potential to widen much beyond the predicted 1.3 cm, with the possibility of even doubling to 2.6 cm. This scenario challenges the surgeon to close a much larger incision, possibly under significant tissue tension and leading to a widened scar.

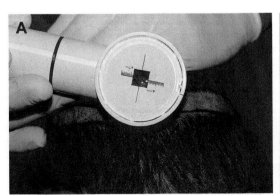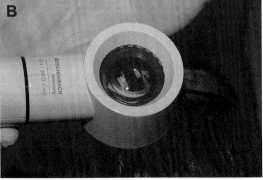

Fig. 3. A densitometer is used to calculate donor density. (*A*) The device has a precise one-square-centimeter field in which follicles can be counted. (*B*) The device uses magnification to allow easy and rapid visualization of the follicular unit counting zone.

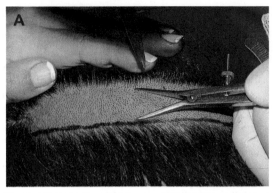
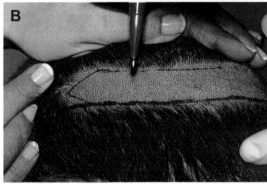

Fig. 4. (*A*) Once the safe donor width has been determined, a caliper is used to precisely define the superior and inferior borders of the donor strip. (*B*) The borders have been accurately marked.

To avoid this problem, one may have to plan on removing a smaller donor strip, thus harvesting fewer grafts.

The donor wound will not spring open if harvesting grafts in an area where punch grafting was previously done. The scarring after punch grafting seems to secure the overlying tissue and the incision width does not routinely increase when the donor strip is removed.

In designing a new donor strip excision, the surgeon should ideally position the old scar at the inferior or superior border and not in the middle of the donor tissue. This makes separation of the scar from the follicles easier for the technicians preparing the grafts. Of note, the follicles adjacent to an old scar often have altered direction, so this should be considered and great care implemented when making the superior or inferior incision along the old scar.

As hair transplantation procedures have become larger and a second, third, or fourth session more common, the appearance of the donor site requires even more attention. It is imperative to leave as inconspicuous a scar as possible at all times, and this can occur only with a conservative approach to the tissue excised.

PREPARING THE DONOR SITE

With the patient either sitting up or prone the donor site hair is trimmed to a length of 2 to 3 mm. Having even this minimal length aids the appropriate direction of the grafts during their insertion phase into the recipient site. There is little need to trim beyond what will be excised, and in fact, long hair above the harvest site will help camouflage the incision. Next, the superior and inferior edges of the donor site are outlined with a surgical marker (**Fig. 6**).

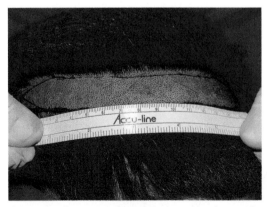

Fig. 5. The donor strip length is determined once the safe donor width and the baseline follicular unit density have been assessed.

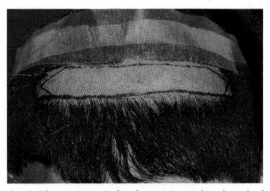

Fig. 6. The entire strip has been trimmed and marked immediately before the donor harvest.

Positioning the Patient

I prefer donor harvesting using the prone position. There is much less chance of a vasovagal reaction compared with the sitting position. This also is a very comfortable position for the surgeon and assistant to work. The patient's head rests in a Pron-Pillow (**Fig. 7**). This pillow is both comfortable and allows air circulation along its periphery so the patient can breathe more easily. Metal hair clips or tape can be used to keep the superior hair out of the field. Harvesting a meticulous strip generally requires about 45 to 60 minutes. Patients have little problem remaining in the prone position for this relatively short time. The head remains stable in the pillow and the patient can move his or her head without any discomfort as the donor strip is harvested from one side to the other. The donor area can be cleansed with a number of antiseptic agents, but one must remember this is a "clean" procedure, not a sterile one. One last laxity check at this point is wise before injecting the local anesthetic, so that any modifications of the planned width can be implemented if necessary.

Donor Site Anesthesia

The superior and inferior edges are injected with local anesthesia. I prefer 1% xylocaine with 1/100,000 epinephrine. A neck vibrator wrapped in a plastic bag is placed over the injection sites to diminish discomfort. An ice cube can also be used to help reduce injection-related pain.

The lateral supra-auricular areas are often more sensitive than the occipital region, and the inferior border injections tend to generate more pain than those placed superiorly. Anesthetic infiltration into

an old scar will also be painful. Thorough anesthetic infiltration along the superior and inferior edges is mandatory because this is where the cuts will be made. Infiltration from these border injections usually suffices to provide anesthesia along the base of the donor strip.

HARVESTING THE STRIP

The key to the donor strip technique is to visualize the follicles and stay parallel to the existing hair shafts to help ensure a negligible transection. I prefer a moderate amount of magnification and use a ×4 OptiVISOR with an attached headlight. This allows me to wear my own prescription glasses and also provides excellent eye protection.

Procedure

- I use a #10 blade to cut through the epidermis, scoring the superior and inferior strip borders. Usually this cut will extend into the upper papillary dermis (**Fig. 8**).

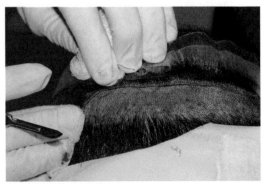

Fig. 8. The superior border has been scored into the superficial dermis with a scalpel. Care is taken to move between adjacent follicular units along the length of the strip.

- Next, delicate double-pronged skin hooks are placed on each side of the incision into the superficial dermis and traction is applied.

Surgical note: The assistant holds one retraction hook while also keeping the field dry. I retract the opposite wound edge with the hook in my nondominant hand and use the #10 blade to gently push through the dermis, visualizing the follicles and separating them from the adjacent tissue

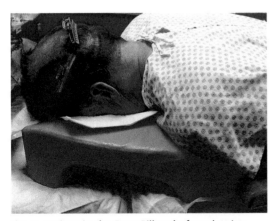

Fig. 7. Patient in the Pron-Pillow before draping.

(**Fig. 9**). The side of the blade is used to gently "push" tissue rather than generating a distinct cutting motion.

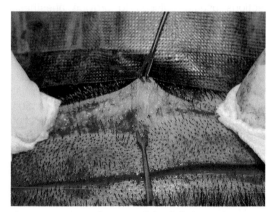

Fig. 9. Direct visualization of the follicles as dissection separates the strip from the adjacent donor tissue.

- Once the superior and inferior dissection is complete, the strip is grasped and sharply freed from the underlying tissue, staying in a plane just beneath the follicles (**Fig. 10**).

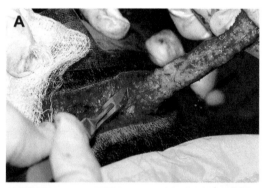

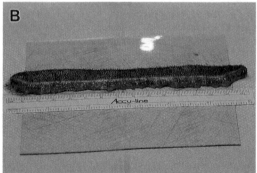

Fig. 10. (*A*) Sharp and blunt dissection in a subfollicular plane frees the strip from the deeper lying aponeurosis and neurovascular bundles. (*B*) The harvested strip demonstrates a clean edge with intact follicular units.

- There are small neurovascular bundles that should be preserved by maintaining the immediate subfollicular dissection, a plane that keeps the blade superficial to these structures.
- Hemostasis can be achieved in several ways:
  - A 3–0 chromic ligature is used when a vessel lumen is encountered.
  - Minor bleeding at the base of the wound can be managed with conservative cautery (**Fig. 11**).

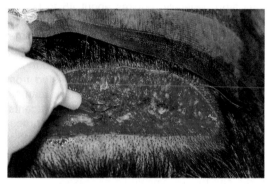

Fig. 11. Conservative cauterization of the deep wound bed.

  - Skin edge bleeding is disregarded for fear of damaging local follicles, but any persistent ooze can often be controlled by injecting a small amount of local anesthetic with epinephrine.
  - The use of any cautery to stop superficial bleeding will invariably damage nearby hair follicles and risks a more noticeable scar devoid of hair.

Surgical note: I prefer to divide the donor area into sections, which allows the width to be altered incrementally depending on the ease of approximation at any given point in time (**Fig. 12**).

- I usually excise 24 to 30 cm of length and 1 to 2 cm of width.
- Beginning laterally, I typically remove 4 to 6 cm at a width of 1 cm.
- The narrowest width will almost always be laterally, as the scalp tends to be tightest in that area.
- I test the closure after removing the small section and, if it is very lax, the strip width may be increased an additional 2 to 3 mm.
- I follow the same approach as dissection proceeds into the occipital area, although the width posteriorly routinely increases to 1.5 to 2.0 cm because of the usual favorable laxity characteristics of that area.

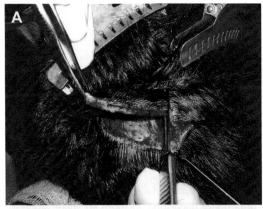

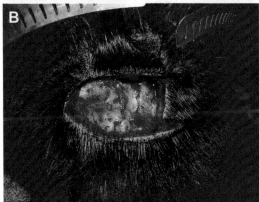

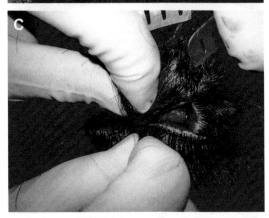

Fig. 12. Segmental donor excision helps gauge the ease of closure and allows for any necessary adjustment to the donor strip width. (*A*) Beginning laterally, a short donor segment is removed. (*B*) The resulting wound is observed following removal of the lateral segment. (*C*) Wound closure is tested and adjustments are then made if a wider or narrower strip will be required.

Intraoperative Estimation of Graft Total

Another advantage of incremental excision is that the dissecting team can begin preparing grafts quickly instead of waiting for the complete strip

removal. They also can provide the surgeon with information regarding the graft yield from the initial harvest section so that the projections for the remaining harvest can be implemented. One of the surgical assistants is charged with estimating the number of grafts as each section of donor tissue is removed. Obtaining information about the graft yield per centimeter of harvested strip early in the case allows the surgeon to determine how much additional length and width will be needed for the remaining strip to yield the desired number of grafts.

There is routinely a wide variation in graft yield between patients. Typically I estimate 60 to 100 FUs in a single square centimeter of the occipital area, with lower density estimates for the lateral areas. During the strip width decision process, every additional millimeter of width will yield up to 10% more grafts based on my estimation from a 1-cm-wide strip. Of course this remains just an educated guess until the assistant informs me of the actual yield, at which time very precise estimates of graft yield can be made for the subsequent strip dimensions.

Harvesting in a Previously Used Donor Site

Typically there is no problem harvesting in a donor site more than once, but some issues can occur.

- The surgeon should, if at all possible, incorporate the previous scar in the new excision so as to maintain a single scar within the donor site area. If the previous scar is narrow (a few millimeters wide) and the scalp is lax, then this will be no problem.
- Ideally, the old scar will be located along either the superior border or the inferior border of the newly excised donor strip (**Fig. 13**). This is preferable to the scar being in the middle of the new donor tissue because it is easier for the assistants preparing the grafts. They can more easily excise the scar by cutting it away from the edge of the donor tissue, whereas dissection of a centrally situated scar proves more challenging.
- Often, I first remove the donor strip by incising adjacent to the scar and then separately remove the scar. This provides the dissection team with a high-quality strip devoid of troublesome scar. They will, however, later check the scar for any retained follicular units, which will then be separated for grafting purposes.
- If there is excess scar tissue at the base of the wound, it should be removed before closure.

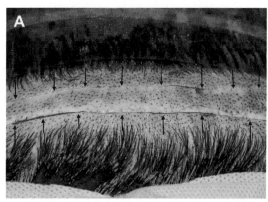
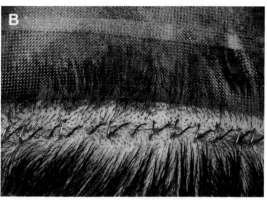

Fig. 13. (*A*) A strip is planned that will remove 2 scars from prior donor harvesting. Incisions are made along the edge of each scar (*arrows*) so as to incorporate them into the donor strip. This maintains an intact row of follicular units along the entire length of both the superior and inferior harvest site edges. (*B*) The result is a neat, scar-free incision line closure.

Surgical Note: One caveat is to avoid neurovascular tissue that may be deep to this dense connective tissue so as to maintain donor circulation and to avoid donor hypoesthesia from inadvertent nerve damage.

As mentioned earlier, in most cases the wound will be wider following a secondary or tertiary strip harvest. It is not unusual to remove a 1-cm-wide donor strip with a resultant gaping wound of 2 cm or more. This can be unsettling, but most will close easily without any undermining if the preoperative laxity estimates were accurate. Yet one should be mindful of this occurrence and thus take a conservative approach to how much width is excised. Again, it is always better to harvest additional tissue after you know with certainty that the wound can be safely closed.

Closure of the Incision

This is a critical part of the procedure. Hopefully appropriate width was removed so the wound can be closed without tension. A telltale sign of a less than elegant hair transplant is a widened visible donor site scar, and this must be avoided. Typically, I close the incision in 2 layers and do not undermine. For the deep layer I prefer using buried, interrupted sutures with 2–0 Vicryl. The purpose of this stitch is to secure the deep fascia or aponeurosis so as to anchor the base of the wound (**Fig. 14**). The deep suture must remain below the follicles to avoid shock loss or permanent follicular damage. Suture approximation draws the opposing subcutaneous tissue and dermal edges to the midline. This suture is critical in its role of removing tension from the skin closure

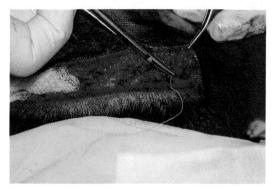

Fig. 14. Placing the deep suture beneath the follicles to approximate the fascia and aponeurosis.

(**Fig. 15**). Following stabilization of the deep layer, the skin then is closed with a running 3–0 nylon "baseball stitch" or surgical staples (**Fig. 16**). The nylon suture or the staples gently approximate

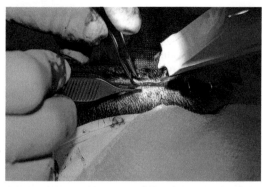

Fig. 15. Proper placement of the deep suture allows skin closure to proceed with minimal to no tension on the epidermal edges.

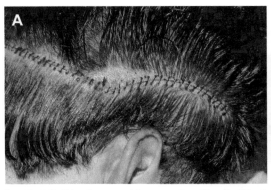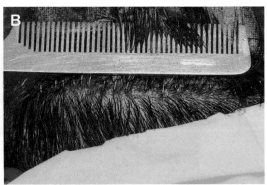

Fig. 16. (*A*) Skin closure with a running "baseball" stitch. (*B*) Skin closure using a combination of staples and sutures.

the skin edges, as there should be no superficial tension at this time. At the end of the case, the donor area is injected with local anesthesia to increase comfort while the patient is traveling home or to a hotel.

Tricophytic Closure

The trichophytic closure has become popular as we strive for imperceptible scars at the donor site. This technique was used for many years to improve the scars of hair-bearing scalp flaps (Juri flaps). It has been used for the past decade in strip harvesting. The basic principle is to alter the edges of the donor site incision so that hair will grow through the scar and thus make it less noticeable.

A trichophytic closure can be used if the wound can be closed without significant tension.

- With this technique, a narrow strip of epidermis is removed from one edge of the harvest site (**Fig. 17**).

Surgical Note: Often this excised tissue will include a small amount of papillary dermis, but it is critical to stay above the sebaceous glands and the follicular bulge. This deepithelializing strip should be no more than 1 mm deep and 1 to 2 mm wide.

- I remove this strip with sharp dissection and ×7 magnification.

Surgical Note: Some surgeons advocate removing this strip from the inferior edge because it may help preserve the acute angle of the hair follicles exiting through the scar. Some surgeons slope the excision and others make a right-angle cut. I am not sure if the various minor modifications

make any difference, but a meticulous skin closure is important to ensure an optimal result (**Fig. 18**).

The method can be deferred if the patient is going to have additional procedures at a later date, in which case the trichophytic closure is delayed until the last session. Another consideration for avoiding this closure method is when a large session is planned, in which case the trichophytic technique will use 1 to 2 mm of donor tissue that could instead be incorporated into the strip to facilitate a higher graft yield. This technique will not work well if one skin edge has scar tissue. To be successful, both edges must have intact hair follicles.

COMPLICATIONS AND TREATMENT
Widened Scar

This is both the most common and worrisome postoperative complication at the donor site. There is always a balancing act between maximizing grafts and leaving an imperceptible scar. Most of the causes of a widened scar are preventable. The most common cause of an enlarged scar is excising too wide a strip and subsequently closing the wound under tension. As stated previously, sequential excision helps prevent a small error in judgment from becoming a large error. It is better to take too little than too much, because one can always go back and remove more donor area with a second smaller strip.

Certain patients seem more prone to widened scars. Men in their 20s and 30s seem to heal less favorably, especially those involved in aggressive weight lifting. Patients with extremely lax scalps ironically may also be more prone to postoperative scar widening. I recommend that patients avoid all maneuvers that stretch the donor site for 4 weeks, including exercises that

A

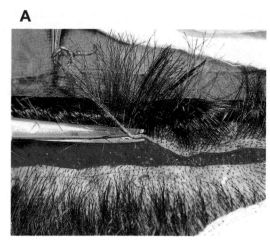

B

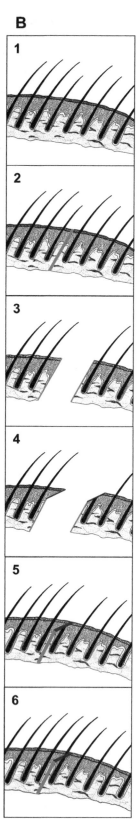

Fig. 17. (*A*) A trichophytic closure is performed by removing a strip of epidermis from one edge of the harvest site. Care is required to preserve the sebaceous glands and the follicular bulge. (*B*) Illustration of the donor site trichophytic closure technique: (1) Cross-section view of donor hair follicles. (2) Donor incision is made between and parallel to the donor site follicles. (3) Donor site gap following removal of the strip. (4) A tangential cut is made to remove a small section of epidermis and superficial dermis above those follicles that are located along the length of the strip. The opposing edge can be scored to match the deepithelialized skin edge. (5) The skin edges are meticulously approximated so as to bury the deepithelialized segment below the superficial incision line. (6) Final healing results in buried follicles producing hair growth through the donor scar.

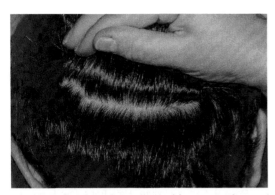

Fig. 18. A fine, nearly undetectable scar is observed following a well-planned and carefully executed donor strip harvest.

stretch the neck and upper back. Conversely, older men and most women usually have excellent scars.

Any maneuver that damages the follicles adjacent to the incision will also cause a wider-appearing scar. Aggressive cautery near the skin edges will likely injure nearby follicles. These tiny vessels usually stop spontaneously and do not require cautery. Occasionally injecting a small amount of local anesthesia will control the oozing. The suture used for the subcutaneous layer closure can also damage follicles, so it is imperative to keep this suture safely beneath the follicles.

The superficial skin suture should approximate the wound edges without tension and remain superficial to the bulge region of the follicles. Some postoperative swelling is inevitable, and if the skin closure is too tight, this can cause ischemic changes in the skin during the early healing phase, which may yield a widened scar. Patients with a snug donor area are encouraged to massage the area for 2 to 4 weeks before surgery to assist in generating local laxity.

Occasionally, telogen effluvium occurs at the donor site. This requires only patience and reassurance for the patient, as it will resolve in 4 to 6 months. Preservation of the donor region blood supply minimizes the risks of postoperative effluvium and problematic scar formation. Careful donor strip dissection in the subfollicular plane is the best method for preserving the local, underlying feeder vessels.

Several factors need to be considered when performing the strip technique in an area with a scar from prior strip harvesting:

1. Removal of an old scar will create a better vascularized skin edge.

2. Excising excess scar in the base of the wound diminishes bulk, which will help improve blood supply.

Everything mentioned so far has focused on the prevention of a widened scar, but when it does occur it can be treated successfully. One should wait at least 6 months before revising an unacceptable scar. Aggressive scalp massage of 5 to 10 minutes at least 6 times per day for 1 month should be done. If one is worried that the scar is too wide for complete removal in a single procedure, then the surgeon should initially remove only half of the scar and then evaluate the remaining closure tension. If feasible, take more small strips of scar as long as the skin tension remains manageable. Undermine only if absolutely necessary, taking caution not to damage the skin flap vascular supply if this maneuver is required.

Infection and Hypoesthesia

A localized pustule may develop along the suture line. The cause may be a stitch abscess or an ingrown hair. Treatment need only be a topical antibiotic and resolution should occur in 7 to 10 days. Any indication of an abscess will require an incision and drainage, followed by antibiotic ointment for 5 to 7 days. Oral antibiotics should be needed only if a cellulitis develops, and this would be exceedingly rare.

Hypoesthesia is common for weeks or even months after the procedure. Patients need to be informed beforehand to expect this and that it will resolve. Complete anesthesia is exceedingly rare and correlated with accidental transection of the occipital nerve. Transection should not be a concern when using magnification and a proper dissection plane superficial to the nerve. There is no treatment for this complication, but often this too will improve over time.

POSTOPERATIVE CARE

The patient can shampoo the donor site the next day and continue this each day. Topical antibiotic ointment should be applied twice a day for 10 days. Light exercise can be resumed in 5 days and more rigorous routines in 14 days. Patients can have their hair cut or colored in 2 weeks. Over the years, I have noticed wider scars in patients who do heavy weightlifting and now encourage them to do lighter weights and more reps for 1 month. I also now restrict doing certain exercises that could stretch the back of the neck for 1 month.

REFERENCES

1. Donor area harvesting. In: Unger W, Shapiro R, Unger R, et al, editors. Hair transplantation. 5th edition. New York: Informa Healthcare; 2011. p. 247–90.
2. Buchwach K, Konior R. The donor site. In: Contemporary hair transplant surgery. New York: Thieme Medical Publishers; 1997. p. 54–79.
3. Mayer M, Pauls T. Scalp elasticity scale. Hair Transplant Forum Intl 2005;15:122.
4. Mayer M, Perez-Mesa D. Managing the donor area to minimize scarring. Int J Cosmet Surg Aesthetic Dermatol 2001;1(2):121–6.
5. Pathomvanich D. Donor harvesting, a new approach to minimize transaction of hair follicles. Dermatol Surg 2000;26:345–8.
6. Marzola M. Single scar harvesting. In: Haber RS, Stough DB, editors. Procedures in cosmetic dermatology, hair transplantation. Dover JS, Series Editor. Philadelphia: Elsevier; 2006. p. 83–6.
7. Marzola M. Tricophytic closure of the donor area. Hair Transplant Forum Intl 2005;15(4):113–6.
8. Rose P. Ledge closure. Hair Transplant Forum Intl 2005;15:113–6.

Follicular Unit Extraction

James A. Harris, MD

KEYWORDS

- FUE • Follicular unit extraction • Donor harvesting • Donor area management
- FUE instrumentation • Body hair grafting • Plug/minigrafts repair

KEY POINTS

- When performing FUE, always wear high-quality magnification of at least ×4.5 to ×6.5.
- If one commits to providing this procedure for patients, then one has to commit to the practice and refinement of the technique before making it a standard procedure in the practice.
- Be sure to explain the procedure to patients, the advantages and disadvantages, and avoid the hype that surrounds this procedure.

INTRODUCTION

Follicular unit extraction (FUE) is a method of graft harvest whereby punches of various types are used to remove follicular units from the donor region one at a time.[1] The principal advantages of this technique to patients are chiefly the lack of a linear scar and more rapid healing of the donor region. In general this technique will allow patients to cut their hair to approximately one-fourth inch or less. For physicians, FUE offers a technique for repairing pluggy-appearing or inappropriately placed hairlines and also the ability to harvest additional grafts in patients who have little or no scalp laxity. Over the past 5 years FUE has gained a degree of popular acceptance by patients such that it is the fastest growing procedure in hair restoration.[2]

There are 2 basic punch types used to perform FUE, sharp and dull tips, and within each category there are manual and powered versions. The sharp dissection techniques typically involve limited depth punch insertion to decrease the risk of follicle transection. The blunt punch dissection technique allows for a deeper level of dissection, thereby decreasing the force required for graft removal.

This article provides the reader an overview of the uses of the FUE procedure with attention paid to donor area management, procedure considerations, and instrumentation.

UTILITY OF FUE
Hair Restoration

There are several indications for using FUE in restorative and repair procedures (**Box 1**). In general, any patient who is a candidate for hair restoration by the strip method is a candidate for FUE, as the cosmetic results in the recipient area are the same as in strip surgery (**Fig. 1**). In addition, there are likely candidates for FUE restoration who are not candidates for strip harvest by virtue of low donor hair density and how short they would like to wear their hair. A patient with very fine donor hair and low donor density may be a poor candidate for a strip harvest, yet may achieve a good result with FUE (**Fig. 2**).

The obvious candidates, and most patients seeking FUE, are those who desire the option of wearing their hair short. Minimal postoperative pain and discomfort is certainly a desired outcome, but it is not usually the primary motivating factor for having FUE. **Fig. 3** is an example

Disclosures: President of HSC Development, a company that produces the SAFE System, a device for performing follicular unit extraction. The author is also a consultant for and a stockholder in Restoration Robotics, the company that produces the ARTAS System for performing follicular unit extraction.
Hair Sciences Center of Colorado, 5445 DTC Parkway, Suite 1015, Greenwood Village, CO 80111, USA
E-mail address: jharris@hsccolorado.com

of a patient postoperative FUE opting for a short hair hairstyle and showing minimal visibility of his donor sites. Patients should be aware that although there is no linear scarring, there will be 2 donor area factors that will not allow most to shave their head after surgery. The first may be visible scarring due to hypopigmentation, and the second is the *appearance* of hypopigmentation, which in reality is the lack of hair in an extraction site that is perceived as hypopigmentation.

Although the amount of postoperative pain after strip surgery is usually not intolerable, many patients who have had a strip procedure and a subsequent FUE note that there is a significant difference in the experience with patients who had FUE often requiring no narcotics and only 2 to 3 days of a nonsteroidal analgesic. The vast majority of patients having FUE also do not experience hypesthesia or sensations of tightness in the donor area.

There are 2 situations in which a combination of a strip harvest and FUE can be used to "expand" donor capacity.

1. Maximize number of grafts obtained from a single surgical session
2. Severe limits to patient's scalp laxity with normal-density donor area

Combination strip harvest and FUE can be considered in a patient who would like to maximize the number of grafts obtained from a single surgical session (a single day or 2 subsequent days). The typical scenario is that first a strip would be obtained and the grafts planted, and this would be followed by an FUE procedure that may increase a single surgery yield by up to 50%. There have been reports of skin necrosis when the FUE is performed inferior to the strip excision site, so this should be avoided.

Combination strip harvest and FUE can be considered in the case of a patient who has received multiple strip procedures and demonstrates severe limits to his or her scalp laxity, but whose general donor area appears to have "normal" density. In this case, FUE may be used to harvest additional grafts. There are cases in which the use of both procedures has allowed the harvest of more than 12,000 grafts without any adverse consequences to the donor region. Obviously this can be a great benefit in Norwood class 6–7 patients and can change the treatment planning significantly.

Body Hair Harvest

FUE has allowed the harvest of body hair without the creation of linear scars on the chest, abdomen, pubis, or submandibular areas. It has also made it possible to harvest areas such as the arms, legs, and back where strip surgeries were never really an option. Although the harvest of body hairs is technically feasible and there is anecdotal information to support its use,[3] there are no studies that address body hair graft survival rates. In my experience, it seems that the use of beard hair may have a higher survival rate than other body donor sites, which may have something to do with either the size of the follicles (generally larger than other body sites) or the length of the anagen cycle. My preference is to harvest hairs in the anagen phase. Anagen hairs may be discerned by

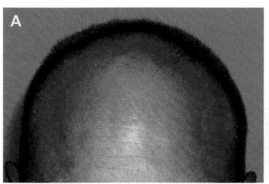
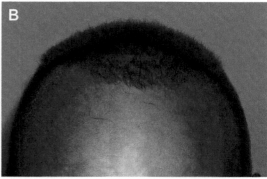

Fig. 1. Showing 2200 FUE grafts. (*A*) Preoperative, (*B*) Postoperative.

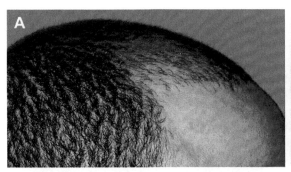
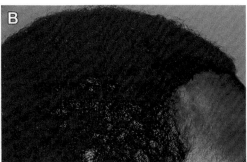

Fig. 2. Showing 1800 FUE grafts. (*A*) Preoperative, (*B*) Postoperative.

either the thickness of the hair shaft or presence of hair pigmentation (in cases of nongray hair), as the telogen hairs will be lighter in color and finer in caliber. One may also shave the donor area approximately 4 to 7 days before the surgery to facilitate identification of the actively growing anagen hair, as the telogen hairs will not have elongated since shaving.

Although many body donor areas, such the arms, legs, beard, and chest, are potentially visible at times, the scarring from FUE has not been problematic in most patients. The scarring on the chest can be visible as small hypopigmented dotlike scars with the chest shaved (**Fig. 4**). The situation is similar for beard extractions, although the natural irregularity of pigmentation and the natural visibility of the hair ostia make the beard donor sites virtually invisible in

most patients. It is prudent to extract only from the submandibular region; however, in some patients who desire more beard grafts, a test session may be performed to see if the scarring above the jaw line or in buccal regions will be visible or problematic for the patient.

The anesthetic administration for beard extractions can usually be accomplished with a wide field block with spot infiltrations for breakthrough sensation. The chest will require a tumescent anesthetic technique similar to that used for liposuction.

In counseling patients, I usually suggest that all scalp donor hair available be harvested before considering body hair FUE. The primary reasons for this are the uncertain survival rate and that the average approximate body region density of 1.2 hairs per graft makes it more difficult to create a dense result. The other possible reason for using scalp hair preferentially is that the quality and characteristics of the hair more closely match the hair in the recipient region as opposed the case of beard hair on the scalp where a texture mismatch is probable. **Fig. 5** shows a body hair (beard donor) transplant result.

Fig. 3. The donor area of a patient who elects to wear his hair short after 2800 extractions. He would be a questionable candidate for strip surgery because of diffuse thinning of the donor area as well as his desire to wear his hair short.

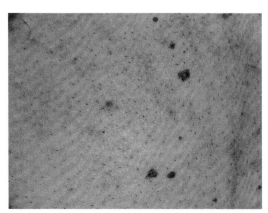

Fig. 4. The small white dotlike scars from FUE performed on the chest.

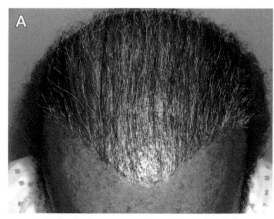
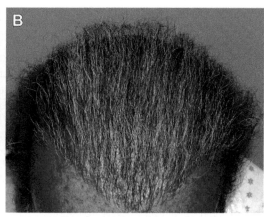

Fig. 5. (A) Preoperative and (B) postoperative appearance after approximately 2000 beard grafts were used over the top of the scalp to increase the density.

Hair Restoration Repairs

FUE can be very valuable in the cases of patients requiring repairs such as inappropriately placed or linear hairlines, multihair grafts in the hairline, or visibly pluggy grafts. In the situation of a hairline placed inappropriately low, the patient's options are to undergo laser hair removal and "waste" the donor hair, or to have the grafts removed and replaced in a more appropriate position. Another indication is the patient who initially had grafts placed in a proper position, but later has additional hair loss and decides to remove the previous grafts and restore a natural pattern rather than have more procedures. The extracted grafts can then be replaced into donor scar if need be.

In the case of a pluggy-appearing hairline due to either minigrafts or multihair follicular units, the offending hairs or grafts may be thinned by FUE. There are 2 advantages of this technique over

simply placing follicular units in front of the offending grafts. The first is that if the hairline is already at the limits of a conservative location, there is no need to lower the hairline any farther. The second is that with the removal of offending units, a single-pass correction with follicular units is often possible.

The technique used in my practice is to first identify the cosmetic issue and then formulate a surgical plan. The plan may be a combination of graft removal and the addition of follicular units. The offending hair or grafts are first identified and trimmed to approximately 1 mm. Now the surgeon may have an approximate "real-time" view of what the FUE can accomplish. This is fine-tuned to the surgeon's satisfaction to either reduce plugginess or to decrease the hairline linearity, and then the hairs or follicular units that were trimmed are removed by FUE. **Fig. 6** shows a reduction in plugginess and linearity in 1 session and **Fig. 7** shows

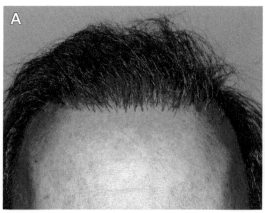
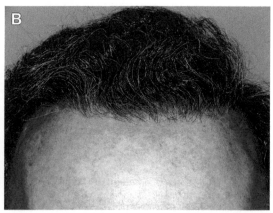

Fig. 6. FUE and additional follicular unit grafting were used to reduce the pluggy appearance and linearity. (A) Preoperative and (B) postoperative appearance.

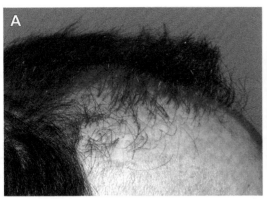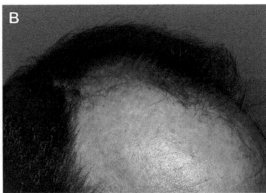

Fig. 7. FUE used to remove grafts to restore a pretransplant appearance. (*A*) Preoperative and (*B*) postoperative appearance.

almost complete FUE removal of unattractive hairline grafts to restore the patient as close as possible to his pretransplant state.

DONOR AREA CONSIDERATIONS

The "safe" donor area for FUE is, in general, the same region used for strip harvest. There are, however, some areas that require special attention or may be used under special circumstances. The lower neck regions and the supra-auricular regions can be used to obtain grafts that contain hair of finer caliber for use in the frontal hairline. A risk of graft loss exists for those hairs obtained from the neck in patients at risk for retrograde alopecia.

In some patients, the hair at the superior aspect of the fringe can appear very thick or "puffy" when compared with the thin or bald area just superior to it or to the thinning hair in the supra-auricular and low neck regions. A unique situation exists here because thinning of the extraction zone following an FUE procedure can further enhance the appearance of a very thick upper fringe region. A possible solution to the situation is to extract follicular units high into the thick fringe region to intentionally thin this disproportionately high-density hair. This method helps to provide a more "blended" appearance throughout the entire donor area rather than creating a more visually distinct transition between a nonharvested upper fringe and the more commonly used inferior extraction zone. There are 2 strategies or techniques that may be followed and both have advantages and disadvantages. The first option is to extract units from the upper fringe, selecting the units that appear to be "permanent" (no miniaturization). This increases the likelihood that they will remain stable in the transplanted area. This

strategy may be less predictable in younger patients in whom the miniaturization process may not have yet started. The potential downside here is that the extraction of permanent hair for stability in the transplanted area risks exposure of the extraction sites at some future time should miniaturization progress over time in the superior fringe. It may be argued that the sites will be virtually undetectable; however, they may be more visible and problematic in some patients. The second option is to remove follicular units from the high fringe that appear to be miniaturizing in the hopes that medical therapy will stabilize them in the transplanted area and the nonminiaturized hairs that are left in the fringe will camouflage the donor sites. With either strategy, the situation may be mitigated by the use of stabilizing medical therapies.

In general, the total number of grafts available using FUE is probably similar to the number available from strip harvesting, but the actual number is dependent on the density of the hair in the donor region. The endpoint for FUE is thinning of the donor hair to a level that is visibly discernible. In a single harvest session it is important to avoid "overharvesting" in a particular area, as the localized trauma may increase the risk of donor area postoperative shock loss. Harvesting approximately 20% to 30% of the available units in a particular area has never resulted in a case of shock loss in my practice and yet allows for the extraction of 2400 to 4000 grafts in a single session if need be.

Care should be taken to avoid overharvesting in a small donor area, as this area may appear significantly less dense than the surrounding donor region, especially if the hair is worn short. An example of this would be harvesting 1000 to 1200 grafts in the occiput alone, as this would increase the probability of creating a low-density area when the hair is worn short. The ideal surgical plan would distribute the FUE sites over the entire donor area at a uniform density relative to the native follicular unit density. Subsequent harvest sessions should be performed in regions not previously harvested to spread the effect of multiple procedures diffusely throughout the entire region.

PERFORMING THE FUE PROCEDURE
Donor Area Preparation

There are several ways to shave the donor area in preparation for the FUE procedure. Normally in patients who elect to undergo FUE because of their desire to eventually wear their hair short (less than one-half inch), the optimal strategy is to shave the entire donor area in preparation for the procedure.

This allows the surgeon to extract diffusely over the entire donor region to avoid focal thinning.

An option for patients who do not want to shave their entire donor area and are unlikely to wear their hair short after the procedure is to perform a "microstrip shave" where 2-mm to 4-mm wide strips are shaved along the donor site. The shaved microstrips are separated by 2-mm to 4-mm strips of unshaven hair so as to leave the donor harvest sites hidden. The limit of this type of preparation is approximately 1200 to 1500 grafts in a single surgical session, as only half of the potential donor area is exposed. Subsequent surgeries should focus the harvest between the previous microstrip harvest regions. Patients must be counseled that should they cut their hair short, distinct "striplike" regions of low density will be visible.

The final shave preparation, as advocated by Cole in personal communications, is to cut only the hair of the follicular units to be extracted over the entire donor area. This will provide a diffuse extraction pattern and diffuse scars, but the technique will require a longer procedure time.

Anesthetic Considerations

The usual method of administration is a ring block in the periphery of the donor region followed by a "bead" of anesthetic along the occipital protuberance to block the greater occipital nerves. The typical anesthetic is a combination of lidocaine followed by a longer-acting agent, such as bupivacaine, or alternatively a single agent, such as articaine. The recipient area is anesthetized in the physician's preferred fashion.

Patient and Surgeon Position

There are 2 basic patient-positioning strategies for FUE.

1. **The surgeon is in a position that is primarily opposite the direction of hair growth.** For the occipital region, the patient is prone and the surgeon is positioned at the head. This allows the surgeon to direct his or her arm motion toward the surgeon's body rather than away. This allows for less fatigue and a higher degree of control. The same strategy is used for the temporal regions, where the patient is positioned in the lateral decubitus position.
2. **The patient is sitting upright and the surgeon positioned to align with the emerging hairs.** This provides the surgeon with the ability to obtain a "line-of-site" directionality to the FUE device. This may cause fatigue for some surgeons and will preclude the patient from being sedated to any great degree. The advantage to this technique is that the surgeon may perform dissections or recipient site openings while grafts are simultaneously being harvested or planted. This method will increase the efficiency of the case.

FUE Methodology

The chief challenge in performing FUE is the uncertainty of the subcutaneous course and configuration of the follicles that may not be represented in the visible hair shafts above the skin surface. These differences may be in the angulation, curvature, or splay of the follicles.

To deal with this discrepancy, 2 strategies have emerged that are related to the 2 major classes of dissection tips available.

1. Sharp punch dissection
2. "Dull" dissecting punches

Sharp punch dissection was first described in the literature by Rassman and colleagues,[4] who noted that follicle transection rates increased as dissection depths increased. To decrease follicle transection, they advocated a limited-depth dissection. However, they observed that that this resulted in some degree of tethering between the follicle and the underlying tissue. This tethering had to be overcome by grasping and pulling forces that varied by individual. Cole developed a manual punch device (US Patent number 2005/0203545 A1, issued September 15, 2005) that featured an adjustable mechanical depth limiter to assist the user in maintaining a more consistent depth of dissection. Various methods for removing the grafts dissected by the sharp punch technique have been developed to address the problem of subcutaneous follicular tethering associated with limited depth dissection. These methods including dissecting the tethering tissue around the unit with needles in a "postage stamp" perforation pattern or grasping the distal follicles with a hemostat like instrument (**Fig. 8**) or forceps.

The use of **"dull" dissecting punches** was developed for dealing with the uncertain subcutaneous course and configuration of the follicles.[5] The proposed mechanism is that the dull tip is less likely to cut the follicles and the tip acts as a "guide" directing the follicles into the lumen of the punch. In addition to providing a low transection rate, the methodology allows a deeper dissection that separates the follicles from the subcutaneous tissue. This method promotes less manipulation and force on the grafts during the extraction.

Both dissection instrumentation modalities, sharp and dull, are available in manual and motorized (powered) systems. The main benefits of the motorized systems are the speed at which dissections can be performed and a decrease in operator fatigue. Surgeon preference, however, will dictate the type of system to be used.

Sharp Punch Technique

As mentioned, the key to the use of a sharp punch (powered or manual system) is that the punch insertion is subjected to depth limitation. This is most often accomplished with a depth limiter, such as a bead or silicone tube on the punch, providing a physical barrier to skin entry. The limiter can be set at various depths, but typically it must be at least as deep as the attachment of the arrector pili muscle, usually 2.0 to 2.5 mm, to allow graft removal. Some practitioners advocate a deeper dissection at least to a level where the follicles remain in a bundled configuration.

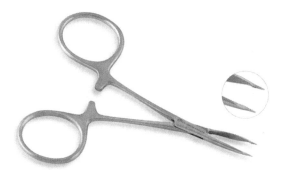

Fig. 8. ATOE (Aide to Extraction) instrument for removing dissected follicular units.

Transection rates increase dramatically if one goes beyond the region where follicle splay begins.

Stabilization of the skin is very important. The sharp punch has to be accurately "aimed" along the course of the follicles and the follicles must remain immobilized to minimize follicular damage. The skin is usually stabilized by the use of tumescent fluid in the target areas. The problem encountered by some practitioners is that excessive tumescent fluid injections into a region can cause the harvest area to become "mushy" and make subsequent dissection attempts in the region difficult.

Once the skin has been injected with a tumescent solution, the surgeon, wearing adequate magnification loupes, assumes his or her preferred position to perform the dissections. The punch is aimed such that the emerging hair is centered and the angle of entry is matched to the emergence angle of the hair. The punch is inserted, usually with a twisting motion in the case of a manual punch and directly into the skin using a powered punch. Another extraction variation is first inserting the punch tip at an angle close to 90° to the skin and entering just enough to score the skin. Following the scoring incision, the punch angle is adjusted to the hair angle. This method creates a wound that more closely approximates a circle than an oval. The punch is then inserted to the depth limiter and the grafts are removed and inspected. The depth controller can be adjusted depending on the length of the follicles, the position of the sebaceous gland, the ease of extraction, or the degree and position of splay in the follicles. These variables can change in different scalp regions so a continuous evaluation is conducted so that adjustments can be made.

Manual sharp dermal punches are available from a variety of suppliers. The most common sizes for FUE are 0.8 mm to 1.0 mm. The powered versions are also available from several hair restoration suppliers. There are specialized versions, such as the Neograft (Neograft Solutions, Dallas, TX) device, which has a suction apparatus that assists in harvesting and planting grafts, and a device called the PCID (Cole Instruments, Alpharetta, GA) (**Fig. 9**), which is a programmable device that oscillates or rotates the punch depending on the surgeon's requirements.

Dull Punch Technique

The general process for using a dull punch technique involves a few distinct steps that differ from the sharp punch technique. There is also

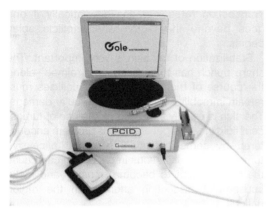

Fig. 9. PCID (Power Cole Isolation Device) for sharp punch powered FUE.

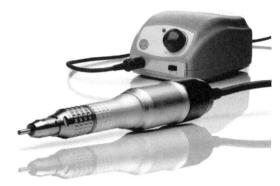

Fig. 10. SAFE system for powered dull punch FUE.

a technique difference between the manual and the powered dull punch versions. The manual dull punch technique, called the SAFE System (HSC Development, Greenwood Village, CO), is essentially a 2-step dissection process that was first described in 2003 at the International Society of Hair Restoration Surgery meeting in Vancouver and published in 2006.[6] The first step is "scoring" the epidermis and dermis to a limited depth of approximately 0.3 to 0.5 mm to allow entry of the blunt dissection punch. The blunt punch is then oriented to the approximate angle of the emerging hairs and inserted into the scoring incision. It is then rotated or oscillated by hand to a depth of approximately 4.2 mm, the depth of a "hard stop" on the punch, after which the follicular unit is removed. The chief criticism of this technique is a graft burial risk of approximately 7%. Although most buried grafts are recoverable, there remains an unrecoverable rate of 1.4%. In 9 years of performing FUE, there have been 3 instances of hair-bearing inflammatory cysts that required an excision procedure.

The powered version of the dull punch device,[7] the Powered SAFE System (Fig. 10), is a single-step dissection process that requires a defined technique to ensure success. After the donor area hair is shaved to the desired length, a 3-cm^2 to 4-cm^2 area is infiltrated with 1 to 2 mL of a dilute epinephrine solution in the subcutaneous fat for the purpose of hemostasis. Traction is placed opposite the direction of hair growth and the rotating dull punch is then positioned over the emerging hair at the approximate angle and direction of hair growth. Slight pressure *perpendicular* to the skin surface is placed

on the punch handpiece to allow the punch edge closest to the skin to "engage" or enter the skin. Using continued pressure in the same perpendicular direction, the punch will dissect the unit free. The punch can be inserted to the shoulder (depth approximately 4 mm) or the punch can be inserted to a submaximal depth if it is determined that a limited depth dissection will work. When the punch is inserted, there should be an audible and visual slowing of the punch rotation, as this will minimize transection rates. The absence of slowing following insertion should indicate to the operator that a decrease in the rotation speed is required. The amount of slowing may be decreased as the surgeon gains experience.

Robotic FUE

This technique is accomplished with the ARTAS System (Restoration Robotics, San Jose, CA), a robotic device (Fig. 11) used under physician control.[8] The technique involves the placement of a skin tension device which stabilizes the skin. This skin tension device houses fiducial markings on the periphery to define the active donor region and provide data for the assessment of the angles and directions of the hairs emerging from the scalp. The physician directs the robot to either dissect random grafts a given distance apart, to select follicular units with a given number of hairs, or to dissect those grafts that the physician designates.

The robot uses a 2-step dissection process similar to the 2-step manual dull punch system described previously. Once the robot has selected a target graft, an inner sharp punch will score the skin to a depth of approximately 1 to 2 mm. This is followed by a 1.2-mm rotating dull punch that is inserted to a depth of

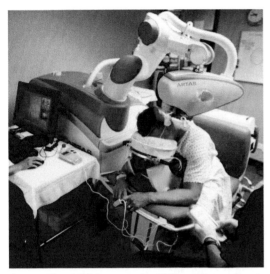

Fig. 11. The ARTAS system for FUE and its configuration in the operating room.

approximately 4 mm to dissect the follicular unit free from the skin. Adjustments to the insertion depths of the 2 punches, the speed of rotation, and the angle of insertion are essentially automated. The operator, however, can make fine adjustments as needed based on observations of the dissection process. Once the system has completed the dissection with the skin tension device, it is moved to the next donor area and the process is repeated until the desired number of dissections has been complete. The follicular units are then removed from the donor area.

Graft Handling and Planting Considerations

Once the grafts have been dissected and removed from the donor area with care to avoid crush injury, they are immediately placed into the holding solution of choice. Because most of the grafts are devoid of investing fat, an effort must be made to ensure that their time outside of the holding solution during the counting or sorting process is minimized. Additionally, the planting process must also be conducted with care to prevent graft desiccation and overmanipulation. The planters should limit graft exposure during their insertion to less than 2 minutes.

A team without extensive graft-placing experience places a high risk of overmanipulation and graft damage, which could easily result in suboptimal clinical results. In cases of an inexperienced team, consideration should be given to using one of the implanter devices available on the market.

Postoperative Considerations

The recipient areas can be treated the same way that one would treat the area after a strip harvest. Although the nature of an FUE procedure usually results in significantly less pain and discomfort than a strip harvest, the patient should have a narcotic and possibly a sleeping aid prescribed. The donor area can be dressed the first evening with an occlusive dressing and antibiotic ointment; however, this is optional. The continued application of an antibiotic ointment can be used if the patient would like to

---

Pearls: Performing FUE

After having observed many doctors attempting to perform FUE, there are several suggestions that will make the adoption of FUE easier.

- One of the most important factors is that the doctor learning the technique **should invest in high-quality surgical loupes with magnification in the range of ×4.5 to ×6.5.** I have observed physicians, claiming that ×2.5 or ×3.0 magnification is perfectly adequate, attempt to center a punch over the emerging hair and miss the target more than 50% of the time. If the punch cannot be centered, there is little likelihood that a successful graft extraction will be possible.

- **Performing FUE requires excellent eye-hand coordination, patience, stamina, and commitment.** The physician interested in performing this procedure needs to critically assess his or her qualifications in these 4 areas. If there is an issue, then a realistic decision needs to be made whether or not to pursue FUE. If the surgeon is lacking in the first 3 areas but has a high level of commitment, then consideration of the ARTAS System may be reasonable.

- **A surgeon interested in FUE must practice with his or her instrument of choice.** A suggestion for this is to perform FUE on every patient undergoing a strip procedure and attempt to remove 25 to 50 grafts. Once this can be accomplished in 3 to 5 minutes with a transection rate of 10% or less, the surgeon is ready for FUE cases in the range of 250 to 500 grafts. Of course if the surgeon would prefer not to become proficient at a manual technique, automated or not, there is the option of obtaining an ARTAS System. With this system, the surgeon may, after a day or two of training, extract at a reasonable rate with low transections.

have the scabs separate as rapidly as possible. Strenuous activity may be started after 3 to 4 days, as there is minimal or no risk of hematoma formation.

SUMMARY

FUE can be a valuable addition to a surgeon's repertoire, as the demand for this procedure is growing. Granted, there are details that have yet to be worked out, such as optimal extraction densities, scarring issues, dealing with donor area depletion, and strategies for combining strip and FUE for maximal graft availability. However, the technique has provided excellent results for thousands of patients.

What is certain is that some patients want a procedure that will not only provide excellent results but also minimal scarring, rapid recovery, and the ability to wear their hair short if they desire. Surgeons willing to take the time and effort to learn the procedure will be able to offer this segment of patients a procedure that will meet their needs. FUE has proven valuable in patients that require repairs and for former strip patients that require additional surgery. Those physicians not offering FUE to patients will surely be perceived as lagging behind the technology curve.

REFERENCES

1. Harris J. Conventional FUE in hair transplantation. In: Unger W, Shapiro R, Unger R, et al, editors. Hair Transplantation. 5th edition. London: Informa Healthcare; 2011. p. 291–6.
2. International Society of Hair Restoration Surgery: 2011 Practice Census Results, July 2011.
3. Cole J. Body to scalp in hair transplantation. In: Unger W, Shapiro R, Unger R, et al, editors. Hair Transplantation. 5th edition. London: Informa Healthcare; 2011. p. 304–6.
4. Rassman WR, Bernstein RM, McClellan R, et al. Follicular unit extraction: minimally invasive surgery for hair transplantation. Dermatol Surg 2002;28: 720–8.
5. Harris JA. Follicular unit extraction: the SAFE system. Hair Transplant Forum International 2004; 14:157, 163, 164.
6. Harris JA. New methodology and instrumentation for Follicular Unit Extraction (FUE): lower follicle transection rates and expanded patient candidacy. Dermatol Surg 2006;32:56–62.
7. Harris JA. Powered blunt dissection with the SAFE system for FUE (Part I and II). Hair Transplant Forum International 2010;20:188–9, 2011;21:16–7.
8. Harris J. Robotic-assisted follicular unit extraction for hair restoration: case reports. Cosmet Dermatol 2012; 25:284–7.

Management of Advanced Hair Loss Patterns

Michael L. Beehner, MD

KEYWORDS

• Forelock • Hair loss • Hair transplant • Forelock pattern • Hair miniaturization

KEY POINTS

- The male patient with a very large area of alopecia relative to the amount of donor hair is best served with a frontal forelock approach, in which front-central density is emphasized along with a gradient of diminishing hair density to the sides and back of the central forelock area.
- All young men should be transplanted in a manner that assumes and prepares for the "worst-case-scenario" in order to avoid creating an unnatural appearance later in life for the patient.
- The lateral gaps off to the side of the forelock can be transplanted using a "hump" concept, which brings the lateral fringe up to the projected "crease" line area, or it can simply be filled in with a "mirror image" approach using sparely spaced FU grafts.
- The vertex area is virtually ignored in most of these very bald patients, since the overriding priority is the frontal and midscalp regions.
- I recommend using the "oval" forelock pattern for the patients with the worst degree of alopecia. For those in whom there is a moderate amount of donor hair and a bi-itemporal width of 12–14cm, I recommend using the "shield" forelock whenever possible.

INTRODUCTION

A fair number of the men who consult a hair surgeon have such a large area of alopecia that filling in the entire region or even the entire top plane of hair loss is impossible.[1–9] Because the area of baldness is large, the corresponding donor area is necessarily reduced. Because the chief surgical goal for these patients with extensive alopecia is to frame the face and have the final result appear natural, the best way (in my opinion) to accomplish this is to create gradients of density, such that the final distribution of hair captures a stage of hair loss that people naturally see in men of that age, namely, that of a frontal forelock. In this article I describe a couple of approaches that can be taken, in which a modest amount of donor hair is used to create the effect of much more hair having been placed on the head and in an area that strongly creates a framing of the face.

Another equally important group of men are those younger patients in their 20s and early 30s who have various clues in their physical examination and history to indicate they might go on to extensive alopecia in the future.

I describe in detail my 2 favorite forelock patterns, the shield forelock (**Fig. 1**) and the oval forelock (**Fig. 2**). In addition, I briefly discuss a third pattern, the rounded arrowhead pattern (**Fig. 3**), which I use rarely.

For the small group of female patients who have extensive balding, the same principles apply, namely the priority of creating front-central density. In women, the useable donor area is often confined to the occipital region. A magnified examination of this occipital hair is key in determining if hair transplantation is likely to be successful for a given patient. If there is some degree of miniaturization in these hairs, then sometimes it is futile to even begin

Disclosure Statement: I have no financial connection to the makers of any product or instrument mentioned in this article.
Saratoga Hair Transplant Center, 60 Railroad Place, Suite 102, Saratoga Springs, NY 12866, USA
E-mail address: mlbeehner@saratogahair.com

Facial Plast Surg Clin N Am 21 (2013) 385–395
http://dx.doi.org/10.1016/j.fsc.2013.05.008

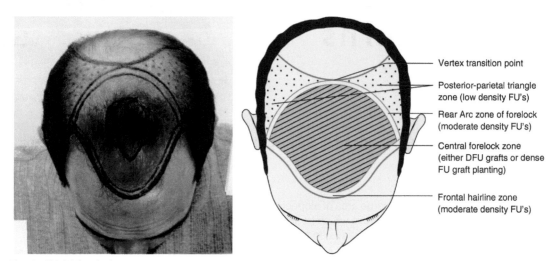

Fig. 1. Shield forelock pattern.

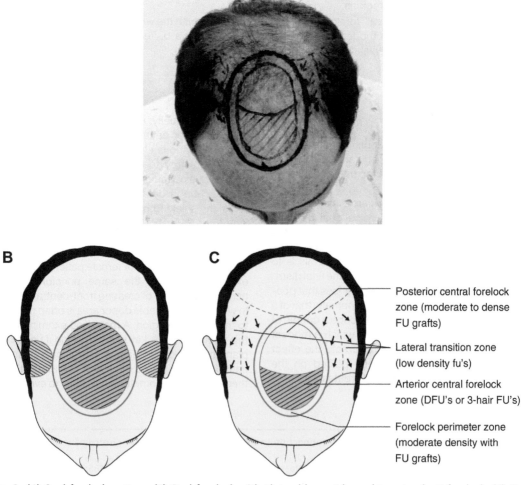

Fig. 2. (*A*) Oval forelock pattern. (*B*) Oval forelock with "lateral hump" brought up to abutt forelock. (*C*) Oval frontal forelock.

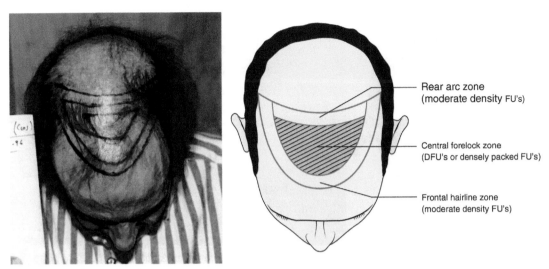

Rear arc zone
(moderate density FU's)

Central forelock zone
(DFU's or densely packed FU's)

Frontal hairline zone
(moderate density FU's)

Fig. 3. Rounded arrowhead pattern.

hair transplantation. Often, a nonsurgical hairpiece is a better solution to achieving the look of a full head of hair. When these women with extensive hair loss are transplanted, usually a single styling pattern is agreed on, and the transplants are preferentially placed where they can be styled to create the best visual density of hair.

THE CONSULTATION AND INITIAL PATIENT EVALUATION

Everything begins with the consultation. That is when the all-important rapport and sense of mutual trust are established between doctor and patient. Also, the surgeon's examination of a patient's scalp with fingers, eyes, and high magnification is invaluable for deciding that person's candidacy for hair replacement surgery. The face-to-face encounter at a consultation is also invaluable for evaluating a patient's level of maturity and whether or not his or her expectations are realistic or not. The use of a high-magnification examination of a patient's scalp enables surgeons to precisely gauge the degree of miniaturization present and the average number of hairs per follicular unit (FU) in the donor area. It is also a great teaching tool for explaining to patients that the strong, terminal hairs seen in the donor area are moved to the recipient area, where patients can see the high percentage of thinner, miniaturized hairs. Most importantly, during the course of the consultation, there is an exchange concerning a patient's wishes and desires for more hair, and this is balanced with the surgeon's realistic assessment of what is possible and best for that patient. The ideal result from the consultation occurs when

patient and surgeon leave the encounter with the same expectations for what the hair transplant process can achieve.

The Younger Man

As noted in the introduction, even though this article deals with what to do with patients with advanced hair loss patterns, I think it is necessary to include in this discussion those young men who have warning signs in their family history and in the physical examination pointing toward possible extensive balding later in life (**Fig. 4**). Among these signs are the following:

- Large area of miniaturization already
- Family history of Norwood class VII male relatives
- Whisker hair above the ear
- Indistinct fringes with extensive miniaturization in the upper inch of the side fringe

Hair surgeons should always be on the lookout for the rare diffuse unpatterned alopecia syndrome (DUPA), in which extensive miniaturization is seen in both recipient and donor areas. As a general rule, men with this syndrome should almost never be transplanted, because the hairs likely will not survive long term and the donor scar someday will be very evident.

It is paramount, when consulting with younger men, to try and visualize the worst-case scenario for them and then use a conservative pattern that still looks normal regardless of how far the fringes may someday fall. Peer pressure is important with men in this age group. Most of them want to quickly regain the exact appearance that all their peers have, which usually includes filling in any

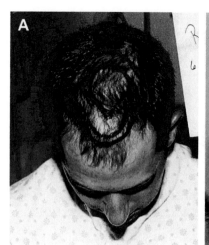
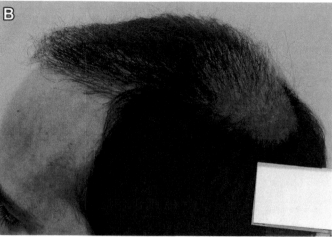

Fig. 4. (*A*) Conservative "shield" forelock pattern drawn on 19-year-old patient's head in 1995. (*B*) Same 19-year-old patient 10 years later, after 3 small hair transplant sessions of 800 grafts each.

thin areas of the vertex and aggressively filling in and flattening the frontotemporal recessions on each side. Also, they often have not emotionally accepted that they are losing their hair and are still angry and bitter about this impending loss. It is wise to defer any surgery in such patients. They can be placed on medical therapy for the time being, some baseline photos can be taken, and they can be asked to return in a year for re-evaluation. Often, with the passing of a few years, they adopt a more mature and realistic set of expectations and become good surgical candidates. Surgeons need to be empathetic and realize that many of these younger men are just starting out their lives and are still in the dating world, trying to attract a suitable mate, or are just getting started on their education or early career. Hair loss is a blow to their self-image and to their overall feeling of self-confidence.

When I am examining a younger man, especially when the bi-emporal width (the distance between the right and left temporal fringe margins) is 12 cm or greater, I almost always use a type of forelock template as the planning pattern. I describe several forelock patterns later.

The Middle-Aged and Older Man

The same goals exist for middle-aged and older men as for younger men, namely, mutual trust must be established between doctor and patient; the expectations for what can be done are seen as the same by both patient and doctor; and a plan is outlined for achieving this result. Patients have a chance to picture what the result will be from viewing photos of patients who presented with the same general degree of hair loss and similar hair characteristics as they possess. A

good medical history is taken, and any significant health issues need to be settled by communication with a patient's personal physician. All medications that patients take must be assessed as to whether they in any way complicate the surgery, especially with regard to anticoagulant types of medication.

Guiding Hair Transplant Patients on Postoperative Considerations

Because most men are still working and living their normal day-to-day lives, they usually ask about how they can best minimize any postoperative evidence that they had the transplant grafts. There are several solutions to help these men: the best situation is when the person is able to wear a cap at work, such as a baseball cap. This hides everything except possibly forehead edema, should that occur. We advise most men with office jobs to plan to not work the week after surgery. For those with a somewhat diffuse amount of native hair still present, use of a camouflage product, such as one with fibers that cling to hairs (Toppik) or of the paint-on-the-scalp variety (DermMatch), can help hide the surgical sites. A few men have for years used a massive comb-over to cover the top of their head, and this can be continued post-operatively, providing the surgeon does not use this hair for donor hair. A hairpiece covers the head, but most surgeons suggest that it not be worn the week after surgery and then worn only as urgently needed thereafter. These men are advised to switch to a clip-type attachment system and to rotate the location of the clips every few months so that the same bundles of hair are not grasped for too long a period of time. For several years I have strongly recommended to my patients the postoperative use of a copper peptide application regimen (Graftcyte) in those men who are very bald and want to return to work 7 to 9 days later in an office situation. For those men whom I sense are private regarding their hair surgery and do not want a soul on earth outside of their family knowing they had it done, I recommend taking 2 weeks away from work. If a transplant surgery features exclusively the use of FU grafts, the scabs fall off sooner and the scalp looks normal sooner. The scabs of any multi-FU (MFU) grafts placed in the more central areas remain for 10 to 14 days. To sum up, some type of plan should be arrived at for what will be done to help camouflage the work and how long a patient needs to remove himself from the general public, if that is an issue for him.

PSYCHOLOGY OF HAIR LOSS IN NORWOOD CLASS VI AND VII PATIENTS

Middle-aged and older men who present with a large square area of hair loss relative to their potiential donor sites are discussed. I observe that there are not many men who reach complete, shiny bald Norwood class VI and VII patterns who come in for hair transplant surgery. Of the men I transplant, 90% are somewhere along the spectrum of losing their hair, and usually at the time of the consultation they have retained at least a modest amount of their native hair on top. I discuss my take on the reasons for this: I think most bald men have comfortably settled over the years with their appearance and it becomes for them their self-image and they are fine with that. The ones who are not fine with it and wish they had a head full of hair do not have the courage to make a change before the world's eyes, especially those of their co-workers, families, and friends, or they subconsciously fear it could end up as a terribly deformed result. Unfortunately, the best work that my colleagues and I produce on patients' heads goes unnoticed by the general public, because these men are simply passed by on the street, whereas the occasional bad, pluggy-looking result screams out to everyone within 100 feet that this man had been transplanted. Thus, the public image of hair transplants for many people is that of hair plugs that are detectable. The artistic advancements over the past 20 to 25 years have helped change that image to some extent, especially because of the prominent use of FU grafting since 1990. Finishing up on possible reasons for very bald men not seeking surgical correction, the considerable financial costs involved have to be considered. For most middle-class families, especially those with children approaching college age, this is an expense beyond what they can spare out of the family budget.

I have just referred to several reasons why I believe many good candidates don't undergo hair transplant surgery. I would now like to refer to some factors that push other men to go ahead with the procedure. A common one is divorce. Many bald men, when faced with the prospect of going into the dating world after all these years, feel disadvantaged by their bald look and seek to look more youthful and attractive to the opposite sex. Another is the man in his 50s who has just paid off the college bills of his last child and tells me, "Now it's time to do something for me!" For many of these men, the starting point is a comment from a doctor or the person cutting their hair, who mentions hair surgery and comments on some patients they have seen who had extremely natural results. Lastly, there is the possibility that very bald men see promotional material from a hair transplant office in the newspaper, on TV, or on the Internet and then come in for a consultation.

SURGICAL PLANNING

Whatever the reason, assume the patient is a man who is at least in his mid-30s and a glance reveals he has already reached or most certainly soon will attain a Norwood class VI or VII level of hair loss. It is fairly easy to quickly estimate if the ratio of available, safe donor hair to the square area of recipient hair loss allows for a side-to-side fill in or not. If the bi-temporal width is 13 cm or less, I think this is possible to accomplish, as long as there is not excessive thinning of the nape area, low donor density, or some other compromising characteristic of the donor hair. It has been my experience that the natural border of strong side fringe hair in the temporal and parietal regions does not drop further as a man ages past 45. I have frequently seen, however, the outer fringes of the vertex continue to expand further outward. Thus, for most of these men, I try hard to undersell what can be done in the vertex and explain that the frontal and midscalp zones are much more important to their appearance. When the width of baldness is more than 13 cm, the position of the side fringe in most men usually is situated lateral to a projection of the lateral canthal line, which is the normal position of the natural crease or separation of hair directions on a man's scalp.

The Patient's Wishes

There are several factors that enter into the final decision as to the surgical planning for a given patient. To start with, there are the patient's own wishes.

What does he want? How does he hope to style his hair? Because, by definition, this article discusses men with a disproportion between their donor supply and their corresponding large recipient area, it often is wise to "cheat" somewhat and load up those areas from which the styling pattern is directed. For instance, if a patient states he would like to have a slight part on the left and sweep his hair toward the right side and slightly to the rear right corner, then he would receive the maximal visual coverage by giving extra emphasis in graft density placement to the left side of the front hairline, the left crease, and the frontal core region, with somewhat of a de-emphasis on the areas of the scalp toward the right side.

In my mind there are 2 polar opposite ways of approaching how to distribute a given amount of donor hair on the head of a man with a large bald or soon-to-be bald scalp:

- The first is to strew the grafts out evenly over the entire recipient area or perhaps the front two-thirds of the balding area.
- The second, and the one I strongly recommend over the first, is to consciously create gradients of density in a predrawn pattern, which features maximal density in the front-central region with gradually diminishing densities going away from that area.

Estimating Donor Hair Available

The next important issue to assess is to estimate as closely as possible how much donor hair can be removed in a session. The density of follicular unit

grafts (FUs) on a patient's scalp and the laxity of the scalp both play an important part in this calculation. Because of the need in this type of patient to obtain as much donor hair as possible, it is usually necessary to extend the donor strip all the way from one temple to the other. Most patients have a second procedure, and the second donor strip is almost always taken directly above and contiguous with the old scar.

Hair Pattern Design

Given the amount of obtainable donor hair and the size of the alopecic recipient area, I then picture in my mind what I can do for the patient, given the area of alopecia present. As I alluded to previously, in most such patients I am leaning toward using a forelock-type pattern. The use of the word "forelock", to describe these patterns is somewhat of a misnomer, but, unfortunately, seems the best available. Most of my forelock patterns usually encompass the entire frontal area plus at least the front half of the midscalp area, if not the entire midscalp. Almost by definition, the vertex is not included in this scheme. The one important feature of all forelock patterns that derives from the forelock term is the emphasis on central density in the frontal core region (**Figs. 5–10**).

After years of trying various shapes and contours of forelock designs, I have settled on using 1 of 2 patterns in recent years: the "shield" forelock (see **Fig. 1**) or the "oval" forelock (see **Fig. 2**). A third pattern that many surgeons use on occasion is what I term the "rounded

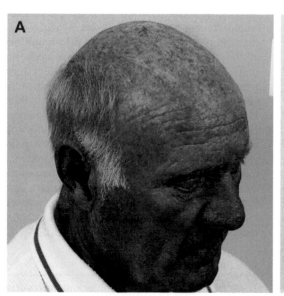
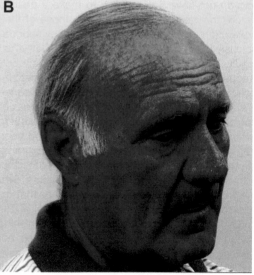

Fig. 5. (*A*) Norwood class VII man who requested small oval forelock in front to frame face. (*B*) Same patient after 2 small sessions of 500 grafts each (1997).

391

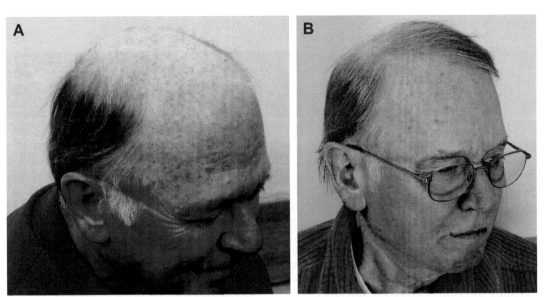

Fig. 6. (A) Norwood class VII patient who received single 1200-graft session (MFU and FU grafts) using shield pattern. (B) Result 11 months after first session.

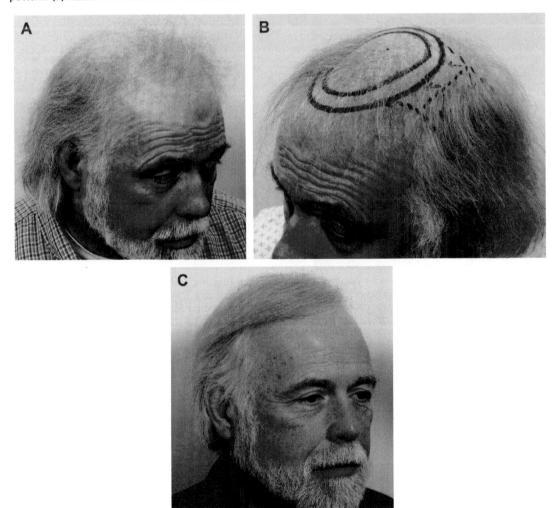

Fig. 7. (A) Norwood class VII patient with salt-and-pepper colored hair. (B) Same patient, with medium-sized oval forelock pattern drawn. Note crease line with hair directed away from it superiorly and inferiorly. (C) Result 2 years after first session of 1500 grafts (FU and MFU).

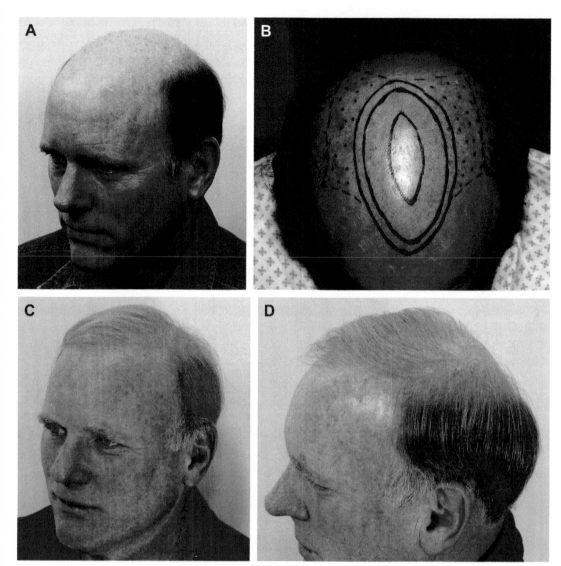

Fig. 8. (*A*) Borderline Norwood class VI/VII patient before surgery. (*B*) Long, narrow oval forelock pattern drawn, and lateral sparse areas with direction of hair noted. (*C*) Result 1 year after 2 surgeries of 1200 grafts each (MFU and FU grafts). Note framing of face. (*D*) Side view of same patient. Denser forelock zone on top contrasts with sparser lateral region between forelock and fringe.

arrowhead" pattern (see **Fig. 3**). This pattern does not work well with a Norwood class VII man with the side fringes set far down the sides of the head. It should not be used in younger patients, because their fringes may drop and thus leave the forelock hair isolated. This pattern looks natural as long as it maintains contact with the temporal fringe. It is not a natural-appearing pattern if wide lateral gaps of baldness are left on both sides.

The oval pattern is a more conservative one and the one I select when there is a tremendous disparity between the meager donor supply and a large bald area. There is no need to connect

the 2 side fringes across the hairline as I usually do with the shield pattern. The size of the oval, which is the center of the entire pattern, can be of various sizes, all the way from a small frontal oval, which does not extend posteriorly past the inter-tragal line, to a fairly large oval extending back to the vertex transition point.

The shield forelock pattern features a flared hairline, which usually connects the fringe on both sides with a front hairline zone. The front-central area is planted with some amount of density, either by placing all of the 3-hair and 4-hair FUs in this region or by using MFU grafts of 4 to 6 hairs. This pattern leaves 2 large triangular areas

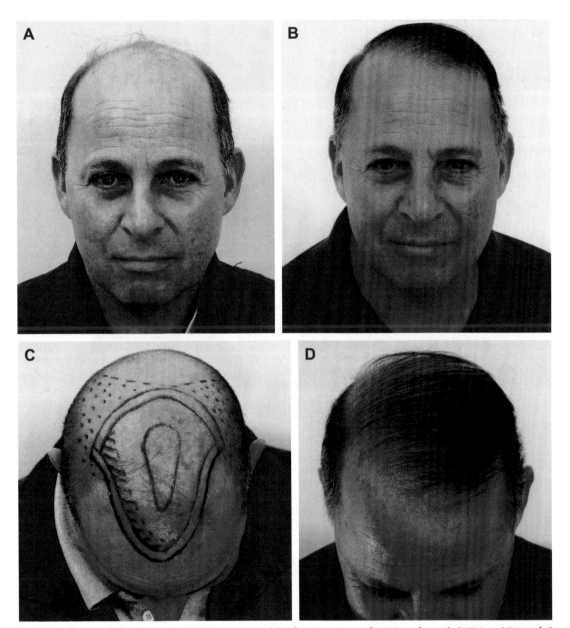

Fig. 9. (*A*) Norwood class VII patient before surgery. (*B*) After 3 sessions of 1500 grafts each (MFU and FU grafts). (*C*) Forelock pattern drawn on same patient's scalp. (*D*) Top view of patient after 3 sessions.

posterolateral to the forelock body, which are filled in with FU grafts with moderately sparse density. As with the oval forelock, I find that the ideal styling pattern is to sweep the hair backwards toward one of the rear corners. This pattern works best when there is a comfortable margin of abundant donor hair to use. If the amount of donor hair is questionable, then the oval pattern is a safer choice.

When viewing any man with extensive hair loss, usually the side fringe curves upward and has an apex, usually above the ear or slightly

anterior. If this fringe hair is weak or lies fairly low, one planning approach is to extend the patient's natural apex and build a "hump" with transplanted hairs (**Fig. 11**), which are directed downward within this area. Ideally, the surgeon attempts to bring the apex of this hump up to the level of the patient's projected crease. The location of the natural crease is best determined by extending a line up from the lateral canthus of the patient's eye and then projecting directly posterior from that line. For patients with residual native hair in the crease region, this is the

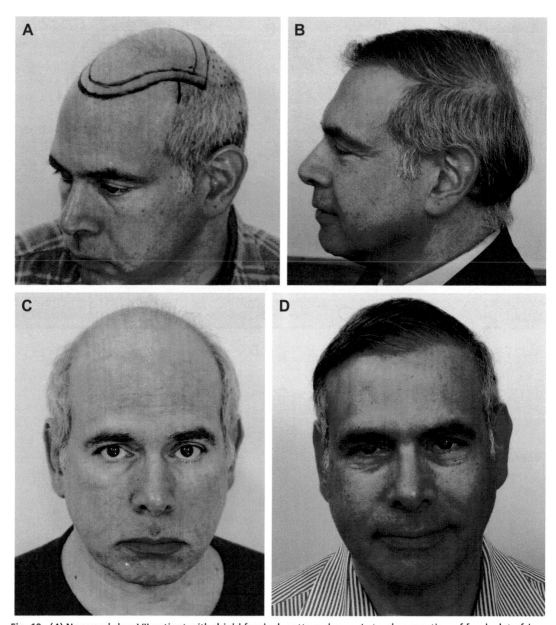

Fig. 10. (*A*) Norwood class VII patient with shield forelock pattern drawn. Lateral connection of forelock to fringe evident from this view. (*B*) After 3 sessions of 1700 grafts each (MFU and FU grafts used). (*C*) Front view of same patient before surgeries. (*D*) Framing of face after 3 surgeries shown.

natural dividing line between hairs that are directed anteromedially and those heading anteroinferiorly. I confess that I only occasionally used the hump pattern, mainly because it requires too much donor hair to fill it in densely. My preference in most cases is to fill the lateral space to each side of the forelock with FU grafts planted somewhat sparsely. Using far fewer grafts, this artistically "blurs" that space and helps reduce any "isolated" appearance for the forelock.

The other alternative to using the hump concept in planning the lateral area of the scalp in these patients is to simply draw in a crease line and then sparsely fill in the side area, with hairs directed either anteromedially or anteroinferiorly, depending on where the projected crease line is. I find that this approach does not require much donor hair and satisfies the artistic task of blurring the lateral space between the strong forelock area and the side fringes, thus not rendering the forelock isolated in appearance.

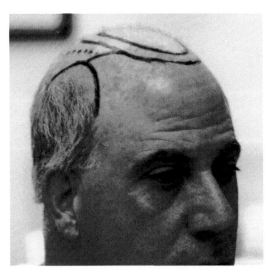

Fig. 11. Inverted C-shaped surgical marking above the temporal fringe shows where the lateral hump will be created by transplanting the bald zone between the existing fringe and the curved mark.

CONCLUDING REMARKS

For me, when there is limited donor hair and an extensive area of alopecia, it is necessary to use a conservative planning approach, which uses the limited hair available to create a result that looks natural and captures a naturally occurring stage of hair loss that some men go through. The 2 chief goals are

1. Framing the face
2. Having the hair appear natural

In my opinion these goals are best achieved by using a forelock-type approach in men with extensive balding. By doing so, there is virtually no one who cannot be helped in some fashion by hair transplantation. As long as the goals and the plan are clearly communicated and patients adjust their expectations in line with them, then happy patients are usually the result for years to come.

REFERENCES

1. Beehner M. Update on forelock approach of hair transplantation. Hair Transplant Forum Int 2007; 17(1):11–4.
2. Marritt E, Dzubow L. The isolated frontal forelock. Dermatol Surg 1995;21:523–38.
3. Beehner M. The frontal forelock concept. Int J Cosmet Surg 1998;6(1):35–42.
4. Beehner M. Frontal forelock concept in hair transplantation. Am J Cosmet Surg 1997;14:12–8.
5. Beehner M. A frontal forelock/central density framework for hair transplantation. Dermatol Surg 1997; 23:807–15.
6. Schell B, Stough DB. Cadre de cheveux. Am J Cosmet Surg 1995;12:317–9.
7. Norwood O. Patient selection, hair transplant design, and hairstyle. Dermatol Surg 1992;18:386–94.
8. Beehner M. The front forelock. Hair Transplant Forum Int 1995;5(1):1–3.
9. Beehner M. Isolated frontal forelock. In: Unger W, Shapiro R, Unger R, et al, editors. Hair transplantation. 5th edition. New York: Informa; 2011. p. 178–82.

Management of the Crown

Jean Devroye, MD

KEYWORDS

• Hair transplantation • Crown • Donor-recipient • Halo of baldness • Scalp reduction • Vertex

KEY POINTS

- The vertex is a complex zone with hair that is arranged as a whorl and is potentially subject to complete baldness.
- It is often virtually impossible to predict with absolute certainty the final degree of vertex balding before ages 40 to 50 years old.
- Due to the unpredictable nature of androgenetic alopecia, vertex treatment must be carefully considered and integrated into a global strategy.
- Ideally, it is preferred to finish treating the frontal and midscalp zones before treating the vertex.
- For most patients, a surgeon should not attempt to achieve maximal vertex coverage but instead restore an acceptable density that maintains donor supply reserves for future needs.
- An unnatural halo of baldness could appear around a vertex transplanted zone if future hair loss progresses.
- There are 2 distinct treatment philosophies for the vertex: (1) minimalist covering and (2) maximalist covering.

INTRODUCTION

The vertex, commonly referred to as the crown, is a complex zone with hairs that are arranged in a radial fashion. This zone is subject to more or less complete baldness. The evolution of vertex balding typically starts from the center and evolves at a variable rate toward the periphery. It is no easy task to treat the vertex for several reasons, discussed later.

Balding is often an uncertain situation with evolutionary patterns that may be hard to predict and with a potential for hair loss that is often widespread. The thinning often includes the frontal zone, the midscalp, and the vertex. It is essential to take into account the donor-recipient area ratio. Unfortunately, this ratio is evolutionary. It is never easy to choose the best strategy, knowing the vertex is a secondary zone in comparison with the anterior and median zones.

I describe exclusively vertex alopecia in men. It is exceptional to treat vertex baldness in women. Women almost never have enough graft reserve to treat the vertex.

ANATOMIC DESCRIPTION OF THE VERTEX

The vertex literally means *the highest point*. It is a round or oval zone, surrounded at the back and on the sides by the borders of the permanent zone. It is defined as the most posterior part of the area affected by male pattern baldness (MPB). Its limits are the midscalp on the front and the parietal and occipital fringe on the back and on the sides. Hair is arranged there as a whorl or swirl, starting from 1 or 2 centers.[1]

In order to define the limit between the midscalp on the front and the vertex on the back, an anatomic mark, the vertex transition point (**Fig. 1**), is used. The vertex transition point is the

Disclosures: None.
Belgium Board of Medicine, 180 Avenue de la Chasse, Etterbeek 1040, Belgium
E-mail address: officedevroye@aol.com

Facial Plast Surg Clin N Am 21 (2013) 397–406
http://dx.doi.org/10.1016/j.fsc.2013.06.005

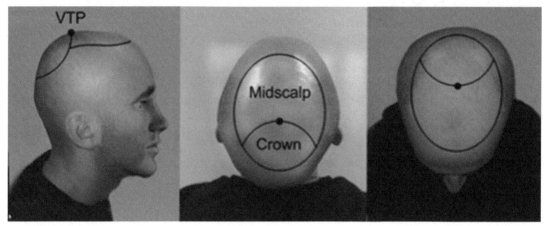

Fig. 1. Anatomic description of vertex transition point (VTP).

point where the horizontal part of the skull starts sloping downward to become oblique and then vertical toward the back. From this point, a concave curved line is drawn downward that joins the side limits. It is not always easy to locate this point because the surface of the skull is often round without any real point of visible transition. Unger[2] further describes the crown: "… in most men with Type IV and Type V MPB, the anterior outline of the vertex area usually naturally ends at the posterior border of the 'mid-parietal bridge,' or the remnant thereof. In the majority of men with vertex Type III as well as Types IV and V MPB, this designated 'vertex' area occupies the classic 'tonsure' position, thus straddling both the horizontal and vertical planes of the scalp. In balding men with the more severe Norwood Types VI and VII patterns, the vertex has a large, circular (or somewhat oval) shape that rather than straddling both the horizontal and vertical planes, occupies essentially only the vertical plane. This is because its posterior border extends further inferiorly than in Types IV and V, and, therefore, the anterior border of its anterior mirror image is farther posterior than in Types IV and V MPB."

The vertex transition point does not correspond to the center of the whorl (**Fig. 2**). It is situated several centimeters above. It is necessary to be precise when discussing treatment of the vertex or crown. A transplant of the posterior part of the scalp, centered on the whorl, often includes not only the vertex but also the posterior part of the midscalp.

The posterior and side edges of the vertex, the occipital and parietal fringe, do not correspond to anatomically precise entities because they are at the evolutionary limit between the thinning zone and the hair-bearing area. These borders are an important area because they move over time.

It is useful to try to foresee as precisely as possible the future peripheral limit of the balding of the vertex. The current surface to be transplanted or the potentially bald one is often large. When baldness is advanced, it can be identified as the area where the hairs of the donor zone give way to predominantly miniaturized hair. When balding is incomplete, it is often easier to determine this limit in a macroscopic manner by wetting hair and by using a good light to visualize the skin through the hair. This region is often named, *the evolving area* (**Fig. 3**).

There are anatomic variations, in particular, the existence of 2 swirl centers. There is often a small

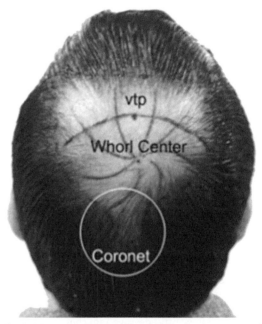

Fig. 2. Vertex transition point (VTP), whorl center, and coronet.

area of loss in the low part of the occipital fringe, inferior to the larger crown pattern, that Arnold named, *the coronet* (see **Fig. 2**).[2] It is important to take the coronet into account because it encroaches and thus reduces the safe donor zone.

The exit angle of the vertex hair compared with the skin is also variable and high in the center of the swirl and becomes more acute toward the periphery.

HOW DOES VERTEX BALDNESS EVOLVE?

Vertex balding is a part of general baldness. Most of the time it appears later than balding of the anterior and midscalp zones. According to age, hair loss on the vertex is generally perceived as of greater importance (younger patients) or of lesser importance (older patients). Vertex balding is present in stages III vertex, IV, V, VI, and VII of the Norwood scale (**Fig. 4**).

A study of 999 men by Norwood[3] correlated the incidence of vertex MPB and found a consistent progression based on patient age.

Male pattern vertex baldness: incidence by age, according to Norwood	
Ages in Years	**Incidence**
Between 18 and 29	5% (9 of 185 Individuals)
Between 30 and 39	21% (35 of 165 Individuals)
Between 40 and 49	33% (55 of 165 Individuals)
Between 50 and 59	42% (65 of 156 Individuals)
Between 60 and 69	56% (84 of 149 Individuals)
Between 70 and 79	54% (55 of 102 Individuals)
Over 80	65% (50 of 77 Individuals)

A study by Unger[4] showed that men above 60 years old had a prevalence of vertex baldness from 65% to 73%.

Patients rarely lose their hair only at the level of the vertex. Hair loss of the vertex begins mostly from the center and propagates toward the periphery. It evolves in the form of a circle or an oval, which grows gradually toward the outside. The surface of a circle evolves exponentially with the increase of its diameter. For this reason, it is necessary to be cautious when judging an unfinished hair loss. The surface area of an emptied vertex of 5 cm in diameter quadruples when it grows to a diameter of 10 cm.

CLINICAL EXAMINATION

It is thus important to observe exactly the situation of the vertex before any decision making. The use of the cross-section trichometer is recommended.[5] It allows quantifying exactly the scale of loss. Also, a fine observation of the emptied zone through quality magnifying glasses of magnification 5 or 6 is recommended to help define the topography of the miniaturization in this area. One should also attempt to highlight the thinning peripheral zone, which frequently begins several years before the definitive balding. Wetting hair and using a strong light is often an effective method.

Unfortunately, before ages 40 to 50, it is often impossible to predict with absolute certitude what degree of balding will be reached. It is necessary to be aware of the unpredictable nature of future hair loss and to explain this risk to the patients so they can approve, in full knowledge of the facts, the final therapeutic choice.

The vertex is not visible in front view, unless patients are seated and slightly bowed forward. On the contrary, from profile and back view, vertex baldness is visible.

ANAMNESIS

A precise evaluation of family history is often useful. It is necessary to try to find the degree of balding of the vertex of the father and the grandparents and of the collateral family, keeping in mind that this comparison is not always reliable. The surgeon should attempt to identify a member of the family having had the same type of evolution in severity and in age. It is patient age that often guides surgical intervention in the vertex region (**Table 1**).

GENERAL REFLECTIONS ABOUT TREATMENT

Requests for vertex treatment vary according to age and situation of patients. The requests of patients who present a pattern affecting any other area than the vertex are variable. Well-informed patients tend to ask first for a treatment of the anterior zone. It is frequent, however, to see patients who want the complete treatment of the anterior and posterior zones. It is less frequent to see patients focusing complaints on the vertex only, because it is the mainly emptied zone or for other reasons, such as fear of a too-radical change of aspect of the anterior area or of not having enough donor zone to cover the entire baldness.

The vertex is hidden from the view of patients. It is rare that they have a perfect consciousness of the size of the thinning zone. They often imagine

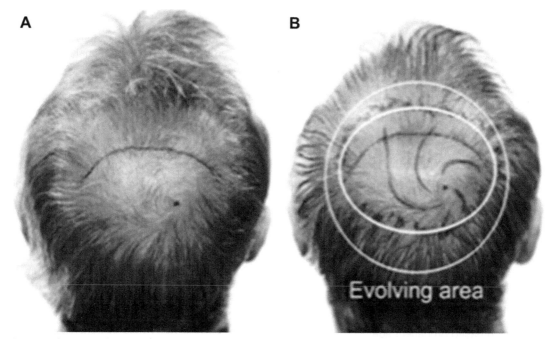

Fig. 3. Defining the balding area with (*A*) dry hair and (*B*) wet hair.

it smaller than it is. This is because the vertex is posterior and vertical and they rarely see it entirely. Patients often imagine that only a few hundred grafts can solve the baldness. It is necessary to spend time clearly explaining the situation to them and informing them about uncertainties regarding the evolution of the donor zone. They have to realize the limit that represents the donor-recipient zone ratio. Patients are often receptive to these explanations. During the first consultation, I detect any unrealistic requests and patient expectations that never will be

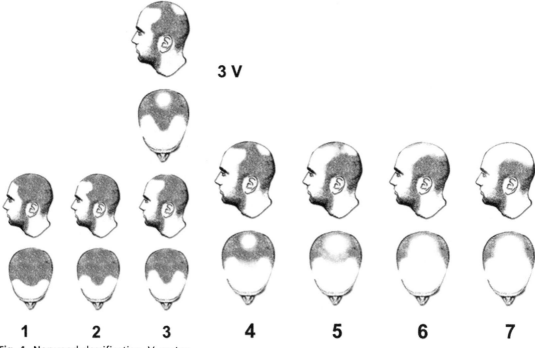

Fig. 4. Norwood classification. V, vertex.

Table 1
Age guidelines for surgical intervention in the vertex region

Age	Recommendation
<30 y old	No operation
30 to 39 y old	Can be operated after a deep observation and a good analysis of the positive and negative factors
40 y old	Can be operated if conditions are suitable Requested conditions: good ratio between donor and recipient area to cover not only the present bald zones but also future ones

Key Point
Vertex treatment must be deeply considered and integrated into a global strategy.

achievable. It is better to give up a surgery than to have an unsatisfied patient.

THERAPEUTIC OPTIONS
Medications

The vertex is a zone that reacts well to medications, such as finasteride and minoxidil.[6,7] When patients are young, and when it is difficult to estimate their evolution, I prefer to first use a medicinal treatment, which allows letting a few years pass before deciding the quantity of grafts to allocate to the vertex. Certain surgeons recommend systematically a 1-year treatment before considering transplant of the vertex on a young man. It is, however, necessary to be aware that the success of a medical treatment is never definitive. It simply delays the inexorable occurrence of the final balding. For a young man, the stabilization of the loss through medication does not give the right to forget the various caution rules expressed in this article.

Scalp Reduction

Not many years ago, scalp reduction was considered the ideal approach to reduce vertex baldness. It consists of removing an oval skin zone in the center of the vertex. The donor side zone is pulled and stretched to cover the bald zone that was removed. Frechet[8] improved the classic technique by the use of an extender, which increases the area of the removed skin. Since the success of the follicular transplant introduced at the end of mid-1990s, scalp reduction gradually lost its indication and few rare surgeons still use it.

The main defects of the scalp reduction procedure are the drastic reduction of the donor zone density by stretching, which can compromise future treatment options of the anterior zone, and a reduction scar, which can widen by a stretch-back phenomenon. Also, the orientation of the displaced hair does not correspond at all to the original orientation; the swirl is replaced by a double-side unsightly orientation. Patients cannot find any hairstyle enabling camouflaging the unnatural appearance of the hair on either side, which grows in opposite directions. Frechet[8] finalized the triple-flap technique, which partially corrects this defect. Finally, it is an aggressive, often painful intervention when extenders are used. These are the main reasons that reductions have fallen out of favor. On the contrary, the general evolution of surgical intervention is the search for soft techniques. The recent advent of follicular unit extraction is a good illustration of that.

Follicular Hair Transplant

Follicular transplantation with dissecting microscopes has revolutionized the practice of hair transplantation. It has become the inevitable baldness treatment. It avoids the pluggy appearance that characterized older grafts. It has the advantage of being able to work with 2 factors: the use of different follicle sizes and composition and the ability to create a density and orientation variation of grafted hair. It gives a natural result that fits perfectly in the existing hair.

Is It Wise to Operate? What are Good Indications?

Surgeons react according to their experience, to the peculiarities of their practice, and to their degree of caution. In his article, "The Paradox of Crown Transplantation," Stough[9] explains the guidelines dilemma in the particular situation of vertex transplant. It is not easy to find infallible rules and there are many exceptions. The danger of guidelines for treatment of the vertex is that they can be used against a surgeon who has made a bad strategic decision. This is why it is always necessary to be careful before deciding to practice transplantation on the vertex.

It is necessary to spend time explaining to patients the risks and the consequences of this intervention. It is also necessary to prepare and sign a precise consent form that explains clearly the uncertainties as to the future evolution of this zone.

Many investigators are reserved regarding treatment of the vertex and refuse to operate before ages 35 to 45 years. There are, however, exceptions to this rule.

What are the arguments in favor of and against surgical intervention on the vertex and the rules to respect for this case?

Arguments in Favor of Surgical Intervention on the Vertex

1. It is necessary to make sure that the donor zone is rich enough to allow covering the crown with sufficient density. It is, thus, necessary to analyze 4 factors: density in terms of number of hairs per square centimeter (hair density), average diameter of hair, texture of hair, and hair color. Donor-recipient area ratio is also important.
2. Patients over age 40 are favored. It is often inadvisable to proceed before ages 35 to 40 years[2] or even 45 years.[9]
3. Ideally, it is preferable to have finished the work in the anterior zones (frontal and midscalp) before deciding to also treat the vertex.
4. Maximal coverage should not be attempted. Instead a conservative but acceptable density is preferred to keep the donor zone viable for the future needs.
5. The surgeon must emphasize to and get assurance from the patient that he understands and accepts the fact that it is impossible to predict with certainty how the donor-recipient area ratio will evolve over time.
6. When treating the frontal zone and the midscalp with a higher density, the surgeon risks increasing the feeling of emptiness at the level of the vertex, mostly if the skin is completely bald at this level. This imbalance may benefit from cautious intervention.
7. The grafted zone may serve to anchor hair coming from the front and brushed to the back.

Arguments Against Surgical Intervention on the Vertex

1. The vertex has little cosmetic impact. When looking at someone face to face, the vertex is unable to be visualized. The aspect of anterior zones is the most important. Limmer wrote, "The most difficult task the consulting physician faces is educating and convincing the hair loss patient that the frontal and midscalp constitutes 90% of the value while vertex restoration produces the other 10 %."[9]
2. The frontal transplants often allow obtaining enough density so that these hairs, brushed to the back, cover the vertex zone. This type of hairstyle is natural and does not give the aspect of the artificial look such as that encountered when the hair is brushed from the vertex forward to cover an anterior balding area.
3. When a vertex transplant has been made and future hair loss progresses, a halo of baldness could appear around the transplanted zone. If, due to a lack of grafts, the vertex is not capable of continuing to be filled in, the result risks being a source of significant dissatisfaction. The halo is made by an island of hair lost in the middle of a completely bald area. A transplant, whatever the concerned zone, stops being natural when it is surrounded by an empty zone. It is perhaps the biggest pitfall of the vertex transplant.
4. It is often advantageous to strengthen a first transplant of the anterior zone and the midscalp by a second transplant. If the global treatment is started with a transplant of the vertex, the possibility of reinforcement during a second intervention may be lost.
5. If patients suffer from an already wide baldness, treatment of the front is going to minimize their complaints concerning the vertex, all the more if they brush the hair backward.
6. The total surface to be transplanted is often big, equal to the addition of the surfaces of the frontal zone and the midscalp combined.
7. The shingling effect is less important at the level of the vertex. The shingling effect, or overlapping phenomenon, is important in the frame of hair transplant. Thanks to the covering provided by shingling of the hair layers, the visible macroscopic density can be distinctly more favorable at the level of the frontal zone than at the level of the vertex, for the same type of work and with the same type of graft density. The explanation is simple: given the fact that hairs scatter according to a swirl, the shingling phenomenon scatters in all directions instead of concentrating in only one. This lack of overlapping is particularly important in the center of the swirl. In spite of the operating subtleties (discussed later), it is often useful to have a second surgery to complete the density at this level.

SURGICAL TECHNIQUE FOR VERTEX

I provide the details of my own technique. There are, of course, other approaches that are also possible.

Preparing the Recipient Zone

- The patient is seated; many pictures are taken. It is often wise to take pictures from the front, with the head lowered forward. To reveal the posterior hair loss and its connection with the front, it is useful to take pictures from the back, with the head extended to the maximum backward.

- I almost systematically shave the recipient area. I convince the patient by emphasizing that the shaving allows a substantial improvement of the quality of the work at all levels. Only a few patients refuse. In cases of refusal, I recommend a short cutting. From time to time, I operate on a vertex with long hair.
- Direct lines are drawn. They follow the main trunk road according to which the existing hairs are arranged (see **Fig. 2**).
- As a general rule, there are enough vellus hairs to guide the reconstruction. I respect scrupulously the existence of the various patterns. It is rare that I have to create a new vertex center. If that is the case, I move the new vertex center away from the original center.
- If a patient wishes to comb counterclockwise, it is better to place the center moved away to the right from the center and conversely for the clockwise direction. By placing the center relatively high, close to the transition line, I increase the overlapping effect on the posterior part and, therefore, the impression of density at this level is improved.

Incisions

There are 2 distinct scenarios that are handled differently:

1. Minimalist covering
2. Maximalist covering

Minimalist covering
Minimal density averages between 20 and 30 incisions per square centimeter. Several circumstances can limit the number of available grafts or, more exactly, the transfer of available hair mass. A minimal density approach can be due to the careful decision of the surgeon to dedicate only a limited quantity of grafts to the vertex, even if the reserve of hair seems sufficient at the moment. It can also be linked to a bad donor-recipient zone ratio, which reduces the number of available grafts for the vertex; to a low average number of hairs per graft; or to a low hair diameter. I also fill this way when, after a previous transplant, the contrast between the anterior hairy transplanted zone and the completely balding vertex requires balance between both areas. In that case, I pursue a light covering density, using approximately 1000 grafts, which also leaves the possibility of strengthening the density of the anterior zone and the midscalp.

The main danger of the minimalist covering approach is having an unsatisfactory pale covering. The second danger is seeing, during the postoperative years, a hair recession with a halo effect developed around the transplanted zone. It is thus recommended to increase gradually the density by starting from the center toward the periphery (**Fig. 5**). The purpose is to give the illusion that the center is thinning while the periphery remains dense. Only the periphery of the emptied zone can be covered without searching to cover the center of the vertex so as to imitate perfectly a natural baldness.

For these minimalist coverings, it is highly recommended to use only small grafts, each containing ideally 1 hair or 2 hairs. The use of larger grafts may give a pluggy unnatural aspect. The presence of small groups rich in hair and separated by a visually perceptible distance signals the surgical origin of this aspect.

Maximalist covering
The strategy is different when patients are lucky enough to be bald only at the level of the vertex, when they are over 40 to 45 years old, or when the decision to proceed to a consequent transplant is taken. As usual, the purpose is to give the best possible apparent density. When the vertex is filled in with an equal density everywhere, the coverture inevitably seems to decrease when the center is approached. This is linked to a reduction of the overwhelming phenomenon (ie, hair shaft shingling), which, by definition, is absent in the center. Managing this issue is a matter of designing a set of incisions, which converge to the same center, while gradually increasing their density. My experience shows that it is much easier to obtain an excellent result by starting from the center and proceeding toward the periphery than trying to do the contrary. In that case, I use in the center a blade cut to size of 0.8 mm to 0.9 mm for 2-hair follicular unit grafts, squeezing as strongly as possible 50 to 100 central incisions (**Fig. 6**). To use bigger transplants in the center often gives a less natural aspect. Be careful, however, that slits do not overlap because the consequence is creating tears of skin of several millimeters.

Going to the periphery, the size of incisions can be increased to 1 mm or 1.1 mm to receive grafts of 3 or 4 hairs each. Incisions are made at 1 cm or 2 cm from the center of the swirl in a way that respects the original orientation of hair. The purpose is double: to integrate perfectly the hair remaining in the middle of the transplanted zone and to assure a perfect connection with the peripheral hair. To avoid the halo, described

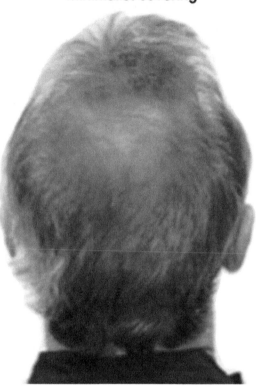

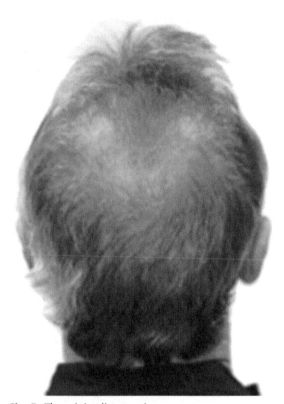

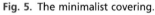

Fig. 5. The minimalist covering.

previously, it is necessary to go deep into the hair-bearing zone with obvious signs of hair loss and to blend the existing hair with the grafts (**Fig. 7**).

For patients whose recipient zone is small and for whom there is a large quantity of grafts, it is logical to privilege the density in the center of the vertex to increase the phenomenon of overlapping hair from the more peripheral zones toward the center. Maximalist covering can achieved by decreasing progressively the density of the incisions from the center toward the periphery. It can also be accomplished by favoring the use of the richest grafts at the center and the less rich grafts in the periphery. The maximalist approach uses a completely different strategy from what has been described for minimalist management.

The Lam method

Lam[10] described a vertex transplant philosophy that focuses on graft size, graft spacing, and graft distribution. Density distribution over the crown is based on zonal priority, with zone 1 having the highest priority and zone 6 the lowest (**Fig. 8**). Zone 1 hair is considered the most important because it serves multiple purposes by contributing coverage to the part, midscalp, and contralateral crown regions. Coverage within zone 6 is the least important because it resides in the lower aspect of the vertex and because there is no shingling effect in this area to supplement coverage over any of the neighboring vertex

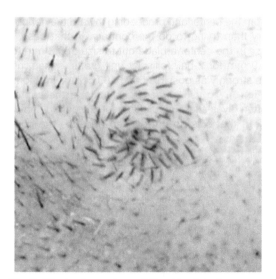

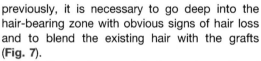

Fig. 6. Maximal coverture of the whorl center.

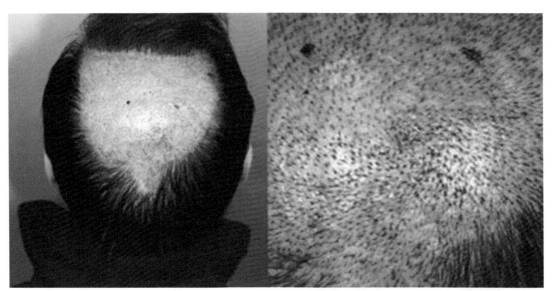

Fig. 7. The maximalist covering. (*Left*) Vertex graft distribution; (*Right*) close-up view.

zones. Density priorities sequentially decrease from zone 1 to zone 6 based on the cosmetic importance and shingling contributions provided by each respective zone. Higher density and closer spaced grafts are favored in high-priority zones (**Fig. 9**).

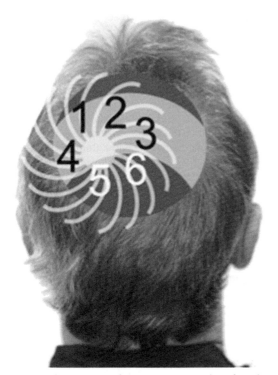

Fig. 8. The Lam graft prioritization plan for the vertex.

Anchoring Zone

When I want the vertex to be an anchoring zone, it is possible to distribute grafts in this key area with a low density. These hairs only serve to anchor the hairs from the frontal zone and the midscalp that are combed backward. Without support, these frontal and midscalp hairs tend to slide on the vertex and reveal more easily the underlying bald scalp. This tendency to slide can often be reduced by the use of only a few hundred anchored hairs.

Exclusive Covering of the Upper Zone of the Vertex

As discussed previously, it often happens that the transplant of a crown contains not only the vertex but also the posterior part of the midscalp. Some investigators, for instance, Unger,[2] recommend filling exclusively this posterior midscalp and the top of the vertex. The purpose is that a portion of these grafts fall backward and cover the untreated part of the vertex. When the vertex is completely bald, the location of the center of the swirl can be changed, such as with a high placement, to increase the quantity of hair covering the lower part of the vertex. The center of the vertex is almost always moved away from the center, most often to the right.

REGROWTH

Some investigators noticed that the grafts on the vertex tend to grow more slowly. I have not observed this phenomenon personally.

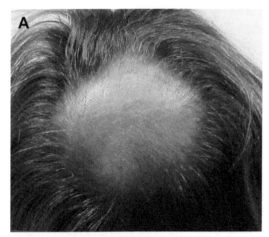

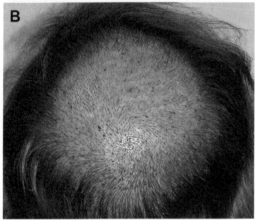

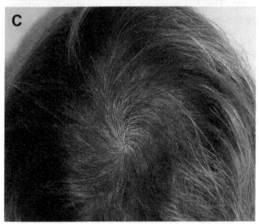

Fig. 9. Surgical hair restoration of the crown—(*A*) preoperative, (*B*) graft placement, and (*C*) postoperative.

SUMMARY

Transplantation of the vertex is not easy. It requires many skills from a practitioner: a good sense of observation, a good sense of anticipation, vast surgical experience, artistic skill, and technical precision. There are often many strategic choices for the same situation. Each situation is determined by surgeon experience, always keeping in mind the famous maxim: *primum no nocere* (first, do no harm).

REFERENCES

1. Ziering C, Krenitsky G. The Ziering whorl classification of scalp hair. Dermatol Surg 2003;29(8): 817–21.
2. Unger W. Surgical planning and organization. In: Unger W, Shapiro R, Unger R, et al, editors. Hair transplantation. 5th edition. New York, London: Informa Healthcare; 2011. p. 106–97.
3. Norwood OT. Male pattern baldness: classification and incidence. South Med J 1975;68: 1359–65.
4. Unger W. Male and female pattern hair loss. In: Unger W, Shapiro R, Unger R, et al, editors. Hair transplantation. 5th edition. New York, London: Informa Healthcare; 2011. p. 36–49.
5. Cohen BM. The cross-section trichometer: a new device for measuring hair quantity, hair loss and hair growth. Dermatol Surg 2008;34(7):900–10 [discussion: 910–1].
6. Kaufman KD, Olsen EA, Whiting D, et al. Finasteride in the treatment of men with androgenetic alopecia. J Am Acad Dermatol 1998;39:578–89.
7. Kaufman KD, Merck Research Laboratories (The Finasteride Male Pattern Hair Loss Study Group). Long-term (5-year) multinational experience with finasteride 1 mg in the treatment of men with androgenetic alopecia. Eur J Dermatol 2002;12: 38–49.
8. Frechet P. Slot correction by a three hair-bearing transposition flap in combination with AR. Int J Aesth Rest Surg 1994;2:27–32.
9. Stough DB. The paradox of crown transplanation. Hair Transplant Forum Intl 2005;15(4):117–8.
10. Lam SM. In: Lam SM, editor. Hair transplant 360 for physicians. New Delhi (India): Jaypee Brothers Medical Publishers, Ltd; 2010. p. 119–26.

Female Hair Restoration

Robin H. Unger, MD

KEYWORDS

- Alopecia • Female hair transplantation • Telogen effluvium • Recipient site • Donor site
- Female pattern hair loss • Scalp

KEY POINTS

- Female hair loss is a prevalent condition with a particularly devastating psychological impact.
- Hair transplantation is the only currently available option to provide a permanent and natural solution for female patients with alopecia.
- Surgery for female patients should be performed in strategic areas to produce the maximum cosmetic impact.
- Grafts containing 1 to 6 hairs can be used to create different zones of density.
- Female patients need to understand the postoperative sequelae and the evolution of female pattern hair loss to ensure a successful outcome.
- When appropriately treated, women are among the most grateful of all hair transplant patients.

TREATMENT GOALS

Unique to female hair transplantation is the advantage that female pattern hair loss (FPHL) does not *usually* cause complete alopecia in any area, rather the affected regions become thinner.[1] Therefore, it is reasonable to focus hair transplant surgery in the most cosmetically significant regions as opposed to the surgical treatment of men that requires a more diffuse coverage of the affected areas that are, or will become over time, totally alopecic (**Fig. 1**). The hair restoration surgeon (HRS) needs to examine patients and have an in-depth discussion to determine exactly which areas this might include. It is best to underestimate the area that can be addressed in a single surgery. The goal is increased density, in other words, patients will still be able to see their scalp, just *less* of it; this needs to be clearly understood. It is also advisable to review and prescribe medical treatments if applicable, which can help to stabilize or slow future hair loss and, in a minority of cases, may even help patients recover some density.

THE INITIAL CONSULTATION

The first meeting with patients should begin with a thorough discussion of the family history of female hair loss and a pertinent medical history of the patients themselves. One of the most important medical issues to review in depth are hormonal disorders or recent changes, including some of the more common ones related to hair loss: polycystic ovarian syndrome, adding/stopping/changing birth control pills, perimenopause, menopause, postpartum hormone changes, thyroid abnormalities, and pituitary abnormalities.[2] Diet changes and changes in medication should be looked at as possible reasons for telogen effluvium, and surgery should not be pursued if it is possible the hair loss may be temporary. In some female patients, the impetus for seeking help may be a recent telogen effluvium coupled with FPHL, in which case surgery should not be performed until regrowth of the recent temporary hair loss has occurred (usually 6 months after the resolution of the inciting event). The reason for this is that hairs in the donor

Disclosures: None.
Department of Dermatology, Mount Sinai Hospital, 710 Park Avenue, New York City, NY 10021, USA
E-mail address: drrobinunger@yahoo.com

Facial Plast Surg Clin N Am 21 (2013) 407–417
http://dx.doi.org/10.1016/j.fsc.2013.05.011

facialplastic.theclinics.com

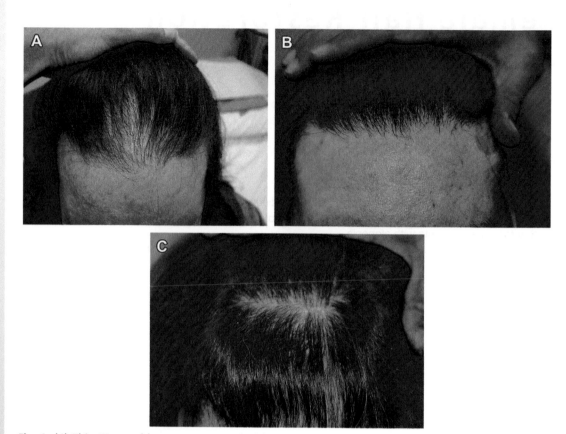

Fig. 1. (*A*) This 47-year-old woman presented with severe FPHL, with the Christmas-tree pattern and frontal accentuation as described by Elise Olsen. The area of greatest cosmetic importance was, therefore, clearly the central frontal region. (*B*) Five years after hair transplantation with the hair pulled back. The surgery performed consisted of 893 follicular units and 455 double follicular units. (*C*) The same patient 5 years after surgery, showing a more critical view of the area treated.

area may have been affected by the temporary loss and would be dormant at the time of surgery; these dormant follicles would be discarded as part of the alopecic tissue between visible hairs, resulting in an unnecessary loss of precious donor hair.

In the author's experience, there have been 2 conditions that warrant special mention with regard to female patients:

1. Lichen planopilaris
2. Alopecia areata incognita (AAI)

Lichen planopilaris[3] is an autoimmune disorder that causes a scarring permanent alopecia; the author has noticed an increased frequency in patients, especially the frontal fibrosing variant. Many of these patients are unaware they have the condition and think they suffer from a particularly severe pattern of female hair loss affecting their hairline and temple regions. It is important to identify this condition, confirm quiescence, and educate patients regarding the recurrent nature of the disease and need for frequent monitoring

by a dermatologist before attempting any surgical correction. This author has had great success in surgical correction of frontal fibrosing lichen planopilaris (**Fig. 2**); however, it requires treating the recipient area as one would any other area of cicatricial alopecia and ensuring there is diligent postoperative follow-up.[4]

The author has diagnosed a much greater number of patients with AAI[5] in recent years. It is unclear whether this increased frequency is caused by better diagnostic tools or a true increase in incidence. This condition is *particularly* difficult to diagnose if patients have an underlying FPHL that is unmasked by the alopecia areata. It is very important to ask questions regarding the onset, duration, and course of hair loss; if patients report that the alopecia has occurred over a relatively short period of time, the physician should have a higher degree of suspicion. The dermatoscope is a tool that has been very helpful in diagnosing AAI. On examination with the dermatoscope, the physician should look for dystrophic or cadaverized or exclamation point hairs, small yellow dots

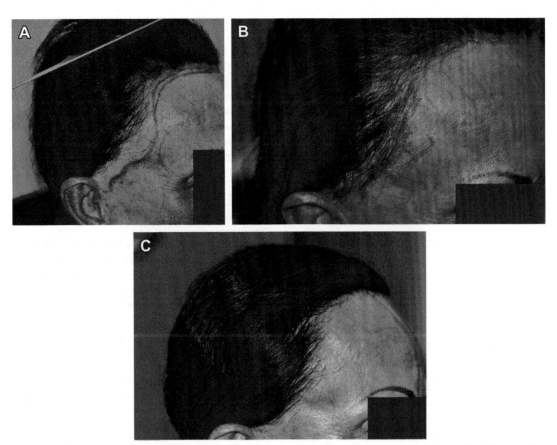

Fig. 2. (*A*) This patient presented at 72 years of age after referral by a physician for hair transplant. On examination, the frontal area showed completely alopecic skin devoid of ostia. She was referred for biopsy to confirm the diagnosis and quiescence of lichen planopilaris (frontal fibrosing variant). (*B*) Excellent early growth 4 months after surgery of 1028 transplanted follicular units. Minoxidil was applied to the recipient area for 5 weeks, starting on the day of surgery. (*C*) The same patient 1 year after surgery to correct frontal fibrosing lichen planopilaris (LPP). The transplant showed excellent survival, and there was no recurrence in the first postoperative year.

within the ostium of both empty and hair bearing follicles, and areas of complete alopecia within intervening areas of thinning (**Fig. 3**). Both the potential recipient and donor areas need to be examined and a biopsy performed if there is any question. Unfortunately, even biopsy results may be unclear.[6] If there is any question remaining, this author prefers to try medical treatment. The treatment of choice for her patients is the use of 0.5% clobetasol cream under occlusion 5 nights weekly for 5 weeks, combined with morning application of 5% minoxidil for 3 months.[7] Results are assessed at 3, 6, and 9 months.

PREOPERATIVE PLANNING FOR FEMALE HAIR RESTORATION

The most important aspect of preoperative planning in females is deciding the size and location of the area to be treated. The donor area should be carefully assessed to provide an estimate of the number of follicular units that can be harvested in one surgery as well as the total lifetime estimate of available donor hair. This assessment will help inform the surgeon's decision regarding which area should be treated in the present surgery and which area or areas might be important to address in the future. Women's long-term donor rim hair is generally less dense and shorter than that seen in men.

Determining Hair Transplant Candidate

There is a great diversity in opinions as to how many women are candidates for hair transplant surgery.[8] The author thinks that the source of this range in perspectives is caused by the HRS's assessment of the available donor hair versus the actual size of the area of thinning. If the HRS' goal is to treat virtually *all* the areas affected by alopecia, then

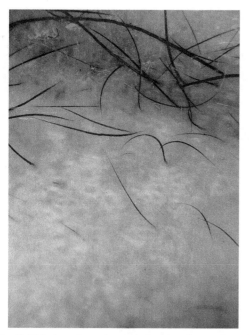

Fig. 3. This is a dermatoscopic image of a region of alopecia areata incognita. Note the yellow dots, dystrophic and club hairs.

make a very significant impact on the woman's appearance and styling options, then many more women can greatly benefit from hair restoration surgery.[9] The author has encountered many women who are, in reality, very marginal candidates in terms of the extent of thinning versus the available donor hair. However, treating the most cosmetically significant area allows these patients to style their hair strategically to cover other areas and avoid wearing a full wig, which is a result that makes a great impact in their lives (**Fig. 4A**).

Styling Hair to Determine Areas for Transplant

It is helpful to try styling the hair in different ways (straight back, central part line, side part line, and so forth) to make the best choice regarding which area is indeed the most important cosmetically. The area to be treated should be outlined with a grease pencil, and photographs should be taken with the patients' hair both wet and dry (see **Fig. 4B**). These photographs should be reviewed with patients and adjusted if necessary to incorporate the patients' goals, keeping in mind the donor limitations and likely future areas of concern. It is vitally important that patients understand that any grafts used in the current surgery will necessarily reduce the number available to address future areas of loss. Ideally, the most important region for the duration of the patients' life should be addressed in the first surgery, and less important

indeed a limited number of women would be good candidates. However, if the surgeon understands that certain areas of hair loss are much more important and increasing the density in those regions can

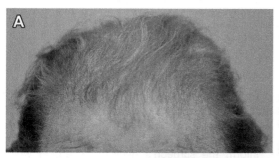

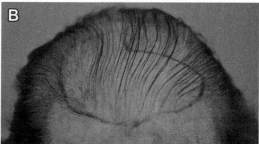

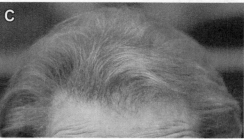

Fig. 4. (*A*) A woman in her 70s presented with very diffuse hair loss, a limited donor area, and very fine hair. It was explained to the patient that she was a marginal candidate for surgery and the hair transplantation would be concentrated in the area of greatest significance. (*B*) The same patient with her hair wet and the surgical area outlined. Given her age and degree of thinning, there was less consideration given to future loss and the need to conserve grafts. (*C*) Early growth at 8 months after the surgery consisting of 1299 follicular units and 400 double follicular units. The patient is very happy with the results.

regions (such as the temple recessions) should be not be treated at all or treated with low density.[10] Preferably, only more mature women with abundant donor hair and a limited region affected by alopecia should have areas of lesser importance addressed in a first surgery. To accept these limitations, the HRS needs to spend a great deal of time explaining to female patients the progressive nature of female hair loss, the relationship to the family history of FPHL, and life events that may cause an increase in the speed of hair loss in the future (very notably menopause).

Examining Female Hairline Design

Hairline design in women is quite complex. There are an endless number of variations; although it may be possible to describe some commonly occurring contours, this surgeon generally creates hairlines based on the individual's unique contour. Many times this contour can be determined by following the miniaturized hairs still evident in the hairline; adding terminal hairs in the same distribution and pattern will create the most natural line. If the hairline is completely absent, an older photograph can direct the surgeon appropriately to create the hairline contour best suited for each patient. The only recurring theme is that the hairline should be *very* irregular, including both macroirregularities and microirregularities.

Determining Hair Transplantation Technique

Donor harvest via strip excision is the most commonly used technique for removing the donor in women; however, there are special situations when follicular unit extraction (FUE) may be of benefit. Specifically, appropriate candidates for FUE are women who have had a previous strip harvest and have areas of chronic paresthesia, those with very limited scalp laxity, and patients who have a history of poor healing. The disadvantages of FUE in women are similar to that in men, with one notable exception: women generally have longer hair and, thus, shaving of the donor area for harvest has a much greater impact and takes considerably longer to resolve completely. Additionally, women frequently have very limited donor hair reserves relative to their large areas affected by alopecia; therefore, it is important to be able to maximize the yield of grafts from the most permanent fringe of hair. The grafts tend to be more fragile and prone to damage, and studies on survival are limited. Furthermore, FUE requires that the extraction sites be surrounded by intact hair-bearing tissue; thus, only every third follicular

unit (FU) can be removed. For these reasons, a strip harvest is usually preferred.

Laboratory Tests Before Hair Restoration

Basic laboratory tests include complete blood count, basic chemistry panel, hepatitis, and human immunodeficiency virus. Medical clearance is obtained when necessary. All patients are prescribed preoperative prophylactic antibiotics and given a list of foods and supplements to avoid. Patients taking anticoagulants for therapeutic reasons are told to continue their medications,[11] whereas those taking baby aspirin as prophylaxis are told to discontinue; clopidogrel bisulfate (Plavix) is the one exception. Provided their cardiologist or neurologist approves of discontinuation for surgery, the patients are told to stop Plavix 5 days before surgery and resume 2 days postoperatively. All patients are advised to start a homeopathic regimen 2 weeks before surgery and continue for 2 weeks after surgery. The regimen includes arnica tablets, arnica gel postoperatively, bromelain, and vitamin C. Although the author does not have scientific proof of efficacy, experience has revealed that this regimen significantly reduces the incidence of postoperative bruising and edema, which is particularly important in female patients who have a greater tendency to bruise and swell in the forehead and temple areas.

PREPARATION FOR HAIR TRANSPLANT SURGERY

Patients who are *not* having deeper anesthesia provided by an anesthesiologist are told to eat a good breakfast and take an antibiotic 1 hour before surgery.

On arrival at the office, patients read and sign the consents for surgery, photographs, and anesthesia. Then the area to be treated is again delineated with a grease pencil and the photographs with dry and wet hair are obtained.

Patients are administered diazepam and the combination preparation of hydrocodone bitartrate and acetaminophen (Vicodin); in situations when anxiety is particularly high, lorazepam is also given. The hair within the prospective donor area is cut to approximately 2 mm in length. Patients are positioned in a prone position for the removal and closure of the donor area and then repositioned in a supine position for the recipient area. In situations that require treatment of the hairline inferiorly into the preauricular areas, patients may be placed in a fetal position on one side and then the other.

PROCEDURAL APPROACH FOR HAIR TRANSPLANTATION
Anesthesia

- In addition to the preoperative medication given to patients, an intravenous line is inserted to provide fluids throughout the day and provide ease of access for additional medications to be administered.
- Just before beginning the local anesthesia, midazolam and fentanyl are injected. A regional block in both the donor and recipient areas is achieved by gradual infiltration of 2% lidocaine with 1:100 000 epinephrine.
- The recipient area block is completed after the donor area has been sutured; a great deal of care is taken to avoid bruising by injecting superficially and avoiding any visible vessels.

Anesthesia note: This author uses small amounts of 1:50 000 epinephrine solution very superficially (usually less than 10 mL for both the donor and recipient regions). Although a recent limited study was done that indicated telogen effluvium was unrelated to the amount of epinephrine used,[12] it is the author's impression that this is one of many factors that accounts for the reduced occurrence of this postoperative complication in her patients. Bupivacaine 0.50% with 1:200 000 epinephrine is used to reinforce the local anesthesia throughout the day.

- An afternoon dose of intravenous diphenhydramine is given to patients who need something additional to keep them sleepy for the afternoon of graft placement.

Donor Harvest

The donor strip is usually 10 to 15 mm in width, as dictated by the patients' scalp laxity and does not extend above the ears in most female patients. The removal is accomplished by excising the strip just below the level of the follicles, to limit the potential for injury to the deeper vasculature and to try to avoid any surface depression in the donor area. The closure is usually accomplished with a single running 3-0 Supramid suture (S. Jackson Inc, Alexandria, VA), maintaining close attention to the approximation of the epidermal layers. Most women wear their hair longer; therefore, a trichophytic closure has limited benefit and increases the tension of closure *without* the added benefit of producing more grafts. It is reserved for patients with a significant hair color/scalp color contrast and those with a previous history of more visible scars. In rare cases of extreme hyperlaxity or tension, a double-layer closure with 4.0 Monocryl

(Ethicon Inc, Somerville, NJ) suture is performed, although this is relatively new in the author's practice, and the benefits of this are as yet unclear. In general, the resulting donor scars are 1 mm or less in width and very difficult to visualize even on close inspection.

Dissection and Graft Size

The tissue is dissected with the aid of stereomicroscopes into slivers and then individual FU or double follicular units (DFU). All naturally occurring multi-haired FUs are left intact, unless there is a requirement for a greater number of 1-haired FU for a particularly long hairline. The DFU must contain a minimum of 4 closely spaced hairs, and the author and her technicians consult as to whether the hair density within the donor strip is appropriate for these grafts. Occasionally, the plan to use DFUs is changed because the spacing between the FU results in DFU that would require larger-than-ideal recipient sites. Very importantly, the technicians carefully select the finest 1- and 2-haired grafts for the hairline zone.

Recipient Site Creation

Early in the author's career, a mixture of FU and DFU was commonly used in female patients. Arguments from colleagues, which seemed to have merit, led to a change in this practice for several years. Although during this time patients remained very satisfied with their results, the author's assessment of before and after photographs revealed a distinct difference in the density achieved with the two approaches. Almost uniformly, the results were superior for surgeries in which FU and DFU were used. In addition to the increased number of hairs per graft and the more complete optical illusion this produces, another possible explanation for the better density achieved with DFU is that some dormant follicles are included in the preserved, *apparently* alopecic intervening tissue, just as earlier survival studies with round grafts revealed that more than 100% yield could be achieved.[13] Thus, the author's current approach frequently involves the use of DFU in areas where high density is desired and always behind a zone of FU in the hairline zone (**Fig. 5**).

In general, the site creation is done in this sequence and pattern:

1. A zone of 3 rows of 1-haired FU is used anteriorly in the hairline (20 Gauge [G] sites).
2. A zone of 2 rows of 2-haired FU (20 or 19 G sites) is used.
3. Three-haired FU and follicular families (18 G sites) are used.

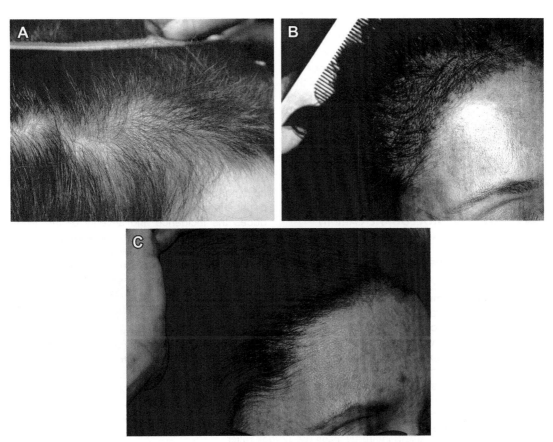

Fig. 5. (*A*) A female patient, aged 54 years, who presented with frontal and temporal hair loss, which is a very common pattern in postmenopausal women. (*B*) The pattern of sites used to achieve a gradient of density, starting with a feathered hairline and becoming denser posteriorly. A total of 1248 FU and 264 DFU were transplanted in the hairline zone and temple areas. (*C*) Two and a half years after surgery, with excellent density and naturalness.

4. Then DFU may be used in central regions (recipient size varies from 1.1–1.4 mm).

Areas laterally, including the temple regions, are usually completed with 2-haired FU, except when patients have a limited frontal zone of thinning and the deeper temple regions can be treated with denser coverage. The most lateral areas of the hairline zone are performed with the bevel oriented face up to create a flap holding the graft in a more acute position and limiting the probability that it may slide upward in the site creating a result in which the hairs are angled more perpendicular to the scalp.

Recipient Site Density

The author's response to the question of what recipient site density is optimal is usually that the question itself is misguided and deceptive. The main focus should be how much of an illusion of density can be created by using the lowest number of grafts in any given area, so as to enable the treatment of the most cosmetically important regions in one surgery. The answer depends on the hair characteristics of each patient, the location and size of the area being treated, the naturally occurring cowlicks, and anticipated future hair loss. As a general guideline, the range is as follows:

- 25 to 35 FU/cm^2 for 1-haired grafts
- 20 to 30 FU/cm^2 for 2- and 3-haired FU
- 15 to 25 DFU/cm^2 (adjust spacing according to the size of recipient site as well as amount of preexisting hair)

Recipient Site Angle and Direction of Preexisting Hair

One of the most important aspects of hair transplantation in female patients is the ability to create the recipient sites at the exact angle and direction of the preexisting hair. This detail is arguably the single greatest technical detail affecting patients' short-term postoperative sequelae as well as their long-term satisfaction with the naturalness and hair density achieved by the surgery. The author has discovered that, rather than producing rows of recipient sites in a lateral or anteroposterior direction, it is most beneficial to follow along the path of the actual flow of the preexisting hair. The tactile sensation during site creation can provide feedback as to whether the direction and angle is correct: As the blade enters, there should be a very smooth sensation; if the surgeon feels something *gritty* or *crunchy*, the angle is most likely incorrect.

IMMEDIATE POSTPROCEDURAL CARE IN HAIR TRANSPLANTATION

Patients are given detailed instructions for the postoperative period.[14]

- In most cases, minoxidil is used in the recipient area after graft placement is completed; telfa (Kendall, Tyco Healthcare Group, Mansfield, MA) gauze with antibiotic ointment and a bandage are applied for overnight.
- Unless there is a contraindication for patients, the following postoperative medications are dispensed: a tapering dose of prednisone, Vicodin, ketorolac, zolpidem tartrate (Ambien) and antinausea medications.
- Patients are advised to take an analgesic the first night *regardless* of symptoms.
- The following morning, the bandage is removed in the office, the hair is washed, and the grafts are checked to ensure that they remained properly positioned overnight.
- Removal of small blood clots on the surface of the skin and some adjustment of the grafts may be necessary.
- Again minoxidil is applied to the recipient and donor areas, followed by the application of a lubricating gel.
- The patients are instructed to wash twice daily and apply minoxidil and lubricating gel; it is recommended to be very gentle in touching the recipient area the first 2 days postoperatively.
- All patients are encouraged to come back to the author's office for a midweek check, suture removal, and a 4- to 6-week follow-up.

RECOVERY, POTENTIAL COMPLICATIONS, AND THEIR MANAGEMENT IN HAIR TRANSPLANTATION

The author tells every patient what to anticipate in the immediate postoperative period and when to expect certain key developments after surgery.

Bruising and Edema

Without knowing whether patients are more likely to bruise or develop postoperative edema, it is safest to tell patients to take a week to 10 days off of work and social activities if they do not want other people to know she has had a procedure. Visible bruising of the forehead and temple regions is more common in women because of their more superficial vasculature and thin skin. In addition to applying ice and taking the oral homeopathic regimen, the author has found that applying arnica gel before bandaging and *hourly* during the first day postoperatively significantly reduces the incidence and severity of this issue. There are patients who can successfully camouflage the surgical area within a few days after the procedure, but this is not usually the case. After 10 days, nothing is visible except occasionally a slight erythema.

Telogen Effluvium

Telogen effluvium may occur in the recipient or donor areas. Patients are told to apply minoxidil 3.5% for 2 weeks before surgery, and it is used in the recipient area before dressing with the bandage on the day of the hair transplantation. Patients are told to continue treatment with the minoxidil for at least 5 weeks after surgery. If shedding does occur, it is recommended to continue with the minoxidil to hasten regrowth. A good HRS should give ample time and reassurance to patients who are affected by telogen effluvium and suggestions for temporary camouflage techniques. The best reassurance for patients is the HRS' own firm conviction and knowledge that the hair loss is definitely temporary in nature.

A recent survey of the author's patients revealed that only approximately 15% of female patients had moderate telogen effluvium, and less than 2% reported fairly severe temporary hair loss. In *every* patient in the survey, the hair loss was temporary and the patients' cosmetic appearance was already improved by 6 months as compared with the preoperative photographs. In the following months, the hair will continue to grow, and density will gradually improve until 18 months after surgery (and occasionally up to 24 months). This timeline is to be given to patients as a rough guide, and it is always explained that some patients may respond more or less quickly and intervening events may affect the pace of growth. For example, the author had one patient whose spouse was very ill within 3 months of surgery, she had very delayed growth of the transplanted hair and diffuse telogen effluvium that most probably was related to severe emotional stress rather than the hair transplantation. Her final result was as expected but did not reach full maturity until close to 2 years after surgery. A great deal of time was required during the interim period to reassure the patient.

Inflammation

The purpose of the follow-up appointment 4 to 7 weeks after surgery is primarily to look for signs or symptoms of inflammation in the donor area, although it also allows the HRS to inspect the recipient area and address any patient questions. If the donor area is erythematous, particularly sensitive, or pruritic, it is injected with a 1:2 solution of triamcinolone/2% lidocaine (**Fig. 6**). Patients who required injections in this initial follow-up visit are asked to return for 2 more visits, spaced 3 to 4 weeks apart, for repeat injections of the steroid solution.

Folliculitis

Folliculitis or ingrown hairs may occur in the first 6 months after surgery. Patients are advised of this possibility and told to apply warm soaks, alcohol, and occasionally antibiotics. Office visits are provided as needed.

Infection and Necrosis

Other complications that can occur, but are extremely rare, include infection and necrosis in the recipient or donor areas.

SPECIAL SITUATIONS FOR HAIR TRANSPLANT IN WOMEN

Most of the female patients seen in the author's practice have patterned hair loss. However, there are patients with cicatricial alopecia, trauma, and a significant number who have an altered hairline following facial plastic surgery (**Fig. 7**). The hairline is reconstructed using old photographs and the HRS' own aesthetic sensibilities as a guide. Simultaneously, even fine scars, which may have resulted from the plastic surgery, can be transplanted and camouflaged successfully. All patients with scar tissue are told that the density of hair may be insufficient after one surgery and may require a second. The density of sites is limited by the vascularity of the tissue. The author does remind patients that scar visibility is caused by both the change in color of the scar tissue itself and the lack of hair. In some situations in which the scar color is particularly altered (hypopigmented or hyperpigmented), tattooing of the scar may be combined with hair transplantation to fully camouflage the scar.

Post Hair Transplant Hair Care and Styling

For the first week after surgery, patients are asked to soak in a tub and wash their hair twice daily. After each washing, they are instructed to apply Aquaphor (Beiersdorf Inc, Wilton, CT) to their donor area and a water-based gel to the recipient region. This regimen helps to loosen and remove any crusting and improves the healing. Patients who tolerate minoxidil also are asked to apply a preparation of 3.5% twice daily to the surgical area for 5 weeks; the improved vasodilation this produces helps reduce the severity of postoperative telogen effluvium. Furthermore, they are instructed to avoid strenuous exercise for 1 week.

Women who have had a hair transplant can start treating their hair as they did before surgery in 2 weeks. This treatment includes hair dyes and other treatments. There is no need to change their

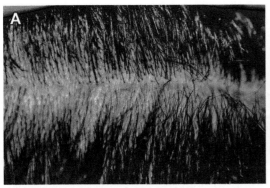 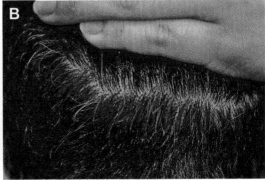

Fig. 6. (*A*) A donor area 5 weeks after strip surgery showing some erythema and hypertrophy. A total of 5 mL of a 1:2 solution of triamcinolone and 2% lidocaine was injected along the entire donor line. (*B*) The same patient 6 months after completing a series of 2 injections of the triamcinolone solution (at 5 and 8 weeks postoperative) in the donor area. The donor scar is undetectable even on close inspection.

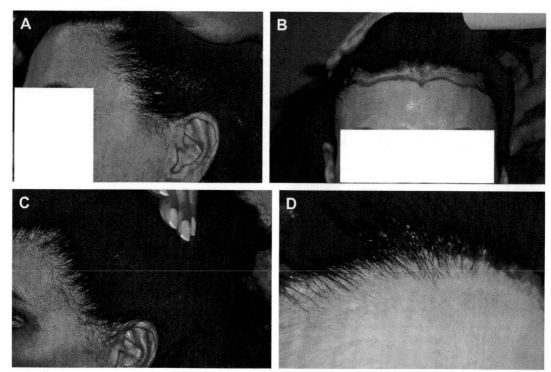

Fig. 7. (*A*) A 57-year-old female patient after rhytidoplasty and brow lift. This view shows the loss of supra-auricular and preauricular hair, a fine preauricular scar, as well as thinning in the lateral hairline, which may or may not have been present preoperatively. (*B*) A frontal view of the same patient showing the scar from the brow-lift anterior to her hairline. The patient was forewarned that the scar might still be visible after hair transplantation because of the hypopigmentation. (*C*) A total of 1766 FU was transplanted into the entire hairline zone and deeper in the central frontal block. This photograph shows the lateral view 18 months postoperatively. (*D*) The brow-lift scar after one session is undetectable. The pigmentation seems to have also corrected itself somewhat after hair transplant surgery.

routine provided they were not using harmful processes before surgery.

The physician should discuss with the patients which processes they used before surgery and advise them regarding their effect on the hair and scalp. Hair extensions are almost uniformly harmful to the hair, causing permanent traction alopecia after a period of time.

The guideline is as follows: *any chemicals used for straightening, relaxing, or dying the hair should not cause itching, burning, or pain*—these are signals that there is damage being done to the scalp and may exacerbate hair loss.

CONCLUSION

Women are becoming more open about the problem of FPHL and therefore there has been an increase in the number of women seeking a means of addressing this issue. Ideally, women should be advised regarding treatments which may slow future loss and informed as to the potential results

they can expect from surgical hair restoration. Surgeries performed with meticulous care and a sound long-term surgical plan are extremely successful and make a significant impact in patients' lives.

REFERENCES

1. Unger W, Unger R. Hair transplanting: an important but often forgotten treatment for female pattern hair loss. J Am Acad Dermatol 2003;49:853–60.
2. Tosti A, Piraccini BM. Diagnosis and treatment of hair disorders: an evidence based atlas. New York: Informa HealthCare; 2005.
3. Wilma B, Dirk E. Lichen planopilaris and variants. In: Elise O, editor. Disorders of Hair Growth. 2nd edition. New York: McGraw-Hill Medical Publishing Division; 2003. p. 370–3.
4. Unger W, Unger R, Wesley C. The surgical treatment of cicatricial alopecia. Dermatol Ther 2008;21(4): 295–311.

5. Quercetani R, Rebora AE, Fedi MC, et al. Patients with profuse hair shedding may reveal anagen hair dystrophy: a diagnostic clue of alopecia areata incognita. J Eur Acad Dermatol Venereol 2001; 25(7):808–10.

6. Tosti A, Whiting D, Iorizzo M, et al. The role of scalp dermoscopy in the diagnosis of alopecia areata incognita. J Am Acad Dermatol 2008;59: 64–7.

7. Gilhar A, Etzioni A, Paus R. Alopecia areata. N Engl J Med 2012;366(16):1515–25.

8. Unger WP. "Female patient candidacy" Lecture delivered at ISHRS Conference. Boston (MA). 2010.

9. Unger RH, Wesley CK. Technical and philosophical approaches influencing perceptions of female candidacy and results in hair restoration surgery. Treatment strategies: dermatology, vol. 1. London: Cambridge Research Ctr; 2011 (1). p. 142–5.

10. Unger R. Planning in female patients. In: Unger WP, Shapiro R, Unger R, et al, editors. Hair transplantation. 5th edition. New York: Marcel Dekker; 2010. p. 182–5.

11. Kirkorian AY, Moore BL, Siskind J, et al. Perioperative management of anticoagulant therapy during cutaneous surgery: 2005 survey of Mohs surgeons. Dermatol Surg 2007;33(10):1189–97.

12. Panchaprateep R, Pathomvanich D, et al. Does epinephrine influence post-surgical effluvium? A pilot study. Hair Transplant Forum International 2012;22(3):98.

13. Unger W. Hair survival in two millimeter round grafts. 8th annual meeting of the ISHRS. Hawaii, 2000.

14. Parsley W, Waldman M. Management of the postoperative period. In: Unger WP, Shapiro R, Unger R, et al, editors. Hair transplantation. 5th edition. New York: Marcel Dekker; 2010. p. 416–9.

Megasessions
Surgical Indications and Technical Perspectives

Steven Gabel, MD

KEYWORDS

- Megasession • Large sessions • Graft survival • Hair transplantation • Follicular unit grafting
- Patient selection • Complications • Patient expectations • Surgical techniques

KEY POINTS

- Megasessions are capable of definitively treating significant areas of the scalp with 1 procedure.
- Careful patient selection and consultation are required to ensure a safe and successful outcome.
- A detailed medical history and evaluation must be obtained to determine whether a patient is an appropriate candidate for a megasession.
- Detailed preoperative planning; meticulous organization; and an experienced, efficient hair restoration team are essential for successful execution and completion of lengthy hair transplant procedures.
- Maximizing graft survival is the key component for successful implementation of a megasession.
- Organizing the grafts into small, identical unit groups; shaving the recipient area; and staining the recipient sites with methylene blue are a few techniques to maximize the efficiency of graft placement.

INTRODUCTION

The term megasession in hair restoration surgery refers to transplanting a large number of follicular unit grafts in a single session. With the abundance of literature available to the general public, patients are educated on advances in hair restoration surgery and what can be accomplished. Even though what is read may not be entirely true, patients have a better understanding of surgical hair transplantation, and, in many cases, have an expectation for a natural result with maximal coverage and minimal downtime. This result may or may not be possible depending on the patient's expectations, medical history, current hair loss pattern, and available donor hair. It is therefore imperative for the hair restoration physician to develop a sound and ethical treatment plan for each patient. Although individuals may not be candidates for a large session, or a clinic may not have the capability to perform large sessions, it is important for the clinician to have a thorough understanding of the procedure and the technical details for a successful outcome.

Megasessions are not unique to hair restoration, and have been described in other fields of dermatologic surgery such as removing a large number of basal cell carcinomas from an individual in a single session.[1] Although no strict definition exists, in 1995, Rassman and Carson[2] described a mega-transplant session as transplanting more then 1000 grafts in a single session. Over the years, as hair restoration has become more refined, the number of grafts transplanted per session has increased. This article refers to a megasession as transplanting greater then 3000 grafts in a single session via the strip method, although larger

Disclosure: The author has nothing to disclose and has no conflicts of interest with respect to the content of this article.
Gabel Hair Restoration Center, 900 Southeast Oak Street, Suite 201, Hillsboro, OR 97123, USA
E-mail address: DrGabel@gabelcenter.com

Facial Plast Surg Clin N Am 21 (2013) 419–430
http://dx.doi.org/10.1016/j.fsc.2013.06.002

sessions are possible. The high numbers of grafts are now possible because surgeons are using naturally occurring follicular units and increasing the size of the donor strip.

In the past, physicians used hair plugs that may have had up to 20 to 30 terminal hairs, each containing 12 to 14 follicular units.[3] These plugs were harvested using a 4-mm punch and were transplanted in rows producing a dolls-head appearance with islands or clumps of hair between larger-than-normal areas of skin. At most, several hundred of these plugs were transplanted per session. Although patients had a significant amount of hair transplanted, the results were not natural and, in many instances, were noticeable to others.

A major advancement in hair restoration occurred with the introduction of the binocular microscope, which allowed natural follicular units, each containing 1 to 4 hairs, to be dissected and transplanted, as first described by Limmer[4] in 1988. By using these smaller follicular unit bundles and spreading them out more evenly in the recipient area to mimic the normal biological appearance of scalp hair, the patient was able to obtain a more natural-appearing result. As strategies evolved for larger donor tissue harvests, the numbers of follicular units transplanted increased, allowing surgeons to transplant a greater area of the scalp.

In the past, the donor strip was removed only in the occipital portion of the scalp (**Fig. 1**).[5] The hair in this area of the scalp is genetically resistant to the effects of dihydrotestosterone, a hormone responsible for miniaturization of hair follicles and hair loss. For the last several years, surgeons have become more aggressive, extending the harvested donor strip from the occipital portion of the scalp to the temporal/supra-auricular area of the scalp (**Fig. 2**). In some cases, this has allowed surgeons to remove donor strips in excess of 30 cm in length, which has the potential to provide a significant amount of donor hair.

GENERAL PRINCIPLES OF A MEGASESSION

There are several advantages and disadvantages of transplanting a large number of follicular units in a single session (**Table 1**). By using a large number of grafts, either a sizable area of the scalp can be transplanted or a specific area may be covered with a high density of hair. The average density of follicular units varies significantly between races,[6] and research by Headington[3] has shown that it can average up to 100 follicular units/cm^2. It is not feasibly for surgeons to transplant hair at this high of density over a significant area because it would require too much donor scalp, which generally is not available in the alopecic patient; however, it can be argued that, in any given area, more transplanted hair gives a fuller appearance and ultimately a better result.

With a megasession, an individual with a Norwood IV/V pattern, who may require 4000 to

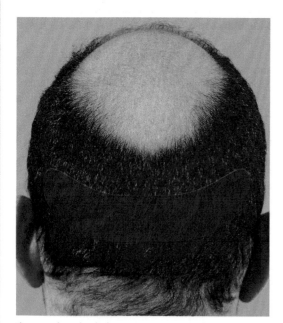

Fig. 1. The shaded area represents the traditional donor region of the occipital scalp.

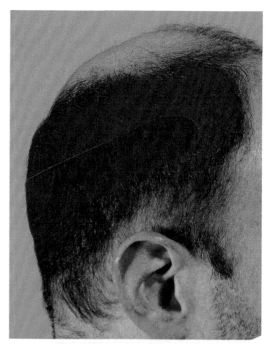

Fig. 2. The shaded area represents the extended temporal/supra-auricular donor region of the scalp.

Table 1 Advantages and disadvantages of a megasession	
Advantages	**Disadvantages**
Treat large area in 1 session	Higher risk for patient
Treat a single area with higher density	Local anesthesia toxicity
Decreased overall downtime	Potential for decreased graft survival
Less scarring in recipient site	Demanding on physician, staff, and patient
Decreased donor site scarring	Donor site scarring with aggressive harvest
Decreased vascular trauma	Increased swelling
—	Long procedure times

5000 grafts to achieve a satisfactory result with 30% natural density throughout the balding frontal and midscalp, can be managed in 1 procedure instead of the commonly accepted protocol that uses multiple smaller sessions of 1500 to 2000 grafts (**Fig. 3**). The same argument holds true for a Norwood II/III patient who desires to have the frontal hairline and frontal zone treated with high-density hair in 1 session. To achieve a more desirable natural and aesthetically pleasing result, the frontal zone requires higher densities with large numbers of microscopically dissected 1-hair and 2-hair follicular units. Transplanting 3000 or more grafts to the frontal hairline region may give the patient the desired appearance of full density with only 1 procedure (**Figs. 4** and **5**). There are also situations in which an appropriate candidate has 2 discontinuous areas of the scalp, such as the frontal zone and the crown, which with adequate donor supply can be treated using a single megasession (**Fig. 6**). Transplantation for patients with any of these hair loss patterns can theoretically be performed with 1 session by harvesting and transplanting a higher number of grafts. However, it is important to always counsel the patient that an additional, smaller touch-up procedure may be necessary after a session of any size to achieve the final results. The advantage of the megasession, is that the bulk of the work is accomplished in 1 procedure instead of many smaller sessions.

Recovery Considerations in Megasessions

With respect to the amount of time that it takes to prepare for and recover from each procedure, it is advantageous for the patient to have a single session versus multiple smaller sessions. Patients who need to travel long distances to the surgical office require an additional 2 or 3 days off for their procedure. After surgery, it takes approximately 9 to 10 days for the swelling to subside and for the grafts to implant with minimal risk of dislodgment.[7] During this time, patients must limit their activity and possibly their ability to work. Afterward, it may take another 6 to 18 months for the hair to grow out to achieve the final results. If patients have to repeat this cycle multiple times to meet their goals, the overall downtime may limit their

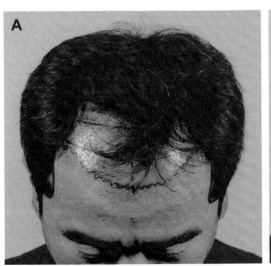 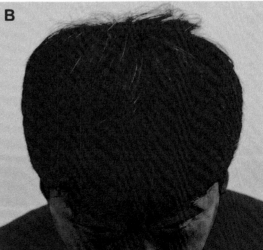

Fig. 3. A total of 3852 follicular unit grafts were placed in 1 megasession. (*A*) Alopecia of the frontal hairline and frontal midscalp before surgery. (*B*) One year after surgery.

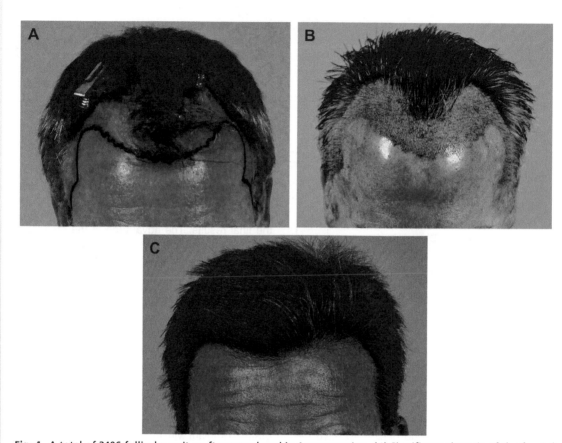

Fig. 4. A total of 3406 follicular unit grafts were placed in 1 megasession. (*A*) Significant alopecia of the frontal hairline and frontal region of the scalp before surgery. (*B*) Immediate postoperative view showing high-density graft placement in the frontal region. (*C*) One year after surgery.

ability or desire to have the transplant performed. Patients want quicker results and do not want to have several procedures when they are aware that larger sessions are available to meet their goals.

The biological effects of surgery on the donor and recipient sites favor minimizing the number of times the surgical areas are treated. Harvesting the donor strip in the scalp results in some degree of hair loss, scarring, and fibrosis of the

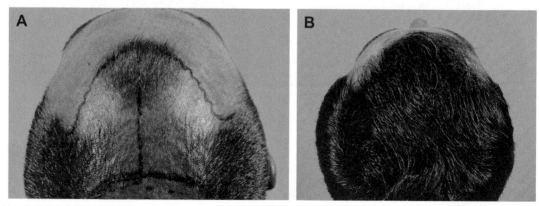

Fig. 5. A total of 3033 follicular unit grafts were placed in 1 megasession. (*A*) Severe alopecia of the frontal hairline and midscalp before surgery. (*B*) One year after surgery.

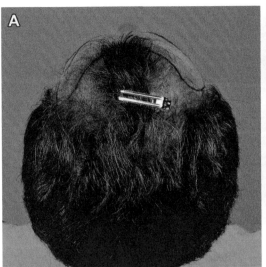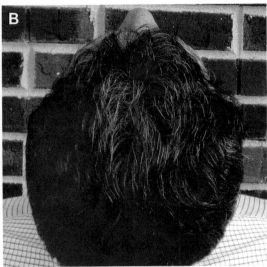

Fig. 6. A total of 4489 follicular unit grafts were placed in several areas of the scalp in 1 megasession. (*A*) Preoperative view showing severe alopecia of the frontal scalp and hairline, and moderate alopecia of the midscalp and crown. (*B*) One year after surgery.

surrounding tissues as the strip heals. Although techniques exist such as beveling the scalpel blade and tissue-spreading devices to minimize transection of the donor hair, there will always be some transection of the hair follicles with each subsequent procedure. Furthermore, as the donor area heals with a scar, the hairs adjacent to the wound edges may become distorted, causing the hairs to exit at irregular angles. These effects may worsen with multiple procedures. By limiting the number of times that donor hair is harvested, the amount of potential donor hair loss and distortion of the adjacent hairs is reduced. The same effect applies to the recipient area as well. In each session in which incisions are made in the scalp, a small amount of scar tissue and fibrosis is formed, which may ultimately decrease the vascularity of the tissues. When fewer procedures are performed in a given area, scarring and vascular damage are lessened.

TECHNICAL CONSIDERATIONS IN MEGASESSIONS
Donor Hair and Tissue

Harvesting a sufficient amount of donor hair is required to perform megasessions. The number of grafts removed is directly related to the dimensions of the strip and the graft density per square centimeter. There are various techniques that aid in harvesting large amounts of donor tissue, including extending the incision laterally into the temple (**Fig. 7**), scalp mobilizing exercises to

temporarily increase the elasticity of the donor area,[8] or even the use of tissue expanders. The second and third of these methods are used to remove a wider strip. Measuring the elasticity of the scalp before (**Fig. 8**) the incision provides the physician with a reference starting point of how much donor tissue is safe to remove, as described by Meyer and Pauls.[9] Once this measurement is made, it is the author's experience that it is best to remove only a few centimeters in the beginning of the donor strip to test the elasticity of the wound edge to ascertain that the closure will be under minimal tension (**Fig. 9A**). If the edges are easily approximated and can be overlapped (see **Fig. 9B**), the incision is widened a few millimeters to maximize the harvest. This step is repeated until the dimensions of the donor strip are such that the greatest amount of tissue is removed while still being able to approximate the edges with minimal tension. In contrast, if there is considerable tension on the wound edges with the initial test strip (see **Fig. 9C**), the strip width is decreased to allow an easier closure. It is imperative that the wound edges are approximated with minimal tension, because this technique helps to minimize the resulting donor scar. However, there are situations in which the wound edges are difficult to close. If patient has been promised, and is expecting, several thousand grafts to be transplanted, it puts additional pressure on the physician to accomplish this. The physician may subsequently become overly aggressive in harvesting the donor strip. If too

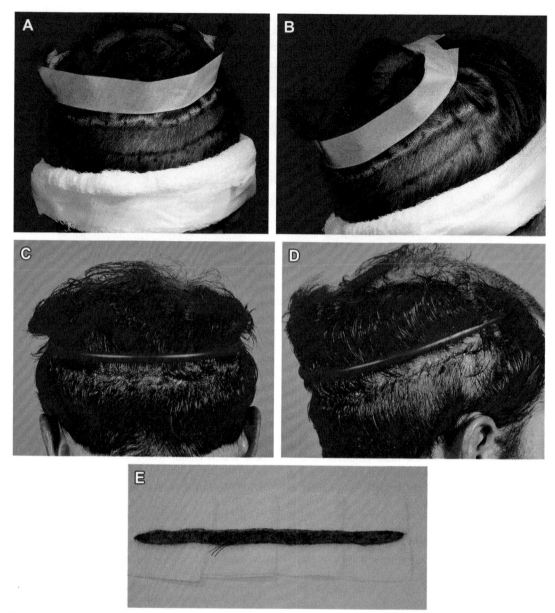

Fig. 7. Extended donor harvest. (*A, B*) The posterior and lateral harvest area is marked out before surgery. (*C, D*) The posterior and lateral sutured incision line after harvesting the donor hair. (*E*) Donor strip measuring 1.75 × 30 cm, which was able to yield 3882 follicular unit grafts.

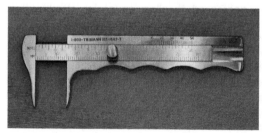

Fig. 8. Surgical caliper used to measure donor site elasticity prior to donor strip incision.

wide a strip is removed and there is difficulty primarily closing the incision, the surgeon may elect to either suture it under considerable tension, which may cause loss of adjacent hair or skin necrosis from lack of circulation, or allow it to heal by secondary intention. Either way, a wide donor scar may form, which is undesirable for both the patient and the surgeon (**Fig. 10**). It is always better to err on the side of conservatism when removing the donor strip to avoid the formation of a wide scar.

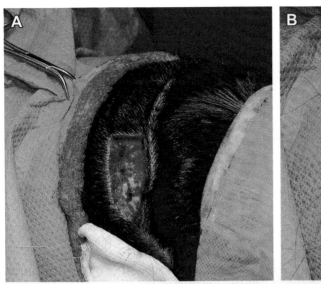
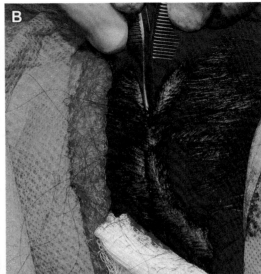
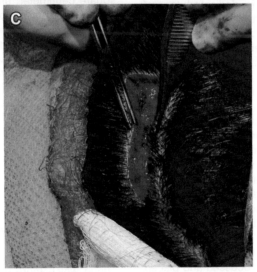

Fig. 9. The importance of measuring the elasticity in the first few centimeters of strip. (*A*) Five centimeters of strip are initially harvested. (*B*) The tissue edges are grasped to show that the edges are easily overlapped. In this example, the width of the donor strip may be increased to increase the overall yield of the strip. (*C*) The tissue edges are not easily approximated, showing poor laxity. In this example, the width of the strip must be decreased to avoid excessive tension with the final wound closure.

Graft Survival

Graft survival is a key component to consider when performing a megasession. The time it takes to complete the procedure is variable; however, as the number of grafts transplanted increases, the time required to finish the procedure also lengthens. Several studies have shown that graft survival decreases when follicular units are subjected to longer durations out of the body. Limmer[10] performed an in vivo study using chilled normal saline that showed 95% survival at 2 hours, 90% survival at 4 hours, 86% survival at 6 hours,

88% survival at 8 hours, 79% survival at 24 hours, and 54% survival at 48 hours. Given these data, it is crucial that the grafts be placed into the scalp in a timely manner.

There are several strategies that physicians and clinics have put in place to minimize the time that the grafts are out of the body:

- First, it is imperative to have a sufficiently large and experienced hair restoration team to be able to prepare all the grafts and at the same time place them into the patient's scalp. It is common to have at least 4 to 5

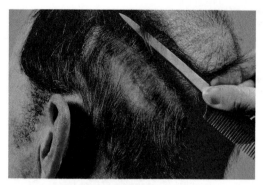

Fig. 10. Large postoperative scar after closing the wound with excessive tension. There is also hair loss around the incision site from poor postoperative vascularity.

people dedicated to graft preparation and another 3 or 4 people dedicated to graft placement. This team approach allows the individual members to rotate in and out of the session in order to maintain the high level of intensity required to complete the procedure.

- Second, there are multiple approaches available for planning the timing of the strip harvest, which can ultimately affect the out-of-body time of the grafts (**Box 1**). Physicians have the option of harvesting the strip in 1 sitting (the most common method), harvesting it in multiple segments throughout the day's session, or planning the procedure over more than one day. The type of approach used depends on several factors. Harvesting the strip in the beginning of the session sets the tone for the day because there is no ambiguity about how much donor material needs to be processed and placed. Although it is easier for the team to harvest the strip only once, it may be detrimental to the grafts that are placed toward the later part of the session because they may be subjected to prolonged out-of-body exposure time. In contrast, if only half of the strip is harvested, processed, and placed during the first part of the session, and the second half of the strip is harvested and placed in the

later part of the session, this method reduces the out-of-body time of the grafts and, ultimately, graft survival.

- Third, there are some physicians who advocate a staged 2-day procedure in which half of the planned donor strip is harvested and placed in one day, and the second half of the strip is harvested and placed the following day. Although there will be some edema in the donor and recipient areas (**Fig. 11**), this approach reduces the strain on all involved because the procedure becomes more manageable for even a modest-sized staff.

Harvesting the strip in multiple segments, whether in over 1 or 2 days, provides the surgeon with a great deal of information pertaining to the case, such as the number of grafts obtained per square centimeter, and how easy or difficult the grafts are to place. For example, if the first half of a donor strip yielded more grafts then anticipated, the physician is able to make an adjustment and decrease the dimensions of the second half of the strip to accurately obtain the planned number of grafts for the session. This additional information allows the surgeon to execute the surgical plan more precisely and provides a template to make adjustments for the second half of the session.

Anesthesia

Consideration must also be given to the amount of local anesthesia injected throughout the procedure. Most hair restoration physicians use lidocaine, whereas some also use bupivacaine for its long-acting properties. For the longer procedures during which more anesthetics are needed, it is important to monitor the amount of local anesthesia that is administered because the patient may be given doses approaching the total daily dose, which for lidocaine is 4.5 mg/kg (maximum 300 mg) without epinephrine, or 7 mg/kg (maximum 500 mg) when used in combination with epinephrine.[11] Although in hair restoration surgery the total daily dose of lidocaine is often exceeded, it is important for the physician and staff to be aware of this and to recognize the signs and symptoms of lidocaine toxicity (**Box 2**).[12] The use of bupivacaine may help in this situation because it is a longer acting local anesthetic than lidocaine and has a half-life of 2.7 hours.[13]

PATIENT SELECTION FOR MEGASESSIONS

Patients must be carefully evaluated to determine whether they are appropriate candidates for a

---

Box 1
Timing strategies for harvesting of the donor strip

- Single harvest, single day
- Multiple harvest, single day
- Multiple harvest, staged over 2 days

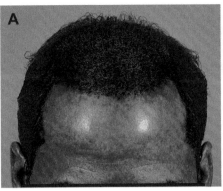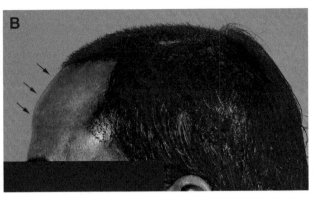

Fig. 11. (*A, B*) Edema formation (*arrows*) of the forehead on the first postoperative day.

challenging megasession, which may last more then 10 hours during which time their heads must be kept in an immobile position for graft placement. Although completing the procedure in 1 session may be appealing to some, others may find this length of time arduous, or have a relative contraindication (**Box 3**), and elect to have it performed over multiple sessions. Some patients have a tendency to become agitated from sitting in the operating room chair for prolonged periods of time and/or nauseated from the narcotic pain medications, if required. Anxiolytics and antinausea medications may help in these situations, but the overall experience for the patient may not be worth the discomfort. Also, if the patient is maintained in a sitting position for long periods of time, there is an increased risk for medical complications such as a deep vein thrombosis[14] (DVT). Patients who have had DVTs or coagulation disorders are better suited for shorter sessions. Patients with chronic medical problems, anxiety disorders, or pain issues may not be ideal candidates for a lengthy procedure because they may require frequent breaks or have difficulty maintaining their heads in a motionless state, making it impossible to complete the procedure.

Patients who have had a prior hair transplant or scalp reduction may have excessive scarring, tension, or even vascular compromise of the scalp, which may prevent harvesting a significant amount of donor tissue. In addition, poor donor hair density and/or excessive follicular unit miniaturization are contraindications for a megasession, or even a hair transplant. Therefore, it is imperative for the physician to evaluate all aspects of a patient's medical history with a detailed examination of the scalp to determine whether they are medically and/or physically appropriate candidates for the transplant procedure. If there is any doubt about their ability to safely undergo a lengthy megasession, it is in the best interest of both the patient and physician to use smaller sessions.

STAFF CONSIDERATIONS IN MEGASESSIONS

Megasessions are inherently more complicated and demanding because of the increased size and length of the procedure. A detailed plan and experienced surgical team are required to be able to manage all aspects of the procedure including the patient's needs, assisting in harvesting of the donor strip, preparation of the follicular

Box 2
Effects of lidocaine on the central nervous system

- Mild sedation
- Analgesia
- Slurred speech
- Lightheadedness
- Drowsiness
- Respiratory arrest
- Euphoria
- Sensory disturbances
- Nausea
- Dysphoria
- Diplopia
- Disorientation
- Muscular twitching
- Seizures
- Uncontrollable tremors
- Coma

Box 3
Relative contraindications for megasessions (not inclusive)

- Chronic back pain
- Chronic pain issues
- Movement disorders
- History of deep vein thrombosis

- Type 1 diabetes
- Bladder insufficiency
- Claustrophobia
- Anxiety disorders

- Excessive scalp scarring
- Miniaturization of donor hair
- High scalp tension
- Anticoagulation medications

---

units, and the proper placement of the thousands of grafts into the scalp. Once the last graft is placed, time is needed to check the recipient and donor sites, place any bandages, and assist the patient in departing the office. The staff also must be prepared to handle situations that extend an already long day, such as extra bleeding and/or popping of the grafts. This extended period of time must be taken into account before attempting a megasession because it can be demanding even for the most experienced clinicians. Therefore, it is essential that the team is organized and members are well versed in their particular areas of responsibility to maximize efficiency throughout the day.

Selecting a Strategy

There are several strategies that can be used by the clinic to improve the speed and efficiency of the procedure (**Box 4**). The most important asset to completing the procedure is the hair restoration staff, and having a sufficiently large staff is key to being able to complete a megasession. It is important that the team is informed of the details of the surgical plan and that any vital aspects of the patient's medical history are reviewed for

---

Box 4
Strategies for speed and efficiency

- Detailed preoperative planning
- Large, motivated, experienced hair restoration team
- Rotating schedule to allow staff to remain attentive and rested
- Shaving of the recipient site for easier graft placement
- Staining of the recipient site with 1% aqueous methylene blue for better visualization
- Meticulous graft organization for efficient graft placement
- Loop magnification for the graft placers

---

safety purposes. Anticipating a long day, one strategy is to divide the staff members into shifts. so that half of the staff starts in the beginning of the session, and the remainder starts half way through the session. If a clinic has a small staff, the number of grafts harvested may need to be limited and a megasession may not be possible in 1 sitting. In general, there are many scenarios that may be used to minimize staff fatigue and each clinic must determine what works best for its team.

Graft placement is usually the most time consuming aspect of a megasession and there are several strategies to help improve the efficiency of this step. Shaving the recipient area significantly helps to speed up the placement of the grafts because a considerable amount of time may be lost manipulating the hair while searching for empty sites. For planning purposes, the recipient sites may be made before or after shaving the area. In the author's experience, shaving the hair down to 1 to 2 mm before slit placement allows the native hairs to be visualized and serves as a guide in making the proper slit angles. Once the slits are made, the recipient site may be shaved down to the skin, which may also speed up the placing process because the 1-mm length native hairs may be mistaken for a graft. Even with the hair shaved down to the skin, in some cases it may be difficult to visualize the slits. Staining the recipient sites with 1% aqueous methylene blue[15] immediately after they are made can improve visualization of the slits (**Fig. 12**). This technique not only helps to minimize searching for empty slits but also helps ensure that each site that was made is filled with a graft. By the end of the session, most of the methylene blue will have been washed away and any residual color will dissolve a few days after surgery.

Three or more team members are used for graft placement on a rotating schedule to keep everyone alert. To efficiently place the grafts, the graft cutters are responsible for placing the prepared grafts onto Telfa sheets in a medium-sized tray that is saturated with lactated Ringer

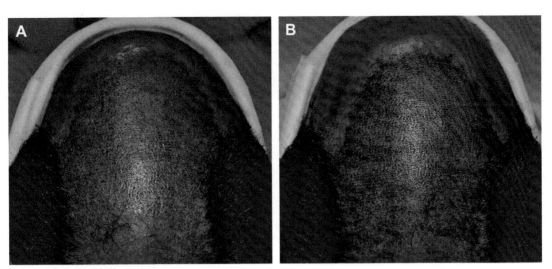

Fig. 12. The recipient sites (*A*) before and (*B*) after staining with 1% aqueous methylene blue.

solution. The grafts are organized into piles of equal-sized follicular units with their hair shafts oriented in the same direction. Each pile has approximately 10 grafts to minimize the potential for desiccation while on the finger of the placer (**Fig. 13**). Each member of the placing team should then have adequate magnification for better visualization of the recipient sites. By using these various techniques, the placers are able to quickly obtain and place the grafts in the most efficient manner to complete the procedure.

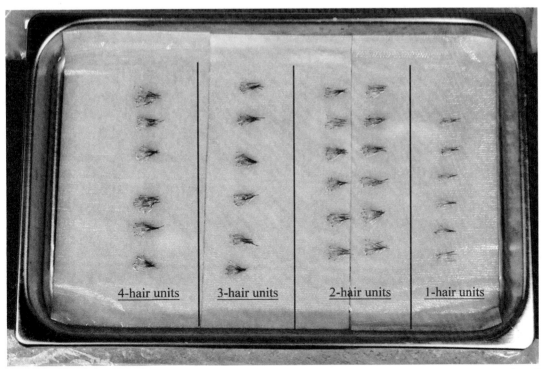

4-hair units   3-hair units   2-hair units   1-hair units

Fig. 13. Follicular unit grafts are organized into groups with 10 grafts each to aid in the efficiency of graft placement.

SUMMARY

Megasessions in hair restoration surgery have the potential to definitively treat a significant area of scalp in 1 procedure, allowing patients to achieve their desired goals while minimizing their overall downtime. Although some may find this appealing for many reasons, patients must be carefully counseled and selected to ensure that they are appropriate candidates for the extended period of time it takes to complete the procedure. Megasessions require detailed planning and organization, and an experienced staff to be able to process and implant the large number of grafts. Strategies to assist in the timing, speed, and overall efficiency needed to complete the procedure should be implemented to maximize graft survival.

REFERENCES

1. Martinez JC, Otley CC. Megasession: excision of numerous skin cancers in a single session. Dermatol Surg 2005;31(7 Pt 1):757–61 [discussion: 761–2].
2. Rassman WR, Carson S. Micrografting in extensive quantities. Dermatol Surg 1995;21(4):306–11.
3. Headington JT. Transverse microscopy anatomy of the human scalp. Arch Dermatol 1984;120: 449–56.
4. Limmer BL. Elliptical donor stereoscopically assisted micrografting as an approach to further refinement in hair transplantation. Dermatol Surg 1994; 20:789–93.
5. Barrera A. Micrograft and minigraft megasession hair transplantation results after a single session. Plast Reconstr Surg 1997;100(6):1524–30.
6. Bernstein RM, Rassman WR. The aesthetics of follicular transplantation. Dermatol Surg 1997;23:785–99.
7. Bernstein RM, Rassman WR. Graft anchoring in hair transplantation. Dermatol Surg 2006;32:198–204.
8. Wong J. Mega session follicular unit transplantation. In: Unger WP, Shapiro R, Unger R, et al, editors. Hair transplantation. 5th edition. London: Informa Healthcare; 2011. p. 363–71.
9. Mayer M, Pauls T. Scalp elasticity scale. Hair Transplant Forum Intl 2005;15(4):122–3.
10. Limmer R. Micrograft survival. In: Stough D, Haber R, editors. Hair replacement. St Louis (MO): Mosby; 1996. p. 147–9.
11. Berde CB, Strichartz GR. Local anesthetics. In: Miller RD, editor. Miller's anesthesia. 7th edition. Philadelphia: Churchill Livingstone/Elsevier; 2009. p. 913–40.
12. Yagiela JA. Local anesthetics. Anesth Prog 1991;38: 128–41.
13. Malamed SF. Clinical action of specific agents. In: Handbook of local anesthesia. 6th edition. St Louis (MO): Mosby; 2013. p. 52–75.
14. Shapiro P. Case history: pulmonary embolism/deep vein thrombosis following hair restoration surgery. Hair Transplant Forum Intl 2008;18(1):11–2.
15. Speranzini M. The use of methylene blue to enhance site visualization and definition of areas by number of hairs per graft. Hair Transplant Forum Intl 2008; 18(2):59.

Dense Packing
Surgical Indications and Technical Considerations

Bessam Farjo, MB, ChB, BAO, LRCPSI, FICS[a,b,*],
Nilofer Farjo, MB, ChB, BAO, LRCPSI[a,b]

KEYWORDS

- Dense packing • Density • Graft survival • Planning • Recipient sites • Maximum density

KEY POINTS

- The treatment goal is to achieve first a natural impression of a full look.
- For advanced hair loss, the best to aim for is a balanced look and to settle on less than optimal density.
- Indications for dense packing are smaller areas of loss, low risk of potential further loss, and high hair/skin color contract.
- A full assessment of hair type and quality, donor hair density, and current and potential future areas of hair loss as well as patient's expectations will help decide the plan.
- Accurate assessment of size and depth of recipient sites for a snug fit is vital.
- The usual approach is 40 to 50 follicular unit grafts per square centimeter for the hairline using single grafts followed by 2 haired grafts with the remainder distributed behind with decreasing densities.

INTRODUCTION

For most practitioners, dense packing is defined as placing hair grafts at a rate higher than 30 grafts per square centimeter in the recipient area.[1–11] Forty to 50 grafts per square centimeter are fairly common (**Fig. 1**); more than that is considered controversial with debatable practicality and graft survival rates.

The general goal of any hair transplant treatment should be to achieve a natural as well as an impression of a full look of hair as possible depending on the degree of baldness and donor hair availability. Naturalness has to be the primary aim. Baldness may not be desirable but it is a natural phenomenon, whereas inappropriate looking hair is neither natural nor desirable, making future planning or allowing for potential future deterioration of the baldness a very important part of the treatment. The potential is the prospect of an ever-expanding bald scalp canvas and a paradoxically decreasing material of hair with which to work. Allocating grafts at higher than 50 per square centimeter in extensive areas in one part of the bald scalp will likely leave the surgeon short of grafts in other significant areas should the patient progress to a Norwood stage 6 or 7. For current or potential future advanced hair loss it is always best to aim for an overall balanced look and perhaps settle on less than optimal density, which is especially relevant as the patient's own expectations tend to lean toward this as they get older.

Ideal Patient for Dense Packing

The ideal patients for dense packing or those who require it the most are those with the following:

- Smaller areas of hair loss surrounded by otherwise dense areas

The authors declare no financial or any conflict of interest.
[a] Farjo Hair Institute, 70 Quay Street, Manchester M3 3EJ, UK; [b] Farjo Hair Institute, 152 Harley Street, London W1G 7LH, UK
* Corresponding author. Farjo Hair Institute, 70 Quay Street, Manchester M3 3EJ, UK.
E-mail address: bfarjo@gmail.com

Facial Plast Surg Clin N Am 21 (2013) 431–436
http://dx.doi.org/10.1016/j.fsc.2013.06.004

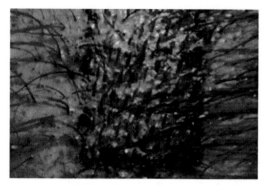

Fig. 1. Forty-five incisions placed in 1 square centimeter.

- Low risk of potential further loss
- High hair-to-skin color contrast (eg, white skin and dark brown or black hair)
- Frontal forelock and hairline zone in most patients
- Those with fine quality hair, as opposed to wiry or curly
- High-density, quality, and quantity donor hair in both occipital and parietal areas

Advantages to Dense Packing

There are obvious advantages to the dense packing approach, which include the following:

- A more natural appearance achieved from the start because of the more even distribution of hairs and less gaps between the grafts
- The obvious higher level of density achieved from a single operation
- Both of the above lead to a higher level of patient satisfaction and help to achieve a more complete result in less time and expense (**Fig. 2**)

Disadvantages to Dense Packing

There are disadvantages as well to dense packing, and these include the following:

- Increased number of grafts per session means more time required for dissection, recipient site creation, and graft placement, increasing the risk of graft exposure and damage
- Smaller incisions are needed in very close proximity, requiring more care and higher magnification
- Increased number of staff who a have the appropriate skill, training, and expertise is required

PREOPERATIVE PLANNING

The patient needs to be assessed fully in terms of suitability for a dense packing approach. A decision needs to be reached to determine whether the patient can have specific areas densely

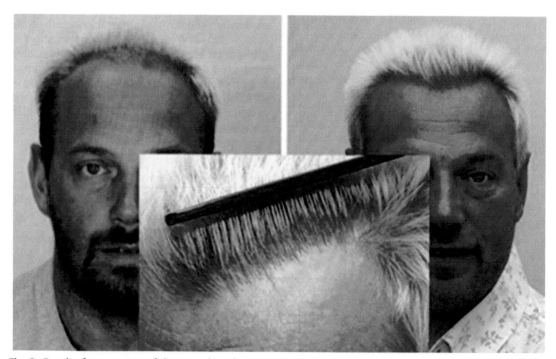

Fig. 2. Result after one pass of dense packing hair transplant.

packed or whether a more general and balanced approach is indicated to achieve more consistent coverage to a current or potential future extensive area of hair loss.

Patient Hair Loss History

The patient's history of his own hair loss is important to determine. The age of onset of the earliest sign of loss should be determined to assess how long it took the patient to get to the stage where he is at now. The next question is whether the hair loss is ongoing or stable and for how long. Finally, a thorough family history of hair loss should be attained, including which side of the family the patient's hair characteristics most resemble. If a 27-year-old patient at Norwood 4 started losing hair at age 20 still becoming worse, and resembles his father who is Norwood 6, then it may not be wise to dense pack his frontal-temporal recessions at this point. He is probably a candidate for the more general balanced approach. On the other hand, if a patient who is 37 years old has frontal loss only that started at 23 in a slow manner and has changed very little in the last 2 to 3 years, then you could be more confident about the dense-packing approach. This reasoning is especially true if his family history does not indicate advanced loss or at least no significant loss in the vertex/crown areas.

Scalp and Hair Assessment

Next the patient's hair and scalp should be physically assessed. Dense packing is most indicated in cases of light-color skin and dark-colored hair, high number of hairs per square area in the donor area, or patients who have a fine quality to their hair. Patients with thicker caliber hairs or those with wiry or curly hair have the potential to achieve the look of density with fewer hairs per square area. Another element to assess is the degree of scalp elasticity if the harvesting is to be done by the strip method, which is important if dense packing is combined with a megasession or gigasession requiring a wider strip than average.

Most patients who are particularly keen on higher densities or low hairline restoration tend to be the least suitable! Because these patients tend to be the very young (early twenties) with early signs of loss, they frequently have unrealistic expectations. Combine this with a family history of likely progression to advanced baldness, and a scenario is created whereby the doctor has a big responsibility to counsel the patient properly and exert wisdom in the treatment approach without losing the patient to a lesser educated, inexperienced, or unscrupulous practice.

Medication Use and Smoking

Another consideration in the patient assessment is whether hair-stabilizing medications, such as minoxidil or finasteride, are being used. Caution should be exercised here when assuming the hair loss is stable because there is no guarantee that these stabilizing medications will continue to be as effective in the future. Indeed, there is no guarantee that the patient will continue to take it. The surgeon should also be wary of heavy smokers when considering dense packing. The patient's viable and healthy circulation in the scalp is heavily relied on to achieve a high survival rate and dense packing places a heavier burden on this. Heavy smokers may potentially have compromised their circulation; if in doubt, it may be advisable to do less grafts per square area per session.

Design Consultation

Finally, all aspects of determining hairline position and design, as well as size of area to be treated, should be discussed and agreed on with the patient at the consultation stage. The authors generally indicate that a session of dense packing will restore a look resembling about 30% of the original in the frontal scalp, but it is more like 25% in the vertex for the same number of grafts per area. The difference is due to the way the hairs fan out away from each other in the vertex. In cases where the transplanted hairs will be placed next to areas of no loss and a high hair to skin color ratio, the patient should always be told that he will very likely require at least a second operation to achieve near visual parity with the denser areas.

PROCEDURE
Dense Packing

In most patients, dense packing is performed in the frontal one-third to two-thirds of the scalp. In these cases, the patient is usually positioned on his back in a reclined manner with the head and neck elevated above chest level using the support of a headrest. As dense packing cases are usually longer procedures, this ensures patient comfort but also ease of access and good ergonomics from the operator's point of view. If the recipient area involves the vertex, then it maybe necessary to recline the patient less (ie, more of a sitting position). The patient may be required to actually sit up without a headrest if access is needed to the lower part of the vertex where the hairs grow in a downward direction.

Incisions

Routine recipient site anesthesia is described elsewhere but there are some points to pay attention to relevant to dense packing and larger and longer lasting operations. A larger number of incisions in very close proximity can be more traumatic, leading to obstructive bleeding and potential postoperative edema. To counter this, the authors routinely use the Abbasi tumescent solution of normal saline containing 1:100,000 epinephrine and 0.4 mg/mL triamcinolone acetate injected both intradermally for vasoconstriction and anti-inflammatory effect, and subcutaneously to move away from the deeper lying neurovascular bundle.

The smallest possible incisions need to be made to fit a large number of incisions per area comfortably and minimize tissue trauma in the process. Mostly 0.8-mm or 0.9-mm size blades or 20-G needles are the best to fit grafts of the neatly trimmed 2-hair follicular unit variety. For the single-hair grafts, 0.6-mm or 0.7-mm blades (22-G or 21-G needles) are required. When it comes to larger grafts of 3 hairs or more each, 1- to 1.2-mm blades (19-G or 18-G needles) are needed to ensure a comfortable fit (**Fig. 3**).

There are variations from patient to patient for the same size follicular unit and graft testing on a smaller number of incisions is recommended before committing to making thousands. The slightest variation could result in graft placing difficulties and increased risk of unnecessary mechanical trauma to the grafts. The authors usually test the 2-hair grafts after 20 incisions or so from 1 to 3 different technicians for both size and depth of incisions before proceeding to make the rest of them. If the incisions are made too shallow, the closely placed grafts will push each other out and may result in popping or healing, with a pimple effect. On the other hand, buried grafts caused by incisions that are too deep may cause skin surface pitting.

The recipient site incisions can be made in 1 of 2 formats according to personal preference and experience:

1. Parallel to the direction of the hair (sagittal)
2. Perpendicular to the direction of the hair (coronal)

The authors make the 1-hair and 2-hair graft slits parallel, and the 3-hair and 4-hair slits perpendicular. The latter aids the better spread of the hairs and a more natural look and also helps distinguish the appearance of these incisions to distinguish them better from the others. The 1-hair and 2-hair grafts probably do not make a significant difference whether placed in parallel or perpendicular incisions.

Grafts

- The usual approach to a case of dense packing in the frontal forelock and the top of the scalp is to create the hairline with single hair grafts of a depth of 0.5 to 1 cm at a rate of 40 to 50 per square centimeter.
- Grafting is continued with a similar concentration further back using the 2-hair grafts but with decreasing density as the top of the scalp is approached at an imaginary line joining the 2 ears. This latter zone is the typical area where the 3-haired and 4-haired grafts should be placed at a density of 15 to 25 per square centimeter, where they are not directly visible to the eye but still provide hair bulk (**Fig. 4**)

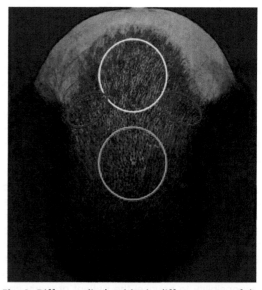

Fig. 4. Different slit densities in different areas of the recipient scalp. Up to 50 per square centimeter front (*yellow/red zones*) and down to 20 per square centimeter in the crown (*green zone*).

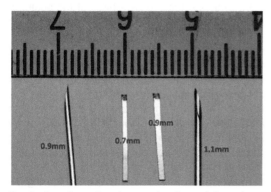

Fig. 3. A variety of tools to make the recipient sites.

Dense packing has the potential to slow down the graft placement process because of the tight spaces between the incisions and the difficulty in finding them when dealing with thousands of sites, therefore increasing the time that the grafts are out of the body. One of the aids in recent years that had certainly helped speed this process is illuminating the incision sites by applying 1% aqueous solution of methylene blue to the skin surface (**Fig. 5**). After wiping the surface clean, the dye remains in the incisions and eventually gets absorbed before the surgery is finished or within a day or 2.

GRAFT PREPARATION

To enable trouble-free dense packing, a large emphasis must be placed on the actual quality and consistency of the grafts so they can be placed predictably and efficiently. A typical session of dense packing involves a large number of grafts and therefore a skilled and properly educated and disciplined team of technicians is needed to ensure graft hydration and viability and a seamless process from the harvesting to the placing into the bald scalp.

POTENTIAL COMPLICATIONS OF DENSE PACKING

Intraoperatively, as discussed, one may get graft popping and recipient site bleeding, leading to significant slowing down of the placing process, thus increasing the risk of graft exposure and dehydration and prolonging the time that grafts spend outside the body. Ultimately this may decrease graft survival.

Postoperatively, decreased yield of the grafts and lower than anticipated appearance of hair density may result. This appearance can result from graft failure and/or compromised circulation

caused by a variety of reasons: overpacking of the grafts, larger grafts dense packed too closely, or incisions that are too large or too deep for the grafts. This last point not only can cause circulatory damage, but potentially may create dead space around the graft, resulting in a lack of sufficient graft oxygenation. Skin necrosis in the recipient area is a rare but devastating complication of such circulatory compromise. Finally, dense packing without the proper preparations as mentioned earlier may produce a higher risk of excessive but temporary bruising and tissue edema to the forehead and face, which may not be particularly harmful to the grafts, but certainly causes cosmetic distress to the patient.

Postoperative care, which is relevant to dense packing in particular, is as follows:

- Help to avoid postoperative edema by recipient area cooling with an ice pack for a few days after the procedure
- Emphasize the avoidance of strenuous activity for a few days
- Advise the patient to avoid heavy smoking
- Advise the patient that in some cases the hair transplant result may be delayed compared with the average transplant before it fully matures due to the extra demand on the tissues.
- Review the patient at 2 to 3 intervals (eg, 6 months, 12 months, and 18 months) to ensure patient satisfaction and reassurance.

REFERENCES

1. Nakatsui T. Maximum density, maximum vs cosmetic density. In: Unger WP, Shapiro R, Unger R, et al, editors. Hair transplantation. 5th edition. London: Informa Healthcare; 2011. p. 163–5.
2. Keene S. Cosmetic density, maximum density vs cosmetic density. In: Unger WP, Shapiro R, Unger R, et al, editors. Hair transplantation. 5th edition. London: Informa Healthcare; 2011. p. 165–8.
3. Nakatsui T. High-density follicular unit hair transplant. In: Unger WP, Shapiro R, Unger R, et al, editors. Hair transplantation. 5th edition. London: Informa Healthcare; 2011. p. 358–63.
4. Mayer M, Keene S, Perez-Meza D. Graft density production curve with dense packing. International Society of Hair Restoration Surgery Annual Meeting. Sydney, August 24–28, 2005.
5. Seager DJ. The one-pass hair transplant—a six year perspective. Hair Transplant Forum Int 2002; 12:76–96.
6. Nakatsui T, Wong J, Groot D. Survival of densely packed follicular unit grafts using the lateral slit technique. Dermatol Surg 2008;34:1016–25.

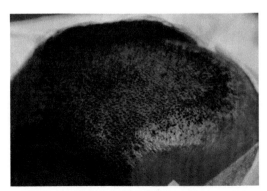

Fig. 5. View of the recipient incisions after methylene blue application.

7. Alhaddab M, Kohn T, Sidloi M. Effect of graft size, angle, and intergraft distance on dense packing in hair transplant. Dermatol Surg 2005;31(6):650–3 [discussion: 654].

8. Bernstein RM, Rassman WR. The logic of follicular unit transplantation. Dermatol Clin 1999;7(2):277–96.

9. Jiminez F, Ruifernandez JM. Distribution of human hair in follicular units: a mathematical model for estimating the donor size in follicular unit transplantation. Dermatol Surg 1999;2(4):294–8.

10. Tsilosani A. One hundred follicular units transplanted into 1 cm^2 can achieve a survival rate greater than 90%. Hair Transplant Forum Int 2009; 19(1):1, 6–7.

11. Headington JT. Microscopic anatomy of the human scalp. Arch Dermatol 1984;120:449–56.

An Analysis of Follicular Punches, Mechanics, and Dynamics in Follicular Unit Extraction

John P. Cole, MD

KEYWORDS

- Follicular unit extraction • Trephine • Serrounded punch • Hair transplant • Hair transplant surgery
- Follicular dissection • Follicular unit punch • Punch size • Follicle transection • Follicle splay

KEY POINTS

- Follicular unit extraction punches are made from a variety of metals.
- The degree of sharpness varies significantly from one punch manufacturer to another.
- Sharp punches require less axial and tangential force to penetrate the skin and dissect hair follicles.
- Minimizing axial and tangential forces helps to reduce the fluid movement of hair follicles during the dissection process.
- Force compression testing allows the degree of sharpness of any punch to be determined.
- Follicular groups consist of between 1 and 6 hair clusters. The frequency of cluster size varies from one person to another.
- The degree of hair splay varies from one person to another.
- Variation in punch size and incision depth allows the dissection of grafts to be customized to the individual patient and follicle transection to be minimized.

INTRODUCTION

Follicular unit extraction (FUE) is the latest major technical advancement in surgical hair restoration.[1–5] The methodology of FUE evolved from the basic principles of circular graft extraction that were introduced more than a half century ago. However, unlike macroscopic plug hair restoration, which used large circular punches, FUE is a refined procedure that requires high-power magnification and uses small circular trephine punches to isolate and extract individual follicular units (Fig. 1). The driving force for developing this technique was elimination of the linear donor scar that accompanies traditional strip harvesting. Shorter hair styles and a greater awareness for cosmesis in the donor site stimulated this movement.

The follicular unit is a delicate structure that is vulnerable to several types of injury during the extraction process. Transection is perhaps the most common injury observed with FUE (Fig. 2). Success with FUE depends on being able to predictably dissect excellent-quality grafts from the donor region. A high-quality trephine punch is mandatory for the accurate isolation of individual follicular units. The hair restoration surgeon must have a thorough understanding of the FUE punch and the nuances of FUE surgical technique to ensure consistent graft quality.

Disclosure: The author owns Cole Instruments, Inc.
Private Practice, 1070 Powers Place, Alpharetta, GA 30009, USA
E-mail address: john@forhair.com

Facial Plast Surg Clin N Am 21 (2013) 437–447
http://dx.doi.org/10.1016/j.fsc.2013.05.009

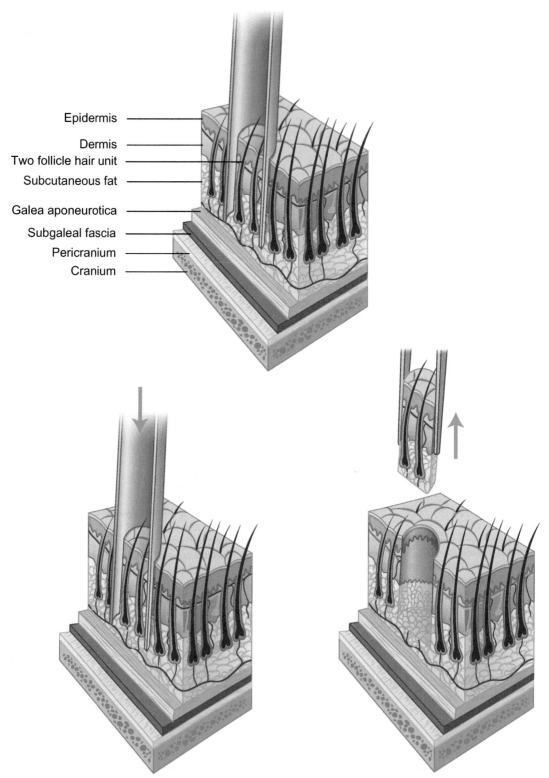

Epidermis

Dermis

Two follicle hair unit

Subcutaneous fat

Galea aponeurotica

Subgaleal fascia

Pericranium

Cranium

Fig. 1. A high-quality trephine punch is needed to accurately isolate an intact follicular unit graft. The ideal punch is small enough to minimize the size of the residual scalp defect and to avoid adjacent follicular unit damage, but large enough to prevent transection of any individual follicle within the isolated unit.

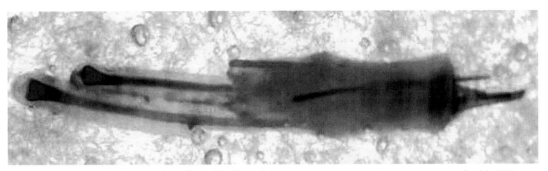

Fig. 2. Transection of follicles within the follicular unit is the most common injury encountered with FUE.

PUNCH METALLURGY

Surgical instruments are made of a variety of types of stainless steel. The type of steel depends on the function of the surgical instrument. FUE is a minimally invasive procedure dependent on a strong material with a sharp edge, thin wall, and small volume. Modern FUE punches are made of a variety of elements including Fe, C, Cr, Ni, Mn, Mo, Si, P, and S. Chromium makes stainless steel corrosion resistant. The other elements enhance other properties of the steel. Some materials, like 303 and 304 stainless steel, cannot be hardened by heat treatment. Other materials, like 17-4, 420, and 465, can be heat treated to harden them to a higher level. Hardness is a measure of the resistance to deformation or indentation. The hardness of steel is often measured using the Rockwell scale, which is a measure of indentation depth under load or indentation hardness.

PUNCH HANDLE AND TREPHINE

Many physical and technical factors affect punch cutting dynamics and their related tendency to produce tissue distortion and graft damage:

- Punch diameter
- Cutting edge location
- Punch wall thickness
- Punch metal type
- Punch edge sharpness
- Punch edge shape (smooth vs contoured)

There are 3 important diameters with respect to an FUE punch:

1. Internal diameter (distance between the internal margins of the punch)
2. External diameter (distance between the outer margins of the punch)
3. Cutting diameter (distance between the cutting edges of the punch) **(Fig. 3)**

The cutting edge is located in one of 3 important locations and the bevel is situated according to each:

1. Inside margin cutting edge with an outside bevel (type 5 punch)
2. Middle margin cutting edge with a middle bevel (type 4 punch)
3. Outside margin cutting edge with an inside bevel (type 3 punch)

The distance between the cutting edges determines the physical location of the incision on the skin. The location of the cutting edge also affects the fluid dynamics on the tissue during the punching process. An outside diameter (inside bevel) is designed to minimize the effect of the fluid dynamics during the punching process as the blunt bevel abuts tissue that has already been cut. The author has found that this design improves tissue cutting, reduces follicle trauma, and is best for high-quality extractions. The inside diameter (outside bevel) punch cuts a narrow hole in which the blunt outside bevel is forced into a hole that is smaller than the outer diameter of the punch. This punch style seems to have the greatest deleterious impact on follicle fluid dynamics and could increase the risk of a lower-quality graft. The middle diameter or middle bevel punch has the cutting edge somewhere between the external and internal punch margins, and seems to have an intermediate impact on adverse follicle fluid dynamics and graft quality.

Tissue distortion is also influenced by the thickness of the punch wall and by the rate of punch insertion. In all instances, a thin punch wall reduces the resistance as the punch is introduced into the skin.

A titanium nitride (TIN) coating helps to improve the life of the cutting edge on punches made of soft steel. However, these punches lack the degree of sharpness that modified hardened steel punches possess. TIN-coated punches are perhaps the most popular of all the sharp punches

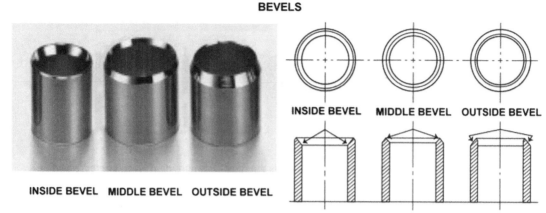

BEVELS

INSIDE BEVEL   MIDDLE BEVEL   OUTSIDE BEVEL

INSIDE BEVEL   MIDDLE BEVEL   OUTSIDE BEVEL

Fig. 3. Punch cutting edge styles.

and they are the least expensive. The punches range from 0.6 mm up to 1.5 mm in diameter depending on physician preference. The internal diameters of these punches decrease after a few millimeters (**Fig. 4**). The internal diameters of punches vary, depending on the arbitrary discretion of the manufacturer and the vendor. However, some manufacturers and vendors label their punches with inaccurate internal diameters. Hardened steel punches have a razor sharp edge that minimizes friction as the punch enters the skin and results in a reduced axial force.

There are multiple handles available that can accept a variety of stainless steel punches. A handle designed to precisely limit cutting depth

is available to further boost the accuracy of the hardened steel punches.

CONTOURED SURFACE PUNCHES

Two contour surface punch designs are available. The triple wave punch is made of 303 stainless steel and titanium nitride coating. It is designed with elevated waves that reduce friction by limiting the total surface area of the punch in contact with the skin. The second is the Serrounded punch (Cole Instruments), which is made of hardened steel (**Fig. 5**). This punch decreases the surface area in contact with the skin, thereby reducing friction and minimizing the axial force required to

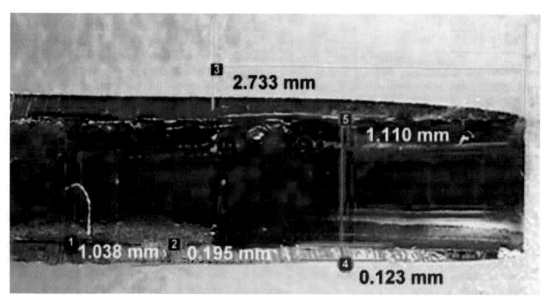

3 2.733 mm

5 1.110 mm

1 1.038 mm **2** 0.195 mm

4 0.123 mm

Fig. 4. A cross section of a TIN-coated cannula punch showing the variation in punch wall thickness, as well as internal diameters, as a function of distance from the cutting edge.

some individual interactions, such as the interaction of the punch and tissue at initial contact.

For example, with a rotating or oscillating punch, a torque is applied to the punch by hand or by a mechanical means. Torque is the rotational equivalent of a force. Just as a force can do work by being applied through some distance, torque can only do work by being applied through some angle. The rotation per minute (rpm) is the rate at which that angle changes, or the rate of rotation.

In the case of a motor power, the torque results from the motor horsepower and the speed. $T = k \times \dfrac{HP}{n}$, where T = motor torque (in lb-ft), k = constant, HP = motor horsepower, and n = speed of the motor shaft in rpm. Also, $T = Ft \times R$, where T = torque in lb-ft, Ft = tangential force, and R = the moment arm (punch radius). The tangential force at the punch cutting edge thus can be determined from the two relations.

Just as a force is a push or a pull, a torque can be thought of as a twist. During dissection, a tangential force is applied on the contact surface and an axial force is applied in the direction of the axis of the punch. The tangential force results from a torque applied to the rotating punch. The torque on the punch produces a force at the peripheral point of the punch. The direction of the force depends on the direction of rotation of the punch. At the initial contact of the punch to the tissue, the punch applies a force in the direction of rotation and the tissue applies resistance to the rotation. In such a case, the following may take place.

- Because of the friction between the punch edge and the tissue surface, a friction force opposing the applied force results. The friction force depends on the applied tangential force, normal or axial force, and the friction coefficient between the two surfaces.
- If the applied force exceeds the friction or resistance force, either the tissue is pulled in the direction of rotation or the punch tends to rotate over the tissue in the direction of rotation.
- If the punch is prevented from rolling, the force results in a shear stress in the tissue. A shear stress is a stress state in which the stress is parallel to the surface of the material. When the shear stress exceeds the shear strength of the tissue, the tissue cracks or fails. Although this is a basic fact, it remains a simplistic analysis because the resulting stresses and the property of the material at contact are complicated.
- The shear stress τ developed is directly proportional to the tangential force Ft and

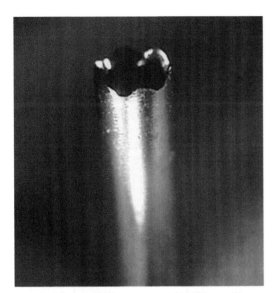

Fig. 5. The surrounded punch cutting edge showing multiple cutting edges.

penetrate the skin. The Serrounded punch has a thinner wall, has more cutting edges, and is sharper than the triple wave punch.

The author typically prefers the contoured punch for mechanical rotation and the standard Cole Instrument (CI) punch for manual extraction. The standard CI punch often seems to work better with oscillation rather than continuous rotation. Sometimes the Serrounded punch yields higher quality grafts using oscillation rather than continuous rotation.

ANALYSIS OF FOLLICULAR DISSECTION

The analysis of tissue cutting in hair transplant surgery is complex, especially for a follicular isolation procedure. The complexity results mainly because soft tissue is composed of layers with different modulus and elastoplastic properties. The mechanical characteristics of homogeneous materials are not applicable to skin. Skin has no unique, single Young modulus (a measure of the stiffness of an elastic material), or shear modulus, because such properties for skin vary depending on the strain applied. Biological materials typically have stress-strain diagrams with an elastic part, which can be linear or nonlinear. In addition, the mode of load application is time dependent and, with a round punch acting at some angle to the surface of the tissue, is complex. The bevel on the punch adds even greater complexity to the cutting procedure.

One approach to help understand punch cutting dynamics is to simplify the properties and analyze inversely proportional to the area of contact A ($\tau = Ft/A$). If the contact area is small, as in the case of a sharp punch, the resulting shear stress is high. Thus, the shear strength of the tissue is exceeded more quickly and the tissue fails or is cut more quickly. A dull punch has a larger contact area, which results in a lower shear stress compared with an equivalent-diameter sharp punch. To exceed the shear strength of the tissue, a higher force is needed with the dull punch. A higher force means a higher torque. A punch with a higher torque results in a higher twist or distortion of the tissue and is also difficult to control and to center about the follicle axis. These variables are the main causes of transection.

FUE requires an understanding of fluid dynamics and the physics involved in the removal of the grafts. A full understanding of these variables is beyond the scope of this article. However, a force applied to the skin results in a reaction by both the various skin layers and the hair follicle(s) comprising a follicular unit. The cutting of skin with a dull instrument requires more force than does cutting with a sharp instrument. The term dull punch is a misnomer in that this device is a punch that is not very sharp (ie, a punch that is incompletely dull). Although it cuts the skin with less force than a completely dull instrument, it can transect hair follicles despite its nonsharp edge. A dull punch or one that is not very sharp requires significant mechanical energy, and the excessive force limits manual control. Any punch driven by a force great enough to cut epidermis and dermis can also cut a hair follicle because the outer root sheath (ORS) and follicle are more delicate than the epidermis and dermis.

Excision of the follicle requires 2 forces: an axial (penetrating force) and a tangential force (rotation or oscillation). Because hair exits the body at an acute angle, the inferior margin of the punch makes first contact with the skin (**Fig. 6**). A large axial force along this inferior margin results in an inferior displacement of the follicle (**Fig. 7**), which can lead to follicle amputation if the displacing force moves the follicles outside the lumen of the punch.

A predominantly tangential force incises into the skin without displacing the follicles as long as torsion of the graft does not occur. A sharp punch minimizes torsion while maximizing the benefits of a tangential force. If a predominantly axial force is used, the surgeon must attempt to achieve an equal force along the perimeter of the punch so as to minimize follicle deflection.

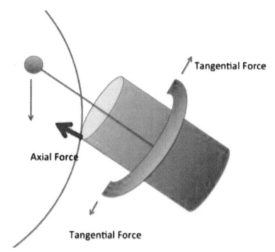

Fig. 6. The acute emergence angle of hair follicles results in a greater axial force on the inferior aspect of the skin. A predominantly tangential force reduces inferior displacement of the hair bulb, whereas a predominantly axial force increases inferior displacement of the hair bulb.

Friction is a resistive force that curtails movement of the punch through the skin. It is a function of the circumference of a punch and the depth of punch insertion (**Fig. 8**). Large punches and deep extractions increase resistance during follicular unit dissection.

FORCE COMPRESSION TESTING

This sharpness testing procedure is needed to evaluate punch cutting edges, to establish reference punch sharpness data, and to monitor the consistency of the quality of the manufactured punch cutting edges. Sharpness testing measures the force required to penetrate through a

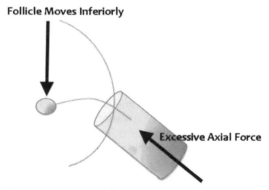

Fig. 7. Excessive axial force results in inferior displacement of the hair bulb and increases the risk of follicle transection.

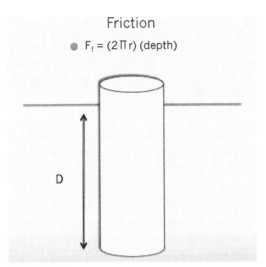

Fig. 8. Frictional force increases as the circumference of the punch and the depth of incision increase.

specimen with known material properties and parameters. A compression force gauge may be used to determine the punching force as a measure of sharpness. The punch is mounted with the axis in a vertical position and the cutting edge facing downwards. A test media of silicon rubber with thickness of 0.8 mm (1/32 in) is placed on a horizontal support surface or substrate. The test media used has a minimum wearing effect on the cutting edge and the support material should give a much lower punching force reading to avoid confusion and prevent punch edge damage.

We lowered each test punch on the test media slowly at constant velocity. If a manual testing machine was used, the feed rate was kept as constant as possible. During testing, the punch cuts through the rubber media into the softer support material. The punching force was plotted against the time or distance of punch travel as it cut through the media thickness. The cutting force increased with increasing travel or time and decreased abruptly when the punch cut through the medium. The punch travel was stopped after seeing the decrease in force value. The maximum force reading on the force-time plot of the force gauge was used as the measure of sharpness. At the beginning of each new test and after each cut through the test media, the medium was moved to a new position and a new punch was replaced. Using these parameters and a Dillon Model GTX force gauge, we assessed a variety of different punches manufactured by different vendors and plotted the force reading for each punch (**Fig. 9**).

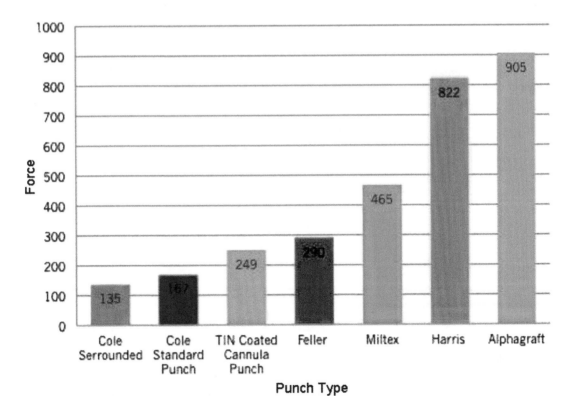

Fig. 9. Surgical punch force analysis compares the sharpness of a variety of commercially available punches.

PUNCH SIZE VARIATION

In 2003, the author conducted a study evaluating the benefits of punches 0.75 mm in diameter. The healing from these extraction sites appeared to be the same as the healing with 1.0-mm extraction sites when intact follicular units were extracted. However, the follicle transection or amputation rate was significantly greater with the smaller punches. After this, the author evaluated punches of 1.25 mm in diameter and discovered that the healing was identical to that of 1.0-mm punches when the intact follicular unit was extracted. Based on this knowledge, the author began to vary punch diameter based on the follicle transection rate. If the rates were high, the author increased the size of the punch. Variation in punch size along with the use of sharper punches resulted in a decline in the mean follicle transection rate from 8% in 2003 to less than 3% by 2006. Some follicular groupings are larger than others, and some follicular groups have more follicular splay. When large groups or significant splay is present, the author discovered that larger punches allowed a lower follicle transection rate with identical healing. However, follicle splay is sometimes so great that even a larger punch size does not overcome all the potential follicle transection caused by the splay.

PUNCH INCISION GEOMETRY BASED ON PUNCH SIZE AND HAIR GROWTH ANGLE
Length of Incision

The incision length created by a punch is based on the angle of punch insertion, which depends on the angle of hair growth. Incising the skin at an angle with a circular punch creates an elliptical opening with a long axis length that is equal to the diameter of the punch divided by the sine of θ where θ is the angle of hair emergence from the skin (**Fig. 10**).

$$\text{Length} = \text{punch diameter} \div \text{Sin } \theta$$

The incision length increases as the diameter of the punch increases and as the angle of hair growth decreases.

Depth of Incision

The punch typically enters the skin along the axis of hair growth. When the punch enters the skin at the acute angle along the axis of hair growth, the inferior margin of the punch always enters the skin deeper than the superior margin of the punch (**Fig. 11**). The acute angle of hair growth creates a disparity in the incisional depths of the superior and the inferior aspects of the punch as it incises down the follicle along the axis of hair growth. This increased depth is equal to the diameter of the punch divided by the tangent of the angle that the punch enters the skin (θ_1).

$$\text{Depth} = \text{punch diameter} \div \text{Tan } \theta_1$$

The cutting depth of the inferior punch margin increases as the diameter of the punch increases and as the angle of hair growth decreases. At approximately 27° to the skin, the inferior margin of the punch incises to a depth twice as deep as the superior margin.

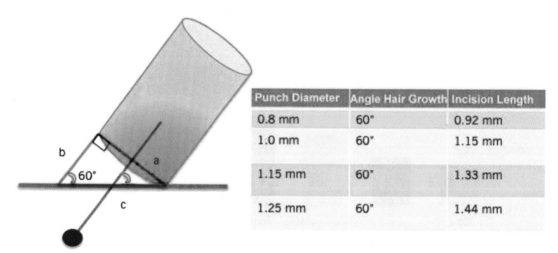

Punch Diameter	Angle Hair Growth	Incision Length
0.8 mm	60°	0.92 mm
1.0 mm	60°	1.15 mm
1.15 mm	60°	1.33 mm
1.25 mm	60°	1.44 mm

Fig. 10. The major axis of a punch wound is proportional to the diameter of the punch (a) and inversely proportional to the angle of incision (Θ). The wound length (c) increases as the punch diameter increases and as the angle of incision decreases. c = a/sin Θ. (b) indicates the direction of hair growth.

Depth of Punch Based on Angle of Hair Growth

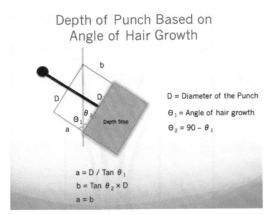

$$D = \text{Diameter of the Punch}$$
$$\theta_1 = \text{Angle of hair growth}$$
$$\theta_2 = 90 - \theta_1$$

$$a = D / \tan \theta_1$$
$$b = \tan \theta_2 \times D$$
$$a = b$$

Fig. 11. A punch following a parallel path to the angle of hair emergence results in the inferior margin of the punch entering the skin deeper than the superior margin. The disparity in depth between the superior margin and the inferior margin increases as the angle of hair emergence decreases and as the diameter of the punch increases.

FACTORS AFFECTING FOLLICLE DISSECTION IN FUE

To best appreciate graft quality problems associated with FUE, the surgeon needs to have a thorough understanding of microscopic follicle and follicular unit anatomy. Each individual follicle is a complex miniorgan formed by multiple mesenchymal and epithelial cell layers. More than 20 distinct cell populations contribute to the formation of individual mature follicles, many of which are arranged in concentric layers that extend out from a central core (**Fig. 12**). The physical properties of each individual cell line vary with respect to cell size, cell strength, layer thickness, and adhesive bond to the neighboring cell layer(s). Variations in these physical properties influence each patient's predisposition to complications relating to the cutting, rotating, and traction forces imposed in and around each follicle.

Follicular groupings tend to exit the scalp similarly to flowers out of the neck of a vase. The follicles are closer together on the surface of the skin, but progressively farther apart as they move toward their position in the adipose (**Fig. 13**). This movement away from one another is termed follicle splay and individual variation is possible. In some, splay is minimal, whereas in others it can be significant. In a few, most follicles follow a similar direction, whereas 1 or 2 follicles in the same surface grouping diverge in a different direction. The degree and type of splay can affect the transection rate of follicles. Using a larger punch often accommodates splay. At other times, the

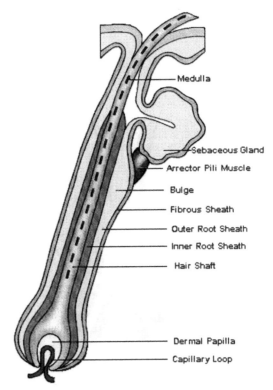

Fig. 12. Follicle anatomy. (*Modified from* Vogt A, McElwee KJ, Blume-Peytavi U. Biology of the hair follicle. In: Blume-Peytavi U, Tosti A, Whiting DA, et al, editors. Hair Growth and Disorders. Berlin: Springer; 2008. p. 4; with kind permission from Springer Science+Business Media.)

physician might use a smaller punch and target only a few hairs within the larger follicular cluster.

Elastic skin often complicates the extraction process. One way to overcome elasticity is to excise the grafts slowly with minimal axial force. Another is to apply tension on the donor area so that elasticity is reduced. Torsion is common with rotating mechanical extractors, but does not occur with oscillating manual extraction. Limiting the depth of the incision minimizes torsion. Another way to minimize torsion is to cut slowly down the direction of hair growth in progressive steps. With each shallow incision, the skin is allowed to relax before incising deeper. Torsion may also be limited by use of an oscillating extractor; however, follicle transection is often higher with oscillating extractors.

Tethering of grafts is a reference to the attachment of the ORS to the adipose. When the attachment of the ORS to the adipose is strong, a deep incision is required to remove the graft from the adipose. When the attachment is normal, the author may limit his incision to 2 mm and refers to this as a zero. When the attachment is strong,

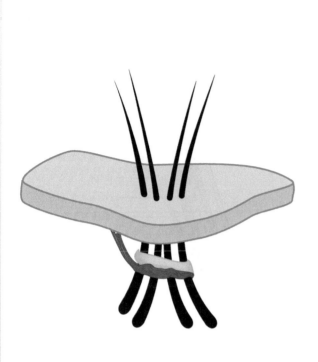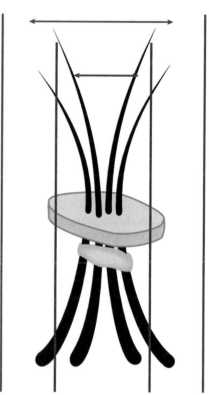

Fig. 13. Follicles can show varying degrees of splay as they extend deeper into the adipose. Blue lines show how a punch width determined by follicular grouping at the skin surface would damage the 2 outer follicles. Red lines show how a larger punch would preserve the unit, albeit at the expense of a larger surface wound.

the incision may require an incision up to 3 mm and the author calls this a +2. When the attachment is weak, the incision may be limited to less than 2 mm, and the author calls this a −1.

Other factors that play a role include the strength of the attachment of the ORS to the inner root sheath (IRS). If this attachment is unusually weak, there is a tendency for the ORS to separate

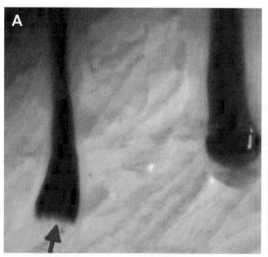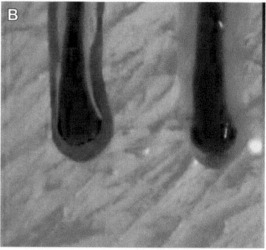

Fig. 14. (A) On the left is a plucked follicle that is missing the dermal papilla (*red arrow*) and the inferior portion of the ORS. The plucked follicle on the right is intact. (B) Orange fill represents the detached portion of the ORS and dermal papilla that remained in the extraction site.

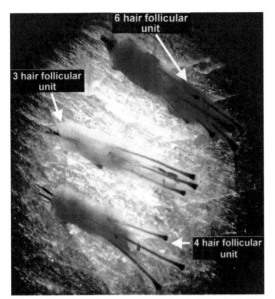

Fig. 15. High-quality multihair grafts are achievable on a consistent basis with the use of proper instrumentation and excellent surgical technique.

from the IRS, in which case the follicle may be removed without the inferior aspect of the ORS and the dermal papilla (**Fig. 14**). A deeper incision is often required to remove the graft intact when this attachment is weak.

Less commonly, the dermal sheath including the ORS and IRS are friable and easily damaged during punch insertion. In such instances, 1 or more follicles within some of the follicular units are missing their ORS and IRS during the extraction process. In this instance, greater caution must be exercised, but there is no specific protocol other than a gentle technique that can prevent the problem.

SUMMARY

Excellent graft quality requires technical expertise, familiarity with punch design, and a thorough knowledge of punch and soft tissue dynamics. With FUE, physicians find that no single punch or method works equally well for all patients, and that versatility is key to ensuring consistently high graft quality from patient to patient. The surgeon should learn both manual and mechanical methods of graft removal because the transection rate is too high when only mechanical devices are used for all patients. The author's success with FUE is a result of variations in punches and incision depth (**Fig. 15**). It is logical that variation in the use of mechanical and manual extraction techniques will also have an effect on individual patient transection rates. By using these strategies it is often possible to achieve transection rates of less than 3%.

REFERENCES

1. Available at: http://www.engineersedge.com/stainless_steel.htm. Accessed February 15, 2013.
2. Available at: http://en.wikipedia.org/wiki/Surgical_stainless_steel. Accessed February 15, 2013.
3. Available at: http://www.wpiinc.com/index.php/vmchk/Surgical-Instruments.html. Accessed February 15, 2013.

FRICTION AND FORCE REPRESENTATION

4. Meriam JL, Kraige LG. Engineering mechanics, SI version: statics. 6th edition. John Wiley & Sons; 2008. Technology & Engineering.
5. Stephenson DA, Agapiou JS. Metal cutting theory and practice. CRC Press; 2006.

Optimal Graft Growth

Jerry E. Cooley, MD

KEYWORDS

- Poor growth • Graft survival • Stereomicroscopes • Graft transection • Graft trauma
- Holding solutions • Ischemia-reperfusion injury • Storage injury • Oxygenation
- ATP-adenosine triphosphate

KEY POINTS

- Achieving optimal growth in hair transplantation is a critical part of obtaining excellent results and high patient satisfaction.
- The most important factors determining graft survival are avoiding physical trauma to the grafts and ensuring that the oxygenation needs of transplanted follicles are met.
- Hair follicles that are physically intact have a much higher chance of survival than transected ones.
- Graft dehydration from loss of intracellular water is very damaging to cells of the hair follicle.
- Grafts that have been roughly handled and crushed by forceps have a significantly lower growth rate than grafts that have been handled gently.
- Variation in scalp oxygenation may be the single biggest factor explaining variability in graft survival.
- The use of liposomal adenosine triphosphate may help replace graft oxygen needs that are not fully met by patients' vascular beds.
- Biochemical injury may occur to the graft tissue while it is outside the body or after it has been transplanted.

INTRODUCTION

Achieving optimal growth in hair transplantation is a critical part of obtaining excellent results and high patient satisfaction. For the purposes of this review, *optimal growth* refers to the highest possible percent survival of implanted hair follicles as well as the quality (eg, caliber) of the resulting hair that grows. Obviously other factors are also critical to the quality of the result, such as hairline design, graft angle and direction, and graft distribution. These concepts are discussed in other articles in this publication.

Many experienced surgeons quietly acknowledge among themselves that graft survival is not consistently as high as is publicly stated, partly because of the natural tendency to avoid publicly admitting to suboptimal results. Furthermore, in the era of follicular unit transplantation (FUT) in which a typical case is 2000 grafts and often

more, it can be very difficult to accurately establish the percentage of grafts that survive. Nevertheless, all surgeons should be aware of the factors related to graft survival and develop their surgical technique accordingly.

This article provides a brief overview of the factors related to graft survival. Relatively little is available in the way of valid, controlled scientific studies. This point may seem surprising to novice surgeons given the advanced stage of development of modern hair transplantation techniques. It is worthwhile to consider the reasons for this lack of quality evidence-based research. Perez-Meza and Shapiro[1] discussed the reasons why tracking hair transplant outcomes is so difficult, and the reader is referred to this excellent review. These reasons include the long time period until a final result is achieved, difficulty in counting hairs among the thousands planted to determine survival rates, and spotty follow-up by patients.

Disclosure: Investigator and investor in liposomal adenosine triphosphate (ATP).
Carolina Dermatology Hair Center, 10650 Park Road, Suite 310, Charlotte, NC 28210, USA
E-mail address: jcooley@haircenter.com

Facial Plast Surg Clin N Am 21 (2013) 449–455
http://dx.doi.org/10.1016/j.fsc.2013.06.003
1064-7406/13/$ – see front matter © 2013 Elsevier Inc. All rights reserved.

Over the years, surgeons have attempted to study factors that might affect growth by performing small study boxes on patients' scalps. Although well intended, these studies lack the proper size and design to eliminate bias and chance as chief reasons for the observed results. Parsley and colleagues[2] have reviewed some of these prior studies.

Nevertheless, important principles can be identified based on the science of transplantation as well as case reports and the opinions of experienced surgeons. The most important factors determining graft survival are avoiding physical trauma to the grafts (transection, crushing, dehydration) and ensuring that the oxygenation needs of transplanted follicles are met. There are other factors that may also be important, and these factors are discussed later (**Table 1**).

PHYSICAL TRAUMA

Hair follicles that are physically intact have a much higher chance of survival than transected ones. This fact is a major rationale for microscopically controlled FUT, first described by Limmer.[3] By using a single scalpel blade for donor excision, transection is minimized along the wound edge. The strip is then slivered and dissected using stereomicroscopes, whereby a 10 × magnification provides for superior visualization of the follicle. A study performed by the author involving multiple experienced surgeons showed that those who used microscopes had half as many transected hair follicles in random samples of grafts than those who did not use microscopes.[4]

Microscopic Dissection

Without the use of microscopes, follicular transection is very likely to occur to varying degrees in all cases. Some individuals have claimed that this is not that important because transected follicles sometimes grow anyway. The probability of follicle regeneration is directly related to the level of transection.[5] If less than half of the follicle is present, regeneration rarely occurs. The author thinks that follicle regeneration is an unpredictable process and that the best way to ensure good growth is to transplant physically intact follicles. In the author's practice, the change to follicular unit grafting with all microscopic dissection has been the biggest factor in increased graft survival.

There are situations in which microscopic dissection is especially critical:

- In patients with extremely curly hair (eg, black patients)
- In those with extensive scarring in the donor tissue from prior procedures

Many of the follicles will be transected if they are not carefully dissected under the stereomicroscope.

There are situations in which the patients' hair characteristics allow for easier dissection and may not require stereomicroscopes. Asians, for example, generally have dark, straight hair, allowing for easier visualization.

Table 1 Factors influencing hair graft survival	
Problem	**Solution**
Physical Trauma	
Transection	Microscopic dissection
Dehydration	Hydration, humidifier (?)
Crushing	Careful, gentle technique
Vascular/Oxygenation Factors	
Baseline blood flow & vascular reserve	Effect of sites on blood flow: size, depth, density of incisions
	Postoperative treatments (?)
	Liposomal ATP
	Other: vasodilators, hyperbaric oxygen
Biochemical injury Storage injury Ischemia-reperfusion injury	Optimized holding solution (eg, HypoThermosol [BioLife Solutions, Bothell, WA]/ATP)
Infection	Clean technique, patient hygiene, antibiotics (?)
Patient disruption	Postoperative instructions
Idiopathic (X factor)	

Many surgeons think that they can have consistently low transection rates with simple loupes and backlighting for all cases. On the other hand, most practices see patients from a variety of backgrounds, and using microscopic dissection on all cases eliminates trying to guess beforehand whether use of microscopes will be necessary. Even in cases when the hair is easy to dissect, the use of the microscope allows closer dissection and sorting of fine hairs for the hairline.

Patients with gray or white hair also present challenges in visualization. Even with the use of the microscope, visualization can be difficult. Some surgeons have found that injecting or soaking the donor strip with methylene blue can be helpful in increasing the contrast between follicles and the surrounding tissue. Others have found that dying the donor hair before harvesting with over-the-counter mustache dye is a useful aid. The author has found the latter approach to be particularly helpful. Many find it helpful to leave more tissue around the follicles to avoid transection. However, this then requires larger recipient sites to ensure a proper fit.

Graft Dehydration

Graft dehydration from loss of intracellular water is very damaging to cells of the hair follicle.[6] With increasingly larger sessions of increasingly more grafts, there is more opportunity for these small grafts to be exposed to the air during dissection and while awaiting placement. There is widespread consensus for the need to keep grafts well hydrated. Achieving this requires constant monitoring of the staff. Some staff, in an effort to cut quickly, leave dissected grafts piled up before putting them in holding solution, increasing exposure time to the air and increasing the risk of dehydration. One factor that can affect graft drying is the ambient humidity in the operatory environment, having an impact especially when forced air conditioning or heat is in use. In the author's experience, having a humidifier running constantly during the surgery helps add moisture to the air and reduces graft drying.

There is some controversy as to whether grafts should be submerged in graft-holding solution or placed at the air-liquid interface on moistened gauze pads. Some strongly advocate the former, whereas other successful surgeons use the latter, both with excellent results.

Graft Crush Injury

Crushing of the grafts during placement is another potentially lethal factor. Given the small size of today's grafts, it is not surprising that the forceps may crush them during placement into small recipient sites, such as 22-gauge needle or 0.6-mm incisions. One point worth highlighting is that the bulb is very sensitive to crush injury. Because of its melanin content, the bulb is often the darkest part of the follicle and may seem sturdy. However, formation of the keratinized hair shaft does not occur until just above the bulb. Grasping the bulb with forceps too aggressively can easily rupture the dermal sheath and cause the dermal papilla to be lost.[7] Grafts that have been roughly handled and crushed by forceps have a significantly lower growth rate than grafts that have been handled gently.[8]

Techniques to minimize crush injury during placement include the following:

- Site dilators
- Implantation devices
- Special forceps
- The 2-forceps technique
- The stick-and-place technique

The last technique, developed by Dr Bobby Limmer, consists of placing the graft immediately after each site is made by a hypodermic needle.[2] Dr David Seager[9] was also a strong advocate of this approach. The author uses a modified stick-and-place technique whereby all incisions are premade. Then the placers will have their forceps in their dominant hand and a dull hypodermic needle (eg, 22 gauge) in their nondominant hand. The dull needle can be used to reopen the incision, if necessary, as the graft is gently placed into the site. The tip of the needle also acts as a tiny fingertip to hold the graft in place as the forceps are withdrawn, which reduces manipulation by the forceps.

VASCULAR/OXYGENATION FACTORS IN HAIR GRAFTS

Grafts must be revascularized to survive after being transplanted. This process takes several days; until completed, the graft must get its nourishment from oxygen diffusion and plasmatic imbibition. The graft imbibes wound exudate by capillary action through the spongelike structure of the graft tissue and through the follicular blood vessels. This process determines graft survival until circulation is reestablished. Revascularization of the graft occurs by a poorly understood mechanism. Vessels in the recipient area sprout and anastomose with the vessels of the graft. Full circulation to the graft should be restored by 7 days after grafting. To survive, the graft must adhere within the site, passively absorb enough oxygen, imbibe sufficient nutrients, and then be successfully revascularized.

Graft Failure to Survive

Grafts may fail to survive because of a failure in the revascularization process. Recipient areas that have scar tissue, whether from previous transplants, scalp reductions, or other trauma, may have an inadequate vascular network to oxygenate the graft during imbibition and revascularization. Stimulating angiogenesis is one of the perceived benefits of advanced techniques including platelet-rich plasma[10] and the use of porcine urinary bladder matrix.[11]

Likewise, patients who smoke tobacco may have inadequate baseline oxygenation of the skin and may be more likely to have poor growth than nonsmokers.

Graft Survival Variability

Scalp oxygenation

Variation in scalp oxygenation may be the single biggest factor explaining variability in graft survival from one patient to another. The author conducted a study measuring surface oxygen on the scalps of more than 80 patients using an oximeter, which is based on visible light spectroscopy (T-stat, Spectros Corporation, Portola Valley, CA, USA) and has been used to predict flap viability.[12] Various points on the scalp and reference points on the fingertip and ankle were measured. Across this patient population, skin oxygen levels showed consistently high values in the fingertip, consistently low values at the ankle, and a broad range of values for the scalp. Furthermore, readings taken in the postoperative period showed marked variations in surface oxygen, with some patients demonstrating increases more than the baseline and others showing a decrease, suggesting the possibility of vascular reserve that may operate in some patients.[13]

Blood supply in recipient bed

In addition to preexisting vascular compromise, the blood supply in the recipient bed can be overstressed by excessive size, depth, and density of incision sites. Some think that placing grafts at a high density (more than 35 FUs/cm^2) with anything larger than a 19-gauge needle overstresses the vascular network and results in poor growth. Others think that the growth rate drops off at densities of more than 35 FUs/cm^2 regardless of the incision size. However, this has been challenged by some who have claimed excellent growth at densities of more than 60 grafts per square centimeter.[2]

Note for the beginning hair graft surgeon: In the author's opinion, beginning surgeons should focus on achieving consistently excellent growth with well-trimmed grafts and smaller incision sites (19-gauge needle size and smaller) placed at moderate densities (20–35 FUs/cm^2). When consistently high growth is achieved, the surgeon can attempt denser packing of grafts (more than 35 FUs/cm^2). All available evidence points to a limit that can be stressed by aggressive site making and implantation of too many oxygen dependent grafts in a given area of scalp.

Incision depth

Besides size and density, the incision depth into the skin may have an effect on the revascularization and survival of the grafts. Most surgeons think that ideally the incision should be just deep enough into the subdermal space to allow the graft to sit in its normal anatomic location without injuring deeper blood vessels. Incisions that are too superficial (ie, within the dermis) or too deep (ie, in the deeper subcutaneous layer) may result in poor growth.

Injecting adequate tumescent solution helps avoid making incisions that are too deep. Most surgeons agree that the tumescence should be injected superficially into the dermal/subcutaneous space, rather than subgaleal. Incisions may be placed parallel (sagittal) or perpendicular (coronal or lateral) to the natural direction of hair growth. Some who have tried the lateral slit technique have experienced decreased or delayed growth. Others claim growth is as good as or better than standard parallel incisions.

Note for the beginning hair graft surgeon: The author recommends that beginning surgeons use sagittal incisions until their technique has been mastered and routinely excellent growth has been achieved. In addition, most experienced surgeons agree that making sites very acutely may have esthetic benefits but that this places a greater stress on the blood supply, and density should be adjusted downward accordingly.

Use of liposomal adenosine triphosphate

One method to replace graft oxygen needs that may not be fully met by the patients' vascular beds, is to use postoperative liposomal adenosine triphosphate (ATP). Ultimately, oxygen is only required as a means for the cell to generate ATP, which then provides for all of the energy needs of the cell. Use of liposomal ATP was shown to enhance graft survival and graft quality when used as an additive to the holding solution and as a postoperative spray.[14,15] The unique liposomal structure of this compound allows for intracellular penetration of the normally hydrophilic ATP. By adopting this postoperative ATP spray, the author thinks that cases of unexplained poor growth have dramatically decreased in his practice and that overall graft survival has been improved in all patients.

BIOCHEMICAL FACTORS IN HAIR GRAFTS

Although physical trauma and graft oxygenation may be the most important determinants of graft growth, biochemical factors likely play a contributing role. This point becomes important when considering which holding solution to place the grafts in before placement. The author has reviewed the variety of available holding solutions and the studies examining and comparing them.[16] Although most clinics use chilled saline, it is worth considering how saline lacks many of the key elements of an ideal holding solution[17]:

1. Correct osmolarity
2. Correct pH and buffering capability
3. Antioxidants
4. Nutrients

In organ transplantation (eg, livers and kidneys), surgeons consider biochemical factors to be critical in predicting graft survival, assuming immunologic rejection has not occurred. A tremendous amount of research has been performed to identify and overcome biochemical injury to transplanted tissue and organs, research that has direct implications for hair transplantation. This biochemical injury may occur to the tissue while it is outside the body (storage injury) or after it has been transplanted (ischemia-reperfusion injury).[18]

Once the donor strip is removed, the cells within the tissue are immediately cut off from their supply of oxygen, glucose, and other necessary nutrients. Oxygen and glucose are required for the production of ATP, the cell's primary fuel. When oxygen is no longer available, the cells switch from aerobic to anaerobic metabolism, which does not produce enough ATP to meet the cell's energy requirements. The lack of energy supplies and the absence of other necessary ingredients lead to apoptosis, or programmed cell death, resulting in storage injury of the tissue. If enough cells within the follicle undergo apoptosis, the follicle as a whole might not survive to produce hair. If only a portion of cells succumb to apoptotic death, then the follicle may survive but produce finer, weaker hair.

Ischemia-Reperfusion Injury

Ischemia-reperfusion injury (IRI) is the biochemical injury to the grafts that occurs after they have undergone a period of low oxygen (ischemia) after harvesting and during preparation and are then implanted in the recipient sites where they are exposed to oxygen (reperfusion). It is an automatic reaction that has been well studied but is only partially understood. What is known is that IRI results from the formation of reactive oxygen species (ROS). Formation of ROS occurs in both the transplanted cells as well as the neutrophils present in the recipient tissue. These free radicals can be thought of as molecular poison that injures the cell. Damaged cells within the hair follicle may result in suboptimal growth or weaker, finer hairs. IRI has been demonstrated to occur in transplanted hair follicles.[18]

Efforts to reduce storage injury and IRI have led to experimenting with different storage solutions. Three broad categories of holding solutions exist:

1. Intravenous holding solutions (eg, normal saline, lactated Ringer)
2. Cell culture media (eg, DMEM [Dulbecco's Modified Eagle Medium], Williams E)
3. Hypothermic holding solutions (eg, HypoThermosol, BioLife Solutions, Bothell, WA)

Many individuals have tried using standard cell culture media, some claiming better results and others seeing no difference compared with saline as a control. Although culture media can provide cells the needed nutrients, it is important to remember that they were designed for use in carbon dioxide incubators, which represents a different holding environment than the ambient air conditions of the operating room.

Furthermore, stored tissue (ie, grafts) is often kept cooled on ice blocks where temperatures are usually 4°C to 10°C. This practice is done to lower cell metabolism and energy requirements. Cooling has been used for millennia by man to preserve food and seems like a logical technique to preserve tissue outside the body. However, it is important to remember that hair follicles are living tissue, not food. At lower temperatures, membrane pumps on the outer surface of the cell do not function properly, resulting in intracellular edema, a lower pH, and an elevated intracellular calcium concentration, all of which are damaging to cells.[15]

It is for this reason that hypothermic storage solutions have been specifically designed to support and protect tissue that is being kept at low temperatures before transplantation. These solutions prevent the pathophysiologic changes that occur with cooling, but it is important to note that they may actually be harmful to tissue at room temperature. In addition, these commercially available solutions (eg, HypoThermosol) contain antioxidants, such as vitamin E and glutathione.

The author performed a study showing less IRI for grafts kept in HypoThermosol compared with saline.[18] A hypothermic storage solution, such as HypoThermosol, may seem to be the ideal choice for keeping hair follicles outside the body before transplantation. However, no comparative studies exist for various storage solutions and it is unlikely that one ever will. Such a study would likely require at least 50 patients in a split scalp study design with follow-up hair counts at 12 months. In the author's opinion, the reason to adopt an optimized hypothermic holding solution (eg, HypoThermosol) is based on scientific reasoning and a desire to use best practices for all cases. Furthermore, the author thinks that postoperative ischemia is the biggest variable in predicting graft growth, something which is largely unaffected by the holding solution. This makes comparative studies of various holding solutions difficult.

UNCOMMON FACTORS IN HAIR GRAFT NONSURVIVAL
Infection in Hair Graft

Fortunately, infections are rare. If they do occur, they will usually be caused by gram-positive bacteria, such as *Staphylococcus*. But other strains of bacteria and even yeast may infect the transplanted sites as well. Whether or not infections affect growth is controversial. Some individuals claim less growth, whereas others have seen even better growth, perhaps because of increased circulation. The issue of perioperative antibiotics is controversial but many surgeons continue to use them.

Patient Disruption

When evaluating patients who claim poor growth, it is important to consider something as simple as patients accidentally pulling several grafts out during the week after the procedure. The author has had a few patients over the years who confessed to bumping their heads and losing grafts in the postoperative period. If they had not admitted to this, the cases would have presented as unexplained examples of poor graft growth. There may be other things patients do (eg, unusual diets, supplement usage, topical products) that may adversely affect wound healing and graft growth. Patients may not admit to this, knowing they were responsible for not achieving the desired results.

Idiopathic Factors (X Factor)

If patients have poor growth from a transplant and all the other factors discussed earlier have been ruled out, this can be called an unexplained or X-factor result. Richard Shiell[19] described this

phenomenon in 1984 and estimated that it occurred in 0.5% to 1.0% of his patients. By definition, this phenomenon would be expected to occur again in future procedures despite a careful surgical technique. Fortunately, the X factor is quite rare.

SUMMARY

Transplanted hair follicle grafts generally survive and grow well. Achieving optimal growth requires attention to several factors. Excellent technique by surgeon and staff will ensure that follicles are not transected, crushed, or allowed to dehydrate during the dissection and placement phase of the transplant. The vascular bed must be respected in terms of incision size, depth, and density. Even with cautious site making, it must be remembered that patients have significant variability in scalp blood flow. The use of a new postoperative scalp treatment containing liposomal ATP may reduce unexplained poor growth and improve overall consistency in graft survival. Adopting the use of an optimized hypothermic holding solution has a sound scientific basis and may yield further improvements in graft survival once postoperative ischemia is controlled. By paying attention to all of these factors, the surgeon will produce consistently excellent results and achieve high patient satisfaction.

REFERENCES

1. Perez-Meza D, Shapiro R. Introduction: practical problems and limitations of hair survival studies. In: Unger WP, Shapiro R, Unger R, et al, editors. Hair transplantation. 5th edition. New York: Informa Health Care; 2011. p. 326–8.
2. Parsley WM, Beehner ML, Perez-Meza D. Studies on graft hair survival. In: Unger WP, Shapiro R, Unger R, et al, editors. Hair transplantation. 5th edition. New York: Informa Health Care; 2011. p. 328–34.
3. Limmer BL. Elliptical donor stereoscopically assisted micrografting as an approach to further refinement in hair transplantation. J Dermatol Surg Oncol 1994;20:789–93.
4. Cooley JE, Vogel JE. Follicle trauma and the role of the dissecting microscope in hair transplantation: a multicenter study. Dermatol Clin 1999;17:307–12, viii. [discussion: 312–3].
5. Kim JC, Choi YC. Hair survival of partial follicles: implications for pluripotent stem cells and melanocyte reservoir. In: Unger WP, Shapiro R, Unger R, et al, editors. Hair transplantation. 5th edition. New York: Informa Health Care; 2011. p. 334–8.
6. Gandelman M, Mota AL, Abrahamsohn PA, et al. Light and electron microscopic analysis of controlled

injury to follicular unit grafts. Dermatol Surg 2000;26: 25–30.

7. Cooley JE. Loss of the dermal papilla during graft dissection and placement: another cause of X-factor. HT Forum 1997;7(1):20–1.

8. Greco J. Is it X-factor or H-factor. Hair Transplant Forum 1994;4(3):10–1.

9. Seager DJ. The 'one pass hair transplant': a six-year perspective. Hair Transplant Forum 2002;12(5).

10. Uebel C. A new advance in baldness surgery with the platelet-derived growth factor. Hair Transplant Forum 2005;15(3).

11. Cooley JE. Use of porcine urinary bladder matrix in hair restoration surgery applications. Hair Transplant Forum 2011;21(3).

12. Cornejo A, Rodriguez T, Steigelman M, et al. The use of visible light spectroscopy to measure tissue oxygenation in free flap reconstruction. J Reconstr Microsurg 2011;27:397–402.

13. Cooley JE. Scalp oxygen levels. Presented at the International Society of Hair Restoration Surgery Annual Scientific Meeting. Las Vegas, 2007.

14. Beehner ML. 96- Hour study of FU graft "out of body" survival comparing saline to HypoThermo-sol/ATP solution. Hair Transplant Forum 2011;21(2).

15. Mathew AJ. A review of cellular biopreservation considerations during hair transplantation. Hair Transplant Forum 2013;23(1):1–11.

16. Cooley JE. Holding solutions. In: Unger WP, Shapiro R, Unger R, et al, editors. Hair transplantation. 5th edition. New York: Informa Health Care; 2011. p. 321–4.

17. Cooley JE. Co-editors' message. Hair Transplant Forum 2005;15(3).

18. Cooley JE. Ischemia-reperfusion injury and graft storage solutions. Hair Transplant Forum 2004;14(4).

19. Shiell RC, Norwood OT. Hair transplant surgery. Springfield (IL): Charles C. Thomas; 1984.

Facial Hair Restoration
Hair Transplantation to Eyebrows, Beard, Sideburns, and Eyelashes

Jeffrey Epstein, MD[a,b,c],*

KEYWORDS

- Eyebrow transplant • Goatee transplant • Mustache transplant • Eyelash restoration
- Repair facelift scars • Beard transplant

KEY POINTS

- Facial hair transplant procedures are best performed using follicular unit grafting, using the smallest recipient sites into which the surgeon and his team are able to insert grafts.
- Angulation is the most critical step in achieving aesthetic results, taking care to make recipient sites at as shallow an angle to the face as possible.
- In the beard, the "danger zone" where bumps can occasionally form is located in a vertical central column extending inferiorly from the lower lip to the entire chin mound.
- Eyelash transplantation should be performed only if the patient fully understands the potential risks.
- For patients who shave their head, follicular unit extraction can be a viable alternative to the strip–follicular unit graft technique.
- The realistic goal of eyebrow and eyelash procedures in not perfection but rather significant improvement.

INTRODUCTION

Refinements in hair transplantation techniques have made natural-appearing facial hair transplants possible. Restoring eyebrows, beards/goatees, and sideburns have all become popular procedures, because of the amount of information readily available and the fact that the results can be outstanding. Eyelash restoration for purely aesthetic, nonreconstructive purposes is a controversial procedure because of the higher incidence of complications and because Latisse (bumatiprost) can safely and effectively make eyelashes look thicker and longer. A variety of factors can cause lack of hair on the face, including genetics, prior laser or plucking, trauma, and the sequelae of prior cosmetic surgery. The scarring and hairline distortion caused by cosmetic surgery can be nicely repaired with hair transplant techniques.

The author has a large case experience with these facial hair procedures, having performed more than 500 eyebrow hair transplants, 700 beard/goatee/sideburn transplants, and approximately 50 eyelash procedures. This extensive experience has provided an appreciation of the aesthetics of these anatomic areas and the best techniques to be used, and a sense of what can be accomplished so as to provide patients with realistic expectations. Although results can truly be undetectable and impressive, patients are always reminded that the goal is an improvement—sometimes conservative, sometimes significant—but perfection is left for Mother Nature, and is something humans can only attempt to emulate.

The author has no disclosures.
[a] Private Practice, Foundation for Hair Restoration, 6280 Sunset Drive, Suite 504, Miami, FL 33143, USA;
[b] Private Practice, Foundation for Hair Restoration, 60 East 56th Street, 3rd Floor, New York City, NY 10021, USA; [c] University of Miami, FL, USA
* Private Practice, Foundation for Hair Restoration, 6280 Sunset Drive, Suite 504, Miami, FL 33143.
E-mail address: jsemd@fhrps.com

Facial Plast Surg Clin N Am 21 (2013) 457–467
http://dx.doi.org/10.1016/j.fsc.2013.05.004

facialplastic.theclinics.com

Provided with realistic expectations, patients are typically very happy with the outcome of their procedures, when performed to the highest aesthetic standards of surgical technique described in this article.

BEARD/GOATEE/SIDEBURN RESTORATION
Treatment Goals

Patients have a variety of personal desires regarding how they want their facial hair to appear. For many men, a strong goatee/mustache is the priority, often complemented by full sideburns. For those willing to have a larger number of grafts, restoration of a full beard is a common request, whereas other men want just a "strap" beard, a narrow band of beard that runs along the jawline.

More common than with eyebrows, patients occasionally choose the FUE (follicular unit extraction) technique for graft harvesting so that the hair can be cut short or even shaved in some cases, because of the absence of a linear donor site scar. Whether the FUE or the strip-FUG (follicular unit graft) technique is used, a scalp donor site is chosen using hairs similar in texture and color to normal beard hairs to help assure the most natural appearance.

Growth of these scalp hairs when placed into the beard is exactly what beard hairs should do, so this is not the potential issue it can be with eyebrow transplants. When performed properly, the number one goal can be achieved: the hairs grow out in a natural direction, angle, and pattern, and once shaved off, the facial skin looks normal and is free of scarring and other obvious signs.

Preoperative Steps

Proper understanding of the patient's goals is critical for having a successful outcome with these facial hair procedures. Because of how these patients have suffered or have been concerned about their undesirable beard/goatee appearance, most tend to have a very good idea of what they hope to achieve. Because my experience has shown the regrowth rate for hairs transplanted into the face to be very high, achieving good to excellent density is typically a realistic goal, provided the patient understands that a large number of grafts may be required. To get an idea of graft counts, to restore sideburns, 250 to 300 grafts per side are usually required. For the goatee/mustache area, this number ranges from 300 to 400 grafts for a mustache to as many as 850 grafts for mustache and full goatee, and 350 to as many as 500 grafts per cheek beard. These numbers can vary depending on how much if any preexisting hairs are present, the thickness of the donor hairs, and of course the exact desired shape and density.

In younger patients particularly, the presence of already existing or risk of future male pattern hair loss must be accounted for and explained to the patient. Performing a facial hair transplant, while providing the masculine look the patient desires, reduces the number of hairs available for transplanting into areas of male pattern hair loss.

Although most patients for these procedures are men with genetically thin facial hair, the occasional case is caused by other factors, including poorly performed or poorly thought-out prior laser hair removal, scarring from a burn (**Fig. 1**) or cleft lip repair, or loss of sideburns from prior plastic surgery (**Fig. 2**). Another small group of patients are female to male gender reassignments seeking the most masculine appearance. Although exogenous testosterone can help regrow some facial hair, usually this hair is of a low quantity, and therefore a transplant can be an important part of the transition.

As with other hair transplants, certain medications and vitamins that can increase bleeding are to be avoided.

Surgical Preparation

After a review of the patient's goals discussed in the original consultation, whether conducted in person or via e-mail (>70% of the author's patients travel in to have their procedure performed after learning about it on the Internet), the areas to be transplanted are marked out. There is no ideal facial hair pattern, because this is a personal decision guided by family history, ethnicity, religion, and the shape of the face and facial features.

Although no rules exist as to what looks natural, the author advises patients that transplants into the central region right below the lower lip (the "soul patch") and into the chin mound are risky, especially in patients with dark or especially thick donor hairs, because small bumps can form at the site of each graft. This "danger zone" is discussed further later, but because of this, the goatee is usually designed to dip down under each lateral two-fifths or so of the lower lip, and not have any hairs in this area at all (see case examples) (**Fig. 3**). If the patient is highly motivated, the author recommends transplanting 20 to 40 test grafts into this area to assess healing. If no bumps form after 6 months or so, then further grafting can be safely performed in this area.

Patient Positioning

If a strip is to be the source of the grafts, the already anesthetized donor area is removed with the

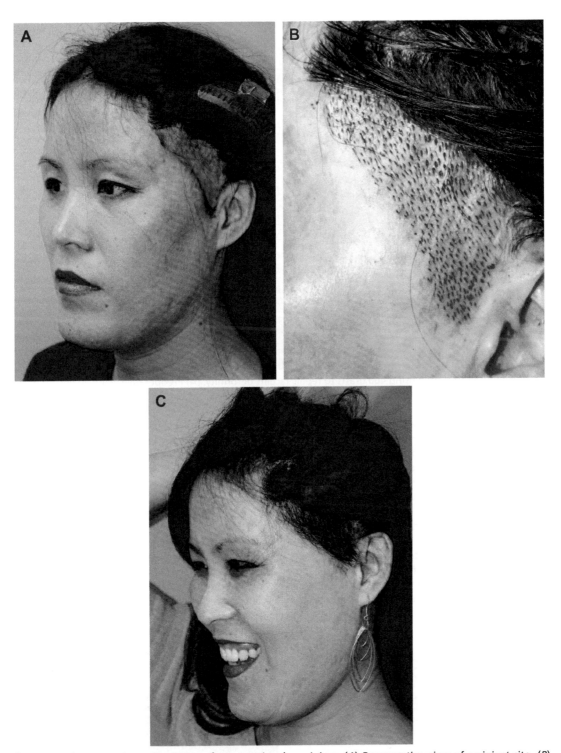

Fig. 1. Temple restoration using 350 grafts to repair a burn injury. (*A*) Preoperative view of recipient site. (*B*) Operative view of recipient site. (*C*) Postoperative result at 5 months.

patient sitting upright, then the area sutured closed. Most patients are given Valium, 10 mg and Ambien, 10 mg. The length of this donor area can vary widely, depending on the anticipated size of the procedure. The donor strip can be as short as 3 cm if only a limited graft number is required for filling in a patchy area or a small scar. Alternatively, procedures of at least 1800

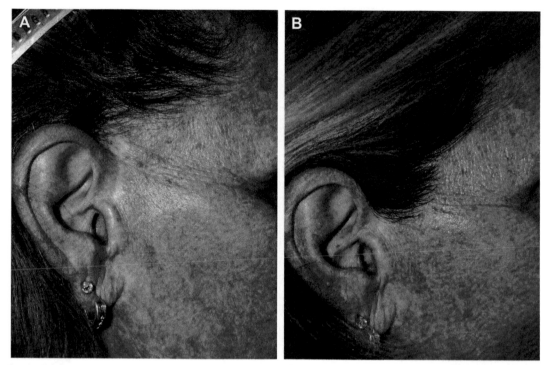

Fig. 2. Sideburn restoration using 400 grafts to repair facelift deformity. (*A*) Preoperative view. (*B*) Postoperative view.

grafts are not uncommon, and require donor strips as long as 12 to 20 cm. In most cases, follicular units containing 1, 2, and 3 hairs compose the grafts; the exception is in patients with thick dark hairs, in whom these naturally occurring 3-hair follicular unit grafts are dissected into single- and 2-hair grafts.

For some patients, particularly those younger than 30 years, in whom a relatively large number of grafts will be transplanted, the author will take 2 separate donor strips from different areas of the scalp. This technique will make the patient's scalp look like it experienced some trauma (eg,

an old hockey injury) rather than was the donor site for a hair transplant. Approximately 25% of these facial hair patients choose the FUE technique, and therefore the areas of the scalp from which the grafts are to be harvested are trimmed. If the occipital scalp is to serve as a major donor source, the patient lies face-down for the first 2 to 5 hours necessary to extract the grafts from the back of the head, then flips over onto his back to so that the recipient site formation and planting can begin. However, for many smaller cases, some or all of the donor hairs will come from the sides, permitting hairs to be extracted

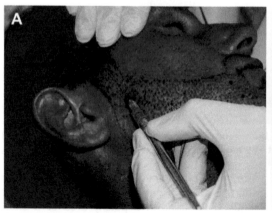
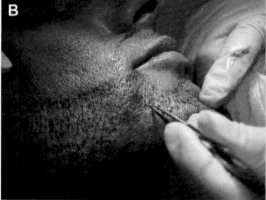

Fig. 3. (*A*) Beard recipient site preparation with 0.7-mm openings. (*B*) Graft placement into beard recipient site.

from one side of the head while the surgeon and assistant sit on the other side, first creating the recipient sites and then inserting the grafts. This efficiency is key for inserting grafts rapidly once extracted, potentially helping to increase hair regrowth.

Procedural Approach

Once all of the FUE grafts from the back of the scalp have been harvested, or as the grafts are dissected out using microscopes from the donor strip, the recipient sites are made. To not have at least some original naturally existing beard hairs present is rare, even if they are fine "peach fuzz" hairs that can guide the direction and angulation of these recipient sites.

- To minimize the chance that the grafts will shift in angulation during healing, the smallest possible recipient sites are made, usually 0.6 and 0.7 mm, sometimes 0.8 mm.
- Each recipient site is made so that the resultant hair direction will be as normal as possible (see **Fig. 3**). Although variations occur, generally the angle the hairs make with the skin is as shallow as possible and the direction of growth is directly downward. On the mustache, the hairs will grow slightly laterally, which usually continues as the mustache extends downward along the lateral aspect of the mouth, where it then becomes the lateral goatee along the jowl region.
- The grafts are then placed, using jeweler's forceps, into each recipient site. This process is performed carefully by highly experienced technicians. Following the plan created by the surgeon, usually single-hair grafts are placed along the borders of the beard/mustache/goatee, whereas 2- and sometimes 3-hair grafts are transplanted into the more central areas of the sideburn and cheek beard, and 2-hair grafts are placed into the mustache to achieve the desired density.
- Because the immediate results are very close to what will be the final result, this allows the patient to assess the shape and density of transplanted areas, permitting feedback and making desired alterations before the procedure is completed.

Potential Complications and Their Management

Angle of hair growth

Given the author's experience treating patients who are dissatisfied with prior work performed elsewhere, the biggest challenge is achieving proper angulation of hair growth. All too often these hairs grow out too perpendicularly from the skin, giving an unnatural appearance. The areas of the face where this is most difficult to avoid is the mustache, followed by the lateral goatee region, but this can occur anywhere. In the author's experience, the key to avoiding this cosmetic problem is to create the smallest possible recipient sites and angle them as flat as possible to the face, which is achieved using a long blade that permits the blade handle to lay flat to the face. To repair these unaesthetic results, the poorly directed grafts can be removed using FUE techniques, allowing the remaining small holes to heal through secondary intention rather than through suturing, which leaves essentially no perceptible scarring.

Bumps around transplanted hair

Tiny bumps can form in the soul patch and chin mound. These bumps seem to occur because of the different texture of the skin in this area, the chin mound in particular being more "meaty." Although who exactly is at risk for this happening is unclear, nearly every instance the author has seen—in 3 patients when the author first began to perform these procedures and on a few others who have been in contact—has been in a patient with dark and, in particular, thick donor hairs. These bumps seem to form as the thick hairs emerge from the skin, raising it up. Shaving or lasering these bumps is not usually curative; rather, the entire hair must be removed, which, because of the poor healing qualities of the skin in this area, can result in scarring. As a result of this experience, the author advises any patient desiring hairs in these zones to undergo a test procedure to assess healing.

Immediate Postprocedure Care

- For the first 5 days, the areas transplanted must be kept dry. This allows the hairs to set properly, helping assure the maintenance of proper angulation of hair growth.
- Antibiotics and analgesics (for the donor area) are given for several days.
- Shaving is not permitted until the eighth day.
- Donor site sutures (3-0 Prolene) only need to be removed on patients who live locally; otherwise, dissolvable 4-0 Caprosyn sutures are used.

Long-term Follow-up and Care

Pinkness in the area usually resolves by the second week, but occasionally can last for as long as several months, for reasons that are unknown. Transplanted hairs start to regrow by the fourth month, and can be shaved or allowed to grow out. Because of the high percentage of hair regrowth, most patients are more than satisfied with the coverage and do not request touch-up fill-in procedures (**Fig. 4**).

EYEBROW TRANSPLANTS
Treatment Goals

As with all of these facial hair transplant procedures, the goal in eyebrow restoration is to come as close as possible to restoring the density, direction, and angle of growth, and the distribution of hairs to how they grow naturally. Because of their highest reliability in regrowth, hairs from the scalp typically serve as the transplants, and, because they continue to grow, need to be trimmed on a regular basis. For most patients, the linear scar from a donor-site strip is acceptable, easily concealed by hair longer than typically a half inch. However, for patients who prefer to have a shaved head, the follicular unit extraction procedure avoids this linear scar. The 2 downsides to using FUE grafts are that they seem have a lower percentage of regrowth, and that the natural curvature of the hairs, which can be used to help guide the placement of the grafts, can be more difficult to assess because the hairs must be trimmed short for extraction.

Although the donor area is almost always the scalp, the author has used hairs from other areas of the body. Viable hairs can sometimes be obtained from the legs and chest, but patients must be advised that regrowth is not as reliable.

Preoperative Steps

A variety of medical conditions can be associated with eyebrow loss. Although medical conditions constitute a small percentage of cases that present, hypothyroidism must be ruled out as a medical cause, and if trichotillomania is involved, it must be resolved, otherwise the transplanted hairs may also be plucked out. More common causes include genetic predisposition ("my father had thin eyebrows"), overzealous plucking, prior laser, and occasionally a tattoo.

Patients must have realistic expectations, and understand the possible limit in density that can be achieved and the typical 10% to 15% incidence of transplanted hairs not growing in the ideal direction in which they were planted. The hairs will need to be groomed and trimmed regularly (biweekly in most cases) to maintain a nice look. Typically no preoperative blood work is obtained, but patients are advised to avoid any medications and vitamins that can increase bleeding.

Surgical Preparation

In the preoperative suite, with the patient sitting upright and actively involved in the process, the eyebrows are marked out. Particularly for women familiar with makeup application, drawing out of the eyebrows themselves is offered, and they are also encouraged to bring in some photos of celebrities with eyebrows they like (Megan Fox has been the #1 choice). Men usually have a less developed sense of what they are seeking, which is fine, because their eyebrows are not so much carefully arched and sculpted as they are "there," forming a relatively horizontal and dense collection of hairs, with some straggling outside hairs.

The author divides the eyebrows into 3 sections:

1. Head (innermost 5–7 mm)
2. Body (central 2.5 cm)
3. Tail (outer 2 cm)

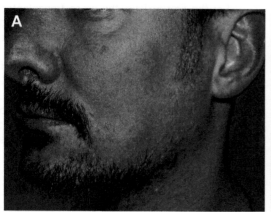
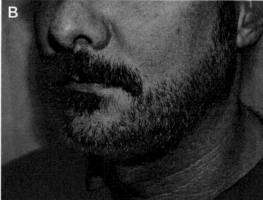

Fig. 4. Beard restoration using 1700 grafts. (*A*) Preoperative view. (*B*) Postoperative view.

In women, the arch, where the body and tail usually meet, is most commonly the highest peaked portion at a point correlating with or just lateral to the lateral limbus of the eye (**Fig. 5**). However, it can vary in its position and its sharpness versus roundedness. In men, the appearance of something resembling an arch is not so much a peak but rather a thickening of 7 to 8 mm of the eyebrow along the area correlating to the lateral limbus.

Patient Positioning

Once the donor area has been anesthetized, the strip is removed with the patient sitting upright. Depending on the number of grafts desired, this strip can range from 3 to 6 cm in length and 10 to 15 mm in width, with the larger size used for procedures of 500 or more grafts. If a lot of gray hairs are discarded in favor of the remaining dark hairs, this strip can be a bit longer. The best location is usually where the caliber and curl of the hairs is the closest match to normal eyebrow hairs, most commonly along the lateral occiput region.

Once the donor strip has been sutured close, the patient assumes an "easy chair" position, lying supine with the head slightly elevated to allow work to be performed on the eyebrows.

If the FUE technique is preferred, the donor grafts get harvested from the back and, sometimes, sides of the head, with the patient lying prone for a few hours until the desired number of grafts are removed.

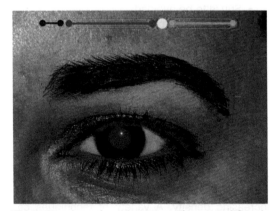

Fig. 5. Female eyebrow anatomy. The natural female eyebrow can be divided into 3 sections: the head (*blue*), the body (*red*), and the tail (*green*). The arch (*yellow*) transitions the body into the tail. It is usually the most superior peaked portion of the brow and typically resides at a point in alignment with or just lateral to the lateral limbus of the eye.

Procedural Approach

- As the donor hairs are being dissected out by the trained hair technicians under microscopes into 1- and, with finer hair, 2-hair grafts, the surgeon prepares the recipient sites in the eyebrows.
- Working within the surgical markings, recipient sites are created one at a time using the smallest possible blades with which the surgeon and/or assistants can place the grafts; in the author's practice, this is 0.5 mm (**Fig. 6**A).

Surgical note on hair growth direction

Usually, existing hairs can serve as a template for direction of growth, although in cases of abnormal hair growth direction, or when no prior existing hairs are present in a regions of the eyebrows, the surgeon must understand the aesthetics of this process. In the head portion, the direction of growth is generally directly vertical/superior, especially toward the innermost aspect of the eyebrows. Proceeding laterally, this direction of growth rapidly becomes horizontal (first along the upper edge of the eyebrow), so that in the body portion, a cross-hatched pattern is achieved by making the cephalic incisions in a downward/lateral direction and the caudal incisions in an upward/lateral direction. In the tail portion, the direction is primarily lateral, without any cross-hatching at the end.

Surgical note on hair angle

The angle of these recipient sites is also crucial. The flatter the angle these recipient sites make with the underlying skin, the better the hairs will lay and create a natural appearance.

- Once the first set of recipient sites are made, the grafts are inserted using jeweler's forceps, with the planters making sure that the individual hairs are rotated in their recipient sites so that the curl of the hairs complement the desired aesthetic direction of growth (see **Fig. 6**B).
- When 2-hair grafts are appropriate, they are placed into the central aspect of the body of the brows, where they help maximize density.
- In a procedure of, for example, 300 grafts per side, typically 225 recipient sites are first made into each eyebrow and then filled, after which 50 to as many as 125 additional recipient sites are made to achieve both greater density and a symmetric and desired shape, confirmed by the patient sitting upright and inspecting the eyebrows.

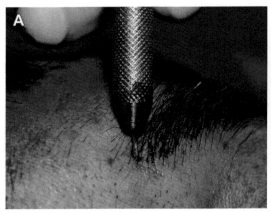 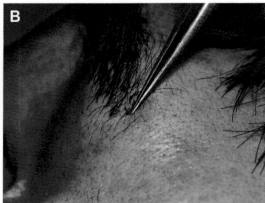

Fig. 6. Eyebrow preparation and planting. (*A*) Recipient site openings made with a 0.5-mm blade. (*B*) Graft insertion into brow slit with a microforceps.

Potential Complications and Their Management

Eyebrow transplants are minimally invasive, and therefore are associated with few medical/surgical complications. Most challenges with eyebrow transplants are cosmetic.

Asymmetry

Once the anesthesia and swelling wears off after 24 to 48 hours, occasionally, despite the best efforts to avoid it, there can be a slight asymmetry to the eyebrows. Probably the most common reason for this is that the anesthesia wears off sooner on one of the eyebrows during the procedure, resulting in asymmetric retraction of the frontalis and/or orbicularis muscle, elevating one brow region higher than the other. If not aware of this, the surgeon can be fooled into making one eyebrow higher than the other. The best way to avoid this situation is to inject anesthesia only at the beginning of the procedure, and then, before more anesthetic is topped off, the eyebrows should be assessed for symmetry and any necessary adjustments should be made.

Lack of hair regrowth

Another cosmetic challenge is a lower-than-expected percentage of hair regrowth. Despite the most careful efforts to keep the grafts moist and cool, and for them to be inserted as atraumatically as possible, often 20% to 25% of the hairs do not regrow on either one or both eyebrows, for unknown reasons. Because the author's practice has performed increasingly more of these procedures, working with only 3 of the top assistants who perform the planting on these procedures every week, the percentage of regrowth has significantly increased, wherein regrowth rates of more than 90% are not uncommon. All patients are advised

that a touch-up procedure of additional grafts in 10 or more months may be desired to achieve greater density. In general, achieving a high regrowth percentage and the desired direction of hair growth is most difficult in the head portion of the eyebrow.

Immediate Postprocedure Care

- Most commonly, the donor site is closed with dissolvable 4-0 Caprosyn sutures, but the alternative 3-0 Prolene sutures are removed at 10 days postprocedure.
- The brows are to be kept dry for the first 5 days, allowing crusts to form and fall off, leaving the transplanted hairs in place until they fall out another 2 or so weeks later.
- Antibiotics and pain pills are given for the first several days.
- Sun is to be avoided.
- Patients may apply makeup to the periorbital region the first postoperative day to help conceal any bruising, and to the eyebrows once all the crusts have fallen off.
- Normal hair washing is permitted the first day after the procedure and full exercise is allowed at 1 week.

Long-term Follow-up and Care

The eyebrows do not start growing in until 4 to 5 months later, after which the hairs will continue to fill in for another 4 to 6 months, gradually increasing density. A variety of techniques can be used to train any misdirected hairs to grow in the desired direction, including the application of gels and other products. The hairs must be trimmed several times a month, something that patients seem to become accustomed to quickly and over which they do not seem to complain (perhaps because they are so happy to have eyebrows). In the author's experience, these patients are definitely among the happiest, being pleased to wake up with eyebrows, and not needing to draw them in every morning (**Figs. 7** and **8**). Any touch-up procedure to achieve more density is put off until 8 or more months later.

EYELASH TRANSPLANTS
Treatment Goals

Restoring eyelashes is more challenging than the procedures described previously and, therefore, patients must be, first, discouraged from having the procedure and, second, provided very realistic expectations.

Any patient who presents with thin and/or short eyelashes is first put on a trial of Latisse to assess whether the results achieved with this medication meet the patient's expectations. However, for patients with a complete absence of eyelashes in whom the procedure is considered at least somewhat reconstructive (which was the original indication for which the author performed these transplants, before beginning to perform them for purely cosmetic purposes), this trial is not necessary. Patients must be told that the goal is not full eyelashes but rather an improvement, and they must be informed of the risks and the maintenance that will be required.

Preoperative Steps

The most common cause of eyelash loss is alopecia areata/universalis, in which hair regrowth can be unreliable, even after a several-year wait period. Scarring from trauma or prior surgery, such as to remove a neoplasm, can be successfully treated with a transplant, so that an improvement in coverage is achieved. Other causes, including trichotillomania and genetics, are usually appropriate indications for the procedure. For the most part, the author will only transplant the upper eyelid, because of the significant challenges in placing transplants in the lower lid to avoid hair growth into the actual globe. However, the author has performed lower eyelash transplants in 3 patients, all of whom were missing a portion of eyelashes because of partial excision of the eyelid. Because the number of grafts that can be placed in a single procedure is limited (typically no more than 60 to 70 grafts per eyelid), patients are advised that a second procedure 8 or more months later may be desired.

Patients with scalp donor hairs that are thick and straight (such as in some Asian groups) or very curly (such as in African ethnicity) are not considered appropriate candidates. In addition, because the grafts are actually threaded into the eyelid, the hairs must be grown out at least 5 cm in length. The FUE technique is not appropriate for harvesting grafts, and therefore patients must be prepared for a small donor site incision. As with eyebrow restoration, patients having eyelash transplants are advised to avoid aspirin and other anticoagulants.

Surgical Preparation

Little preparation is required for these procedures. The donor area is selected based on where the hairs grow with somewhat of a curl, and where the hairs are least likely to turn gray. No hair trimming is performed.

Patient Positioning

Once the donor area has been anesthetized, the strip, typically measuring 3 cm in length by 1 cm in width, is excised with its long hairs and then sutured closed, all with the patient sitting upright. Once the donor area is sutured closed, with the

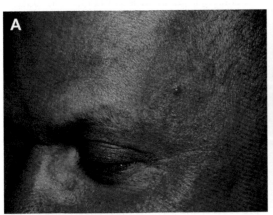
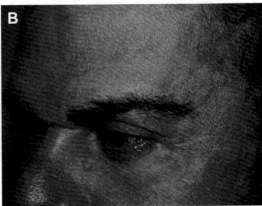

Fig. 7. Eyebrow restoration with 275 grafts into each brow. (*A*) Preoperative view. (*B*) Postoperative view.

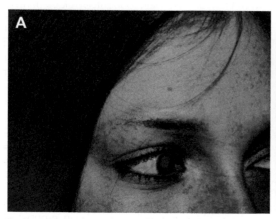
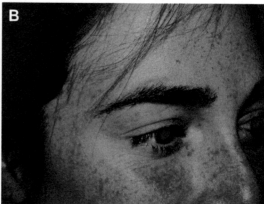

Fig. 8. Eyebrow restoration with 300 grafts into each brow. (*A*) Preoperative view. (*B*) Postoperative view.

patient in a supine position, the upper eyelids from the tarsus to around 15 mm superior are anesthetized, and the area thoroughly prepared and sterilized.

Procedural Approach

- Under microscopic visualization, the single hair grafts are dissected out.
- To minimize the chance of cyst formation in the first few months, as much of the scalp skin around the hair as possible is dissected away.
- Each hair is then threaded through the eyelet of a French curved needle, and the grafts placed in chilled saline to keep them moist.
- One at a time, this needle is then placed into the eyelid approximately 12 mm superior to the lash line, then advanced through the skin to exit out the eyelid where desired. (In cases of absent eyelashes, this exit point is at the lash line, but in cases of eyelashes that are present but where thickening is desired, this point is just above the existing eyelashes.)
- As the eyelet portion of the needle emerges from the exit point, the hair that was threaded through it also emerges. This hair can then be pulled forward until the entire follicle is inserted into the eyelid skin, assuming its desired location. If the procedure is performed properly, the hair emerges so that its natural curl complements the upward desired direction of hair growth, achieving the most natural shape and helping to avoid the hairs going into the globe. The hair can then be trimmed so that it is several millimeters longer than any already-existing eyelashes, making it easier to identify.

- This process is continued until the desired or maximum number of hairs are transplanted, typically 60 to 70 per upper eyelid. Attempting to place more hairs usually has diminishing returns, because these additional hairs displace already transplanted hairs.
- Occasionally, to achieve greater density, 2 hairs can be threaded into each needle eyelet, allowing them to be transplanted into a single recipient site.
- Although not necessary, the use of a corneal shield with ointment can help reduce the risk of corneal injury from inadvertent handling of the French needle.

Potential Complications and Their Management

Several risks and complications are associated with eyelash transplants.

Cyst formation

The most common complication is cyst formation, the incidence of which the author has been able to reduce significantly to less than 20% of patients through thorough trimming of the surrounding skin from the graft. If cysts occur, heat soaks and topical or oral antibiotics can be effective, but occasionally incising these cysts is necessary to eliminate them.

Swelling and bruising

Swelling and bruising are fairly common, but fortunately are usually short-lasting, typically resolving by 3 days. During this time, dark sunglasses can be an effective concealer.

Corneal damage

Damage to the cornea is the main risk of this procedure, and patients must understand the seriousness of this potential complication. It is the reason why the author rejects patients with thick straight or exceedingly curly hairs as surgical candidates. Although surely difficult to accomplish, transplanted hairs growing into the cornea can be surgically removed.

Inconsistent regrowth

Regrowth of the transplanted eyelash hairs is somewhat inconsistent, but patients seem to average 70% to 80% regrowth. Touch up procedures, with the patient made aware of the likely need for them, can effectively overcome this.

Immediate Postprocedure Care

- The patient should be advised to keep the eyelids as dry as possible for the first 5 days and inform them that the dry crust that forms around the skin is holding their grafts in place during this initial healing period.
- Trimming and curling of the eyelashes, so that they do not grow downward but rather assume the natural upward curl, can be performed at 1 week.
- Oral antibiotics and analgesics for donor site tenderness are given for the first several days.

- The donor site sutures dissolve at approximately 3 weeks, but the hair can be washed normally the very next day after the procedure.

Long-term Follow-up and Care

Once the eyelashes begin regrowing at 3 to 4 months, these transplanted hairs will need to be curled and groomed on a regular basis. A variety of mascaras can be used to help hold these hairs in place. Occasionally, the hairs can be permed and/or tinted to achieve the desired appearance. The hairs usually need to be trimmed every 4 weeks.

FINAL THOUGHTS ON EYELASH, EYEBROW, AND BEARD HAIR RESTORATION

These facial procedures are all effective when performed properly on patients who have informed and realistic expectations. Achieving consistent results requires adherence to careful technique and the assistance of experienced hair technicians. As someone who has specialized for the past 10 years in transplants to these areas, the author has found the results to be exceedingly rewarding and the surgeries challenging.

Use of Body Hair and Beard Hair in Hair Restoration

Sanusi Umar, MD[a,b],*

KEYWORDS

- Body hair transplants • Beard hair • Scalp transplantation • Eyebrow transplantation • FUE
- Follicles

KEY POINTS

- Body hair (beard, leg, chest, and other areas below the neck) can be used by itself or in combination with scalp hair to provide coverage in cases of severe baldness, to aesthetically improve hairlines and eyebrows, restore facial or other body hair, and camouflage scarring.
- Body hair retains some of its characteristics but the recipient site can also modify them minimally; thus, matching likely final hair characteristics is important.
- Leg and chest hair does not typically grow to the same length as scalp hair and short hairstyles may be needed.
- The skill level and time needed for successfully transplanting body hair is higher compared with conventional follicular unit extraction.
- Potential patients, regardless of gender, must be hirsute or have sufficient hair for the surgery to be successful.

INTRODUCTION

Conventional follicular unit hair transplantation often leaves linear scars at the donor site. In some instances, the scar is not acceptable and may require camouflage or subsequent revision using trichophytic closure or controlled tension at closing.[1,2] In contrast, when individual hair follicles are transplanted using the technique of follicular unit extraction (FUE) the result is minimal scarring.[3] Moreover, FUE offers other options in cases where the head hair donor supply is limited.

Typically, the average safe donor area (SDA) of the occipital scalp contains about 12,500 potential, transplantable hairs[4] but because two to three hairs are usually associated with each follicular unit, this means only about 6000 follicular units can be transplanted.[5] In individuals who have moderate to severe baldness (Norwood baldness scale of 6–7) at least two to four times as many follicles are required for reasonable coverage. As a result, the choices of using exclusively head donor hair can be inadequate. In these situations, it is possible to use nonhead hair sources, including the beard, chest, and legs in hirsute individuals, which increases the potential follicle supply. Moreover, because leg hair is much finer,[6] it can also be used to create a softer, more natural-looking hairline, particularly if miniaturization of hair follicles has occurred as a result of androgenetic alopecia.[6,7] Besides fixing unnatural hairlines and filling in donor scarring from previous hair transplantation procedures, restoring eyebrows, eyelashes, and moustaches is also possible using nonhead hair transplantation.[2,5,6,8,9]

Disclosures: S.U. is the founder of DermHair Clinic.
a Dermatology Division, Department of Medicine, University of California at Los Angeles, Los Angeles, CA, USA; b DermHair Clinic, 819 North Harbor Drive, Suite 400, Redondo Beach, CA, USA
* DermHair Clinic, 819 North Harbor Drive, Suite 400, Redondo Beach, CA.
E-mail address: drumar@dermhairclinic.com

Facial Plast Surg Clin N Am 21 (2013) 469–477
http://dx.doi.org/10.1016/j.fsc.2013.05.003

Transplanting nonhead hair using FUE is more demanding of the patient and is technically challenging for the surgeon. In addition, one has to deal with the consequences of donor dominance, defined by Orentreich[10] as the "retention of donor hair characteristics at recipient sites," in which beard hair is coarser, whereas chest and leg hair are shorter, finer, and tend to be curlier than scalp hair. Although several studies suggest that transplanted hair is influenced by the recipient site (eg, growing slightly longer and becoming straighter over time),[11–13] my experience performing hundreds of body hair-to-head transplantations is that the recipient influence seems to be cosmetically insignificant.[5,6]

This article focuses on the use of body hair and beard in hair restoration, which has not been widely described in the literature. The reader can expect to know the indications and effective techniques for performing hair transplants using nonhead hair donor sources. Pitfalls and risks are also discussed.

TREATMENT GOALS
Definition of Process, and Distinction from FUE Using Head Hair Donor Sources

FUE traditionally involves restoring balding areas of the head by extracting grafts *in vivo* from the SDA one follicular unit at a time. It is a minimally invasive process involving little pain and is performed with patients receiving local anesthesia and a mild sedative. Depending on the number of grafts to be transplanted, most procedures can be scheduled over the course of several back-to-back work days with additional work for extensive cases scheduled months later. Microsurgical techniques allow patients to usually return to most normal activities the day after surgery is completed with healing ranging from 3 weeks to 4 months.

The use of nonhead donor hair in FUE requires several considerations related to follicles. Hair follicles renew themselves through a cycle consisting of three distinct phases: (1) anagen, (2) catagen, and (3) telogen. Research into a fourth phase, commonly called the exogen phase, is ongoing.[14] Although 85% to 90% of scalp hair is anagen hair, between 40% and 85% of body hair can be in the telogen phase, and the anagen phase of body hair is much shorter, a few months compared with several years for head hair.[15–17] Consequently, it is not only desirable to change these proportions before harvesting grafts but also develop a method where late-phase anagen hair can be identified, because early phase anagen and telogen hair are unsuitable for transplantation (being much more fragile and susceptible to transection during the extraction processes). The characteristics of the recipient hair have to be matched to the donor hair, taking into account hair diameter, color, curliness, typical rate of growth, and shaft angle. However, the slight modifications of these parameters by the recipient area may occur but are generally of minimal cosmetic significance.[5,6]

Indications for Use of Nonhead Hair Donor Sources in General

In hirsute individuals, the use of nonhead donor hair is considered in situations of a relative or absolute lack of head donor hair supply. Head donor supply may be rendered inadequate because of a severe bald state. An example of this scenario is a Norwood 6 to 7 patient requiring global coverage with only a total head donor hair supply of 6000 to 7000 follicular units. Another situation is a patient who has undergone prior hair transplants that have resulted in a depletion of head donor supply but who still has a significant amount of bald areas that require restoration.[5] Nonhead donor hair can also be used to provide coverage for baldness in conjunction with scalp hair from the occipital region where the level of baldness is not too severe.

Special Indications for the Use of Specific Nonhead Donor Sources

Some hair restoration scenarios can take advantage of the innate characteristics of certain types of nonhead hair to especially produce more natural and realistic results. The following are examples.

1. Because hairs from the extremities, such as legs, are innately finer and shorter compared with hair from the SDA, they are a natural fit for eyebrow restoration. This is also the case for vanguard hair in hairlines and temple areas where leg hair nascent characteristics make for a softer, more natural look. Such an approach could also be especially beneficial for the repair of previously transplanted harsh hairlines.[6] Other individuals who may benefit in this situation include Asians who have thicker hair at the back of the scalp and persons with dark hair and contrasting lighter skin.
2. Patients requiring restoration of upper facial hair, such as mustaches or side burns, could find a more natural fit in using beard hairs from the neck areas of the beard.
3. Beard hair, which is coarser, is a viable alternative for camouflaging a donor scar from a previous procedure.[2]

PREOPERATIVE PLANNING

Planning should include identification of the donor hair sources, approximately how many grafts are needed from each source, and mapping where the donor source hair will be transplanted. It is generally preferable to use a hybrid of hairs from different donor sources in the recipient to create a blended look, which is aesthetically more pleasing than a mosaic look that could result from grafting islands of nonmixed body hairs. By estimating the number of grafts needed and where the grafts will come from, and by assuming that 1500 to 1800 grafts can be transplanted in 8 to 9 hours, surgeons can calculate how many days of surgery are required to achieve the overall treatment goal for the patient.

In my earlier work, I sometimes conducted test transplants to verify outcomes several months later to ensure that the yield and final hair characteristics were reasonable and within patient goals. This is no longer necessary in most cases.

Patient Selection

In general, patients regardless of gender must be hirsute. The quantity, quality (thicker caliber hair preferred), and hair distribution at the donor area are all important considerations in deciding on preferred candidates. Vellus hair has less chance of growth, and is cosmetically inconsequential if it does grow. As in any indication for hair transplantation, all other nonsurgical options must have been explored and found to be nonviable in relation to the patient's goals (although they can still be used in conjunction with hair transplantation).

For potential patients who are African American, it is generally observed that those with tight curls have a higher transection rate that may not produce acceptable outcomes. Anecdotally, I have observed that, apart from the tightness of the curls, another significant factor causing a higher transection rate in this demographic population is the skin texture and graft relationship with surrounding tissue: tougher skin texture and a tighter connection of the follicle to the dermal tissue results in a higher transection rate. Consequently, any at-risk patient seeking head and nonhead FUE should be first tested by extracting 25 to 50 grafts and observing for transections before a large-scale surgery is planned.

Managing Expectations

It is important for patients to understand that the quality of transplanted nonhead hair is not as high as that of scalp hair and that survival rates are not as high for transplanted body hair compared with transplanted head hair. Although the recipient site does seem to influence the characteristics of the donor hair minimally, with the exception of beard hair, transplanted body hair may not grow as long or fast as head hair. Consequently, patients are advised, at least initially, to keep their hair cut short. Body hair could also initially be a different color than head hair, although over time sunlight and other factors can bleach exposed transplanted hair in the scalp. As a result, the body donor hair usually assumes the lighter look of the surrounding recipient site hair. Nevertheless, transplanted gray hair almost always stays gray.

In the case of eyebrow transplants, despite best matching efforts, donor hair taken from different areas of the body can often present characteristics, appearance, and growth rates that are dissimilar compared with existing eyebrow hairs. Thus, patients should be advised accordingly to expect a need for more frequent trimming of the transplanted eyebrow. However, leg and arm hair, which are innately finer and shorter, require less frequent trimming on transfer to the eyebrows compared with eyebrows that have been transplanted using hair from the SDA.

PREPARATION
Donor Preparation

Anagen hair selection is performed by two maneuvers. In the case of body hair extractions, donor areas are pretreated with 5% minoxidil once or twice daily for a variable period of 6 weeks to 6 months before surgery. This is done because minoxidil shortens the telogen phase by inducing follicles resting in the telogen phase to begin the anagen phase,[18] although no study has reported how effective this is in human body hair. In human scalp hair it has also been reported that minoxidil increases the duration of the anagen phase and hair diameter.[19]

Donor areas are also shaved 7 to 10 days before the first surgical procedure so that late-phase anagen hair is readily identified. This procedure has its roots in the phototrichogram used by Saitoh and coworkers[20] for anagen hair quantification whereby the skin was shaved and growing hairs were counted 2 or more days later.

General Preoperative Instructions

Apart from the lengthy pretreatment with minoxidil, patients are instructed on how to preshave the donor areas 7 to 10 days before the surgery date. Because scalp and beard hair are often in anagen, these anagen hair selection maneuvers are not necessary. Caution is taken to avoid overuse of minoxidil when large areas are involved. Patients are also advised to watch out for hypodynamic and irritant symptoms of minoxidil side effects and to stop further application of minoxidil should any symptom occur.

PROCEDURAL APPROACH

Surgery proceeds more smoothly when the patient, surgeon, and assistants are coordinated in the process. Because sessions can take up to 8 or 9 hours, patient and surgeon ergonomic comfort is of paramount importance. The correct operating table is vital; a table that does most of the postural changes rather than the patient or surgeon is most ideal. An operating table should ideally be capable of tilting sideways in addition to the usual Trendelenberg and reverse Trendelenberg positions. A versatile height adjustment capability, and independent head and back maneuverability, is also very helpful. If leg hair transplantation is to be performed, a table with leg-splitting capabilities is useful, as are maneuverable armboards for arm hair harvests.

I have determined that certain orthopedic tables are better suited for the procedure (**Fig. 1**). For example, a body hair transplant surgery would involve focusing on the head in one moment and yet on the legs in another. Thus, a cool lighting unit hung from the ceiling or wall but with very wide range of movement is helpful.

If any scalp hair is to be transplanted to the recipient area, FUE is done first in this area. For specific donor areas, the following patient positions are recommended. Beard hair extraction is best done with the patient face up and the neck extended to expose the neck and jaws adequately. Chest and abdominal area hair are best harvested with the patient in a recumbent position and the surgeon to the side adjusted for hair direction and surgeon's preferences. Arm and forearm hairs are best harvested with the arms extended out on an arm board. Leg hair extraction is done with a right-handed surgeon sited to the right side of the right leg (legs lying side by side) for right leg hair. For left leg hair extraction the best position for a right-handed surgeon is to be sited in between the two legs facing the left leg (see **Fig. 1**).

The recipient areas of the head are shaved and marked and the donor areas identified. Hair transplantation is performed under local anesthesia by subcutaneous injections of epinephrine (1:100,000) and lidocaine 1%, and bupivacaine hydrochloride 0.25%, in a 5:1 ratio for recipient areas, and a further dilution (5:1) with normal saline for donor areas. Tumescence is not performed in the donor areas.

A rotary tool is used to mount a hypodermic needle (18- to 20-gauge) whose tip has been modified to form a proprietary punchlike instrument (**Figs. 2** and **3**). Although other punch brands could be adapted for the procedure, the author uses the aforementioned proprietary punches that pull the graft up as it cuts around the graft. This reduces the exactness with which

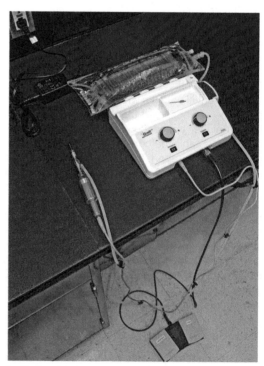

Fig. 2. Equipment set up showing irrigation system in place.

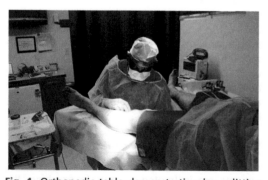

Fig. 1. Orthopedic table demonstrating leg splitting capability and positioning for left leg hair extraction by a right-handed operator.

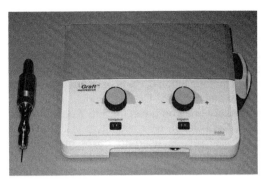

Fig. 3. Close up of console and handpiece used by author.

the operator must trace the angle of the follicle deep to the skin. The axis of the cutting edges of the punch is directed away from the follicles thus minimizing graft damage. The rotation of the punch should be clockwise for optimal effect. Additionally, the handpiece used by the author integrates a controllable fluid irrigation system that hydrates each graft at the time of scoring (see **Fig. 2**). In the absence of such an irrigation armed handpiece, the grafts can be hydrated with a piece of gauze using a 2- to 3-minute interval between the time of scoring and actual removal of the follicles. Individual hair follicles are excised using sharp rotating needle tips to a depth exceeding the bulge area. Freed hair follicles are easily pulled out with occasional aid of blunt needle tip dissection and placed in sterile petri dishes containing chilled Ringer lactate solution or other physiologic solution.

As observed in numerous cases, wounds created by these customized punches widen with depth, so injury to follicles is diminished and wound closure accelerated. The wounds created thus tend to have inverted or straight edges favoring faster healing than in substantially everted wound edges. All grafts are extracted first and then transplanted in order of extraction.

For recipient grafting, slits are created by means of blades custom-sized to the dimensions of the extracted grafts.

PRACTICE PEARLS
Deciding for Each Day's Session Which Hairs Should be Transplanted

Because of limitations of how many hairs can be transplanted for a given patient during a session for each day (typically a 1500- to 1800-hair maximum), it is worth developing a strategy to determine which hairs should be transplanted

(donor and recipient areas) each days when multiple sessions are contemplated for a patient in a given week. This strategy can be modified according to day-to-day experience and is not necessary for a one-time session.

Anesthetic Technique

This is primarily for the patient's comfort and the avoidance of toxicity. The author uses diluted forms to minimize toxicity because compared with head donors body hair extraction surface areas are typically larger. In the neck areas especially, the injecting needle must be kept superficial and in constant motion to avoid delivering bolus doses into major veins or arteries. Factors to consider are length of anesthesia, how anesthesia should be staged during the session, and ensuring that the anatomic areas to be operated on are properly covered.

Minimizing Transection and Maintaining Follicle Integrity

The rotary punch tool developed by the author minimizes transection while allowing a good rate of follicle extraction, but its use does require experience on the part of the practitioner. The punch or other cutting device should permit good alignment with the shaft angle while cutting out an adequate amount of surrounding tissue and minimizing soft tissue trauma.

Create Appropriate Transplantation Angles (Follicles)

When creating recipient slits the angle must be appropriate to the part of the head being transplanted and the overall hair structure (eg, creating a whorl on the crown of the head).

Density of Follicle Transplants

Target density varies from one recipient location to another and can vary from 15 to 60 follicular units per square centimeter depending on location, patient presentation, goals, and what is reasonable given overall donor supply potential. In patients with risk factors for scalp necrosis (eg, smokers or repair patients with prior flap procedure or patients with prior history of necrosis), densities should be kept low per session. Incisions should also be kept small. In some instances, higher density needs are met by scheduling further sessions several months later. Intervals between surgery of greater than 10 months is preferred in these instances.

POTENTIAL COMPLICATIONS AND THEIR MANAGEMENT

When beard hair is the donor source, local anesthesia commonly causes transient, mild paresis of oral mimetic muscles that last 1 to 2 hours. In addition, hypopigmentation at the extraction site of beard hair may occur, especially in darker skin. However, this is usually tolerable for appearance.[2] Uncommon wound complications, such as hypertrophic and keloidal scarring, can occur in susceptible individuals, and good preoperative clerkship is necessary.

IMMEDIATE POSTPROCEDURAL CARE

Nonhead hair donor sites are left open and coated with bacitracin or Neosporin ointment for the first 7 days after surgery twice a day, and triamcinolone lotion 0.1% is used daily for the first 3 days after surgery. Oral antibiotics, although not necessary, may be given for 5 to 7 days postsurgery. Cephalexin, or a substitute in the event of drug allergies, is used to cover gram-positive bacteria. In the absence of minoxidil allergies, the author has recommended that recipient areas are treated with propylene glycol–free oil-based

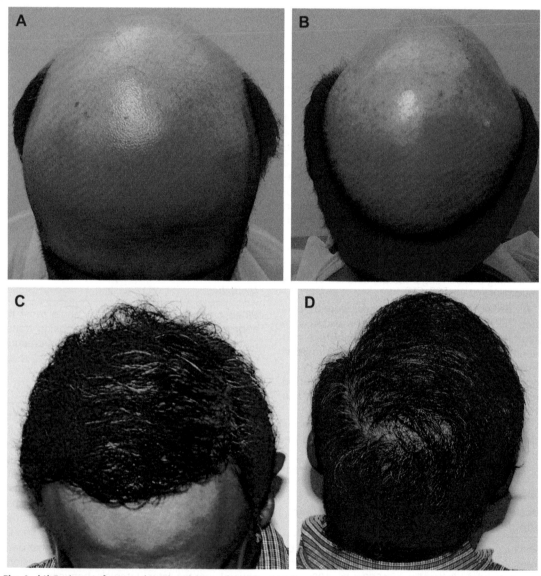

Fig. 4. (*A*) Patient 1: front and top head view of a patient before surgery. (*B*) Patient 1: rear and top head view of a patient before surgery. (*C*) Patient 1: front and top head view after body hair transplantation. (*D*) Patient 1: rear and top head view after body hair transplantation.

minoxidil starting 3 to 7 days postsurgery. The use of minoxidil is advised for 12 months after surgery.

Complete healing, when there are no visible signs of surgery or scarring, typically occurs between 6 weeks and 4 months. Scabs at the recipient site typically resolve in 7 to 14 days. Within 3 to 6 months, the donor extraction site is typically healed without cosmetically significant scarring. In nonhead hair–involved transplants, the author has observed that 10 months is the optimal time to attain results, although improvement could continue into the 18th month.

Beard extractions (especially if carried out below the jaw line) typically heal with a cosmetically excellent profile. This time may vary from 3 to 6 months. The process can, however, be hastened by early laser treatments starting at the second week postoperatively. Laser treatments can be carried out with intervals of 4 weeks. A fractionated erbium or CO_2 laser is suitable if the extraction site is noted to be depressed below skin-level, whereas if redness is dominant, a 595-nm pulse dye laser with a V-beam is used.

Fig. 4A and B show the front and rear of the head of a man with Norwood 7 status. Twelve thousand grafts were transplanted from the head and beard; 1 year later the complete head exhibits full coverage with pleasing aesthetic results (see **Fig.** 4C, D). **Fig.** 5A shows a previously transplanted patient with sparse hair coverage over the entire Norwood 6 area that was restored using 9000 grafts derived from the head, beard,

and chest, which 1 year later demonstrates full coverage (see **Fig.** 5B). **Fig.** 6A shows a patient with sparse eyebrows, whereas at 4 months his eyebrows show significant restoration after grafting with 450 leg-derived hair grafts (see **Fig.** 6B). **Fig.** 6C depicts the patient's right leg a few days after leg hair extractions, which were used for his eyebrow restoration.

REHABILITATION AND RECOVERY

It can take several months or even a year for the full effect of body hair transplants to be seen. During this time, the patient should be instructed on general hair care, especially with hair treatments. When the patient has had severe baldness or problems that require extensive repair (or both), and before surgery the client used wigs or other methods to disguise these issues, it is often difficult for the patient to make the psychological adjustment from using to not using a wig. There is a strong temptation to resume the use of wigs immediately after surgery. I prefer the discontinuation of wigs altogether, although in extreme circumstances the wig could be used for 12 hours of the day and removed overnight. In these instances, clip-on wigs must be used and glues avoided. As discussed in the management of patient expectations, patients should be counseled that in some instances, the hair looks best if kept short, because body hair does not grow as long as head hair.

If beard hair was used predominantly, styling gels may be used to overcome the wiry and unruly

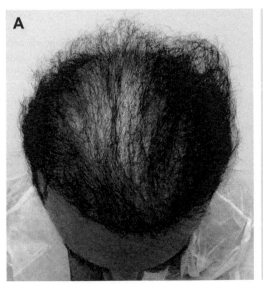
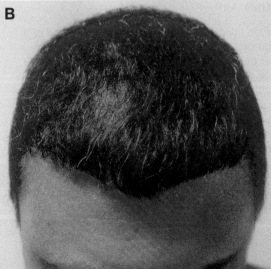

Fig. 5. (*A*) Patient 2: top front view of a patient before surgery. (*B*) Patient 2: Top front view after body hair transplantation.

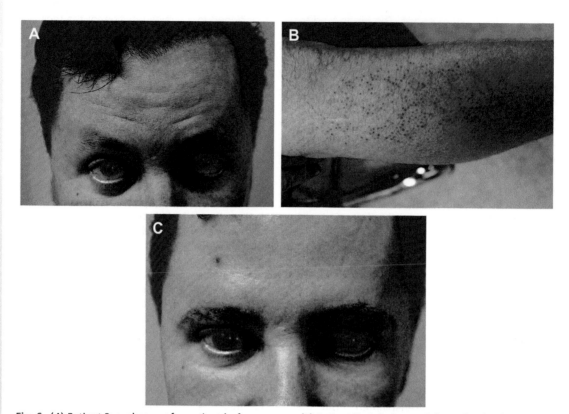

Fig. 6. (*A*) Patient 3: eyebrows of a patient before surgery. (*B*) Patient 3: right leg at 7 days after leg hair extraction for eyebrow grafting. (*C*) Patient 3: eyebrows at 4 months after body hair transplantation using leg hair.

tendencies of beard hair. Hair dyes can also be used to even out hair colors if deemed cosmetically necessary or as dictated by taste.

SUMMARY

When used appropriately, body hair by itself or in combination with hair from the SDA can improve the overall aesthetic appearance of a bald scalp, and especially hairlines and eyebrows. Body hair can also be used to camouflage existing defects from prior hair transplantation surgeries or in situations of relative or absolute lack of head hair donor supply. General limitations in the use of body hair and beard hair in hair restoration include the longer procedure required (often over several sessions); the higher level of skill required on part of the surgeon; more specialized instrumentation and equipment; the variations in hair angulation; the likelihood that the quality of nonhead hair may not be as high compared with donor head hair; the need for sufficient body hair; and the much higher cost than many scalp hair transplants (because of the need for the FUE procedure).

REFERENCES

1. Bernstein RM, Rassman WR, Rashid N, et al. The art of repair in surgical hair restoration part I: basic repair strategies. Dermatol Surg 2002;28: 783–94.
2. Umar S. Use of beard hair as a donor source to camouflage the linear scars of follicular unit hair transplant. J Plast Reconstr Aesthet Surg 2012;65: 1279–80.
3. Rassman WR, Bernstein RM, McClellan R, et al. Follicular unit extraction: minimally invasive surgery for hair transplantation. Dermatol Surg 2002;28:720–8.
4. Bernstein RM, Rassman WR. The logic of follicular unit transplantation. Dermatol Clin 1999;17:277–95, viii [discussion: 296].
5. Umar S. Hair transplantation in patients with inadequate head hair donor supply using nonhead hair: report of 3 cases. Ann Plast Surg 2011;67:332–5.
6. Umar S. The transplanted hairline. Leg room for improvement. Arch Dermatol 2012;148:239–42.
7. Sinclair RD, Dawber P. Androgenetic alopecia in men and women. Clin Dermatol 2001;19:167–78.
8. Jones R. Body hair transplantation to wide donor scar. Dermatol Surg 2008;34:857.

9. Dua A, Dua K. Follicular unit hair transplant. J Cutan Aesthet Surg 2010;3:76–81.

10. Orentreich N. Autografts in alopecias and other selected dermatologic conditions. Ann N Y Acad Sci 1959;83:463–79.

11. Hwang S, Kim JC, Ryu HS, et al. Does the recipient site influence the hair growth characteristic in hair transplantation? Dermatol Surg 2002;28: 795–6.

12. Lee SH, Kim DW, Jun JB, et al. The changes in hair growth pattern after autologous hair transplantation. Dermatol Surg 1999;25:605–9.

13. Hwang ST, Kim HY, Lee SJ, et al. Recipient site influence in hair transplantation: a confirmative study. Dermatol Surg 2009;35:1011–4.

14. Higgins CA, Westgate GE, Jahoda CA. From telogen to exogen: mechanisms underlying formation and subsequent loss of the hair club fiber. J Invest Dermatol 2009;129:2100–8.

15. Ort RJ, Anderson RR. Optical hair removal. Semin Cutan Med Surg 1999;18:149–58.

16. Straub PM. Replacing facial hair. Facial Plast Surg 2008;24:446–57.

17. Randall VA. Androgens and hair growth. Dermatol Ther 2008;21:314–28.

18. Messenger AG, Rundegren J. Minoxidil: mechanisms of action on hair growth. Br J Dermatol 2004;150:186–94.

19. Sinclair R, Patel M, Dawson TL Jr, et al. Hair loss in women: medical and cosmetic approaches to increase scalp hair fullness. Br J Dermatol 2001; 165(Suppl 3):12–8.

20. Saitoh M, Uzuka M, Sakamoto M. Human hair cycle. J Invest Dermatol 1970;54:65–81.

Hairline Lowering

Sheldon S. Kabaker, MD[a,b,]*, Jason P. Champagne, MD[a,c]

KEYWORDS

- High • Hairline • Forehead • Advancement • Reduction • Lowering

KEY POINTS

- The ideal patient for hairline advancement is a woman with a congenitally high hairline and no personal or familial history of hair loss.
- A trichophytic incision is key to scar camouflage.
- Preservation of the occipital arteries is crucial.
- The average scalp can be advanced up to 2.5 cm especially if galeotomies are used.
- A 2-stage procedure with scalp expansion before advancement is required in those with minimal laxity or significantly high hairlines.

INTRODUCTION

Hairline lowering or advancement (also known as forehead reduction), as a stand-alone procedure, has its origins in maneuvers used for scalp reductions and flaps.[1] Although the senior author has performed this procedure for over 25 years, the term "hairline lowering" and its surgical nuances were first published by Marten in 1999 in an article stressing lowering the hairline with foreheadplasty for forehead and brow rejuvenation.[2] The authors' experience is mostly for the purpose of correcting disproportion of the upper third of the face without brow lifting in a younger patient group. The high hairline is more prevalent in certain ethnic and racial groups and is a source of self-consciousness that cannot be overcome with camouflaging hairstyles. Patients perceive the problem as either a high hairline or a large forehead. The hairline-lowering operation is a very efficient and effective method of reducing the forehead with immediately noticeable results.[3] The ideal patient for the hairline advancement procedure is typically female with a congenitally high hairline and no personal or familial history of progressive hair loss. A congenitally high hairline

is one that causes the upper third of the face to be disproportionately greater than that of the middle and lower thirds. To achieve optimal results with a single procedure, potential candidates must meet specific preoperative criteria. Otherwise, a 2-stage procedure is required with scalp expansion before hairline advancement in those with very high hairlines or minimal scalp laxity. This situation occurs in less than 10% of the authors' patients.

PREOPERATIVE ASSESSMENT AND PLANNING

To select appropriate patients for the procedure, the preoperative assessment should include a thorough examination of the scalp with a focus on evaluation of scalp laxity, direction of hair exit, and frontotemporal points and recessions. These key elements are not only important for choosing suitable candidates but also to aid in preoperative counseling and patient decision-making. Forward-growing hairs at the hairline allow for hair growth through the scar and the highest probability of scar camouflage as is discussed in greater detail later in the article. Patients with posteriorly exiting hairs at any point along the hairline, as seen in

Disclosure: The authors have no disclosures.
[a] 3324 Webster Street, Oakland, CA 94609, USA; [b] Department of Otolaryngology-Head & Neck Surgery, University of California, San Francisco, San Francisco, CA, USA; [c] The Champagne Center for Facial Plastic Surgery and Hair Restoration, 10202 Jefferson Highway, Ste. B-1, Baton Rouge, LA 70809, USA
* Corresponding author. 3324 Webster Street, Oakland, CA 94609.
E-mail address: hairflapmd@aol.com

those with cowlicks, are informed that they might require future follicular unit transplantation (FUT) to disguise the scar and achieve optimal results. Likewise, FUT is recommended for individuals who desire coverage of deep temporal recessions or advancement of acutely, downward-facing temporal hairs.

During preoperative consultation, a measurement of the height of the hairline should be taken. To help standardize the measurement, a point should be chosen at the glabella at the level of the interbrow region. From this point, the average female hairline should measure approximately 5 to 6.5 cm, and hairlines greater than this are generally considered high, especially if they cause imbalance with the lower thirds of the face. Once the hairline has been deemed high, adequate scalp laxity can be determined by performing a simple maneuver with the fingers. A point is chosen over the forehead below the hairline and the fingertip is used to move the tissue as far superiorly as possible. The point of maximal tissue excursion superiorly is set to zero at the hairline from the glabella. The fingertip is then used to push the tissue downward from this point as far as possible, and a measurement is then taken between the 2 points. Also, the relative ease of moving the hair-bearing scalp forward and backward and the pinching of forehead skin aid in assessing how much the hairline can be lowered. This distance, which averages greater than 2 cm, very closely approximates the distance that the hairline can be advanced during a single-stage procedure and equates to a 25% reduction of the forehead in someone with an 8 m hairline, for example.

Risks of the procedure as well as potential complications include bleeding, infection, telogen effluvium ("shock loss"), and scalp necrosis. In addition, specific problems relating to the postoperative scar include widening, visibility with future hair loss, hypopigmentation or hyperpigmentation, and the possibility of needing a hair grafting session or scar revision to help camouflage the incision site. These scar problems rarely arise in the authors' experience. All patients are also informed that diminished sensation over the frontal scalp should be anticipated for 6 to 12 months in the postoperative period.

HAIRLINE MARKING

Preoperatively, the hairline should be marked just posterior to the fine vellus frontal hairs in a manner that creates an irregular, undulating pattern similar to those fashioned for routine hair transplantation (**Fig. 1**). As the markings approach laterally to the downward-directed hairs of the temporal tufts, they should be curved posteriorly into the temporal hair for approximately 2 to 2.5 cm and then inferiorly for another 0.5 to 1.5 cm. It is important to create this marking in such a way as to avoid division of the posterior branch of the superficial temporal artery when performing the incision. The desired neo-hairline height is then chosen at a point over the forehead and a marking is made replicating the natural hairline above. A third marking can be drawn 0.5 to 1 cm above the anticipated neo-hairline to allow for a range of acceptable hairlines intraoperatively, and this should be discussed with the patient before surgery.

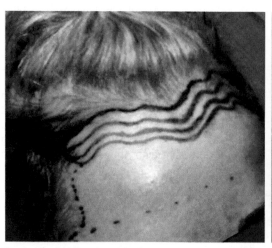 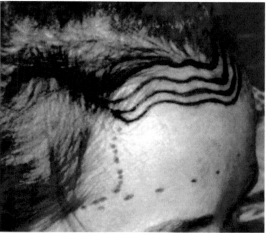

Fig. 1. The hairline is marked just posterior to the fine vellus frontal hairs with an irregular, undulating pattern. Laterally the markings are curved posteriorly for 2 to 2.5 cm into the temporal hair and then slightly inferiorly. The desired neo-hairline height is marked at different levels using a replicating pattern of the natural hairline above.

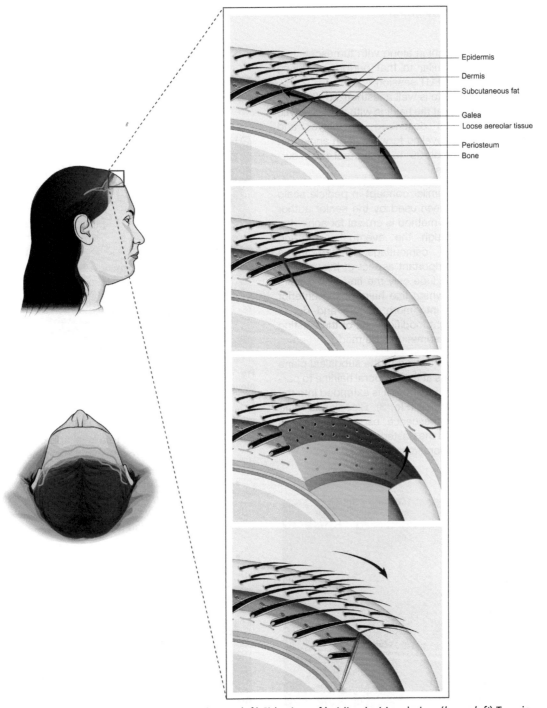

Fig. 2. Trichophytic hairline advancement. (*upper left*) Side view of hairline incision design. (*lower left*) Top view of hairline incision design. (*right, top to bottom*) (1) Hairline-scalp anatomy. (2) Superiorly the hairline incision is made by beveling forward at an angle approximately 90° to the natural exit of surrounding hairs. Inferiorly an incision is made over the forehead with the same beveled angle as that at the hairline (3) Non-hair-bearing forehead tissue including skin, frontalis muscle, and galea is fully excised. (4) The scalp is advanced forward to meet the forehead incision line. Transected follicles along the hairline incision line will eventually grow through the scar to provide camouflage along the length of the hairline.

Labels in figure: Epidermis, Dermis, Subcutaneous fat, Galea, Loose aereolar tissue, Periosteum, Bone

SURGICAL TECHNIQUE

- After hairline marking, the patient is brought into the operating suite and placed in the supine position with the head slightly elevated.

- In the authors' experience, the procedure is well tolerated with a combination of local anesthesia and intravenous sedation. The scalp and forehead are anesthetized in a ring-block fashion along with tumescence in a manner similar to that performed during an extensive FUT session.

- Once the scalp is well anesthetized, the incision is made at the hairline with a trichophytic approach as described by Mayer and Fleming,[4,5] beveling forward at an angle that is approximately 90° to the natural exit of surrounding hairs.

Surgical Note: A similar concept in pedicle scalp flap surgery has been used by the senior author since 1975.[6,7] This method is crucial for achieving hair growth through the eventual scar and providing optimal camouflage in the future (**Fig. 2**). Another important aspect of this incision is that it should include only the first 2 to 3 hairs behind the point where fine hairs of the anterior hairline transition into more coarse and dense follicular units. Slight modifications of the existing hairline shape can sometimes be made.

- The incision is carried to the subgaleal plane and transitions at the temporal hairline to parallel the exiting hairs as it is extended into the posttemporal hair (**Fig. 3**). Bleeding is minimal due to tumescence, especially if care is taken to avoid the posterior branch of the superficial temporal arteries.

- Dissection can then be performed rapidly in the subgaleal, bloodless plane taking care to avoid injury to the occipital arteries posteriorly where visualization becomes more difficult (**Fig. 4**).

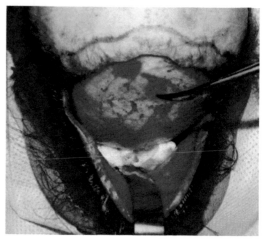

Fig. 4. Subgaleal blunt dissection using sponges and elevators proceeds posteriorly to the nuchal ridge.

- Undermining should take place posteriorly to the nuchal ridge, laterally to the limits of the galea, and anteriorly to a level approximately 3 cm above the brow to avoid lifting the brow in the process of wound closure.
- If the patient desires a brow lift, however, dissection can be easily carried inferiorly to release the brows, and superior advancement of the forehead flap is performed in the usual manner described for brow elevation.
- Once fully elevated, the scalp is advanced, and the use of a D'Assumpção clamp or other flap-marking device helps determine the amount of forehead overlap (**Fig. 5**).

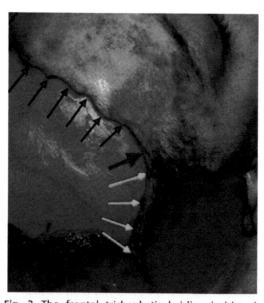

Fig. 3. The frontal trichophytic hairline incision is made by first beveling the scalpel forward at an angle of approximately 90° to the natural exit of surrounding hairs (*black arrows*). The orientation of the scalpel transitions at the temporal hairline (*blue arrow*) to parallel the exiting hairs in the temporal hair region (*green arrows*).

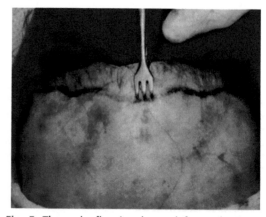

Fig. 5. The scalp flap is advanced forward using a D'Assumpção clamp to establish a safe forehead skin excision. This procedure is repeated after galeotomies and scalp stretching.

- If the planned hairline height is not reached, galeotomies can be performed to allow for additional advancement (**Fig. 6**). These galeotomies are made with the use of a slightly bent, depth-controlled no. 15 blade to reach the more superficial subcutaneous plane while avoiding compromise to the blood supply of the flap. Electrocoagulation blades or needles should not be used for this. Each galeotomy provides a gain of 1 to 2 mm, and therefore, several parallel galeotomies may be required to achieve the desired hairline.

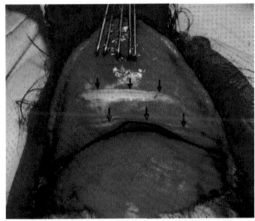

Fig. 6. Galeotomies (*arrows*) facilitate additional scalp advancement.

- After determining the level to which the scalp can be advanced, an incision is made over the forehead with the same beveled angle as that at the hairline while replicating the undulating pattern. Non-hair-bearing forehead tissue, including skin, frontalis muscle, and galea, is then fully excised (**Fig. 7**).

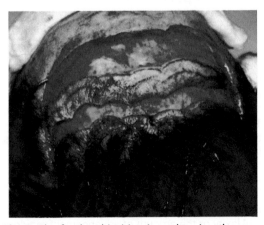

Fig. 7. The forehead incision is made using the same beveled angle and the same undulating pattern as that along the hairline, and then non-hair-bearing forehead tissue is fully excised.

- One or 2 paramedian Endotines are then placed in the calvarium in a reverse direction to the usual placement during a brow lift at a 3 to 4 cm distance posterior to the neo-hairline (**Fig. 8**).

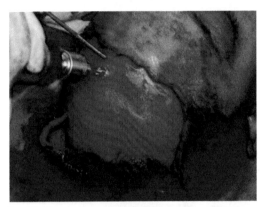

Fig. 8. The midline calvarium is prepared for a reverse-positioned Endotine.

- The scalp is then advanced with the use of 5-prong retractors over the course of 1 to 2 minutes to allow for tissue creep before securing the galea to the Endotines (**Fig. 9**).

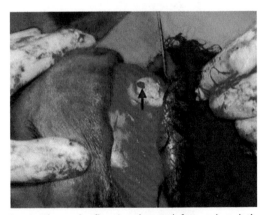

Fig. 9. The scalp flap is advanced forward and the galea is secured onto the embedded Endotine (*arrow*).

Surgical Note: The Endotines, in theory, help to relieve tension at the neo-hairline and work to allow the anterior 3 to 4 cm of scalp to be relatively compressed, thus distributing the subtle stretch of the scalp disproportionately and reducing the possibility of postoperative stretch-back. This anterior compression is thought to minimize splaying of follicular units and help maintain the full preoperative density at the hairline.

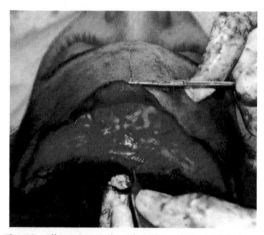

Fig. 10. All tension is placed on the galea which is reapproximated with multiple buried 3-0 polyglycolic acid suture to allow for a tensionless skin edge closure.

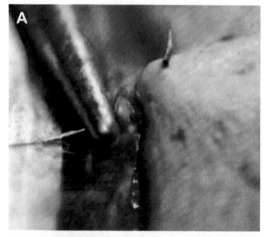

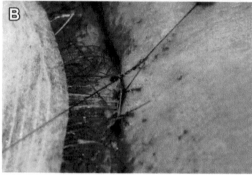

Fig. 11. Skin closure is accomplished with interrupted or running 5-0 or 6-0 monofilament suture. (A) The epidermal sutures are placed using unequal bites with the anterior (forehead) bite located farther from the wound edge than the posterior (scalp) bite. This placement strategy pulls the forehead dermis and epidermis over the denuded hair follicles on the scalp side of the incision line. (B) Meticulous attention to the beveled skin closure ensures appropriate overlap of the de-epithelialized hair follicles.

- The galea is then reapproximated using both 3-0 and 4-0 interrupted polyglycolic acid sutures, often with moderate tension, allowing for a tensionless fine closure at the skin edge (**Fig. 10**).
- The skin is then closed with both 4-0 interrupted nylon sutures interspersed with surgical clips within the temporal scalp and 5-0 or 6-0 nylon or polypropylene sutures over the anterior hairline (**Fig. 11**).

Surgical Note: Meticulous attention is given to the beveled skin closure at the hairline using loupe magnification to ensure appropriate overlap of the de-epithelialized hair follicles. An evacuation drain has not been found to be necessary due to the amount of tension on the scalp and the resultant lack of subgaleal dead space.

On infrequent occasions follicular unit grafts can be performed in the same sitting with donor material harvested adjacent to the intratemporal closure line. These grafts are only used in front of the temple hairs to narrow a wide forehead.

POSTOPERATIVE CARE

- Immediately postoperatively, long-acting local anesthesia is injected along the incision line to provide patient comfort, and a pressure dressing is placed.
- On the following day, the dressing is removed, and patients can resume most nonstrenuous activities within the first 24 to 72 hours.
- Edema is minimal, and periocular and forehead ecchymosis is rare, which is attributed to the strong, layered closure. However, a concurrent brow lift does increase the likelihood of periocular edema and bruising.
- Because tension is borne by the deep closure, removal of skin sutures and clips is permitted within 5 to 7 days.

Due to the initial incision, there is minimal prolonged discomfort from the operation as the scalp is insensate for 6 to 9 months postoperatively, also allowing for the Endotines to be very tolerable. They should be long dissolved by the time sensation returns; hypoesthesia has resolved in all cases to date.

TISSUE EXPANSION

Preoperatively, if the scalp is noted to have minimal laxity or the amount of advancement required to achieve a desirable hairline height is beyond the average 2 to 2.5 cm, a 2-stage procedure is recommended. The 2-stage procedure involves the

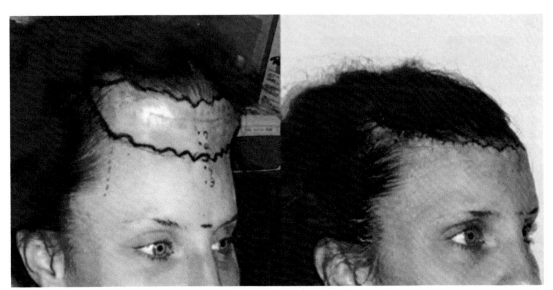

Fig. 12. Tissue expansion assisted hairline advancement. (*left*) A tissue expander had been placed several weeks earlier to assist stretching a tight scalp. (*right*) Results following removal of the expander and final scalp flap advancement.

A   B

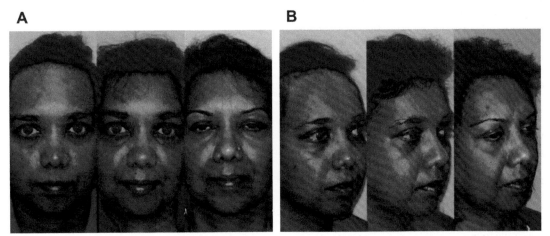

Fig. 13. Hairline advancement procedure using the trichophytic incision showing excellent long-term scar camouflage. (*A*) Frontal view. Preoperative (*left*); 2-week postoperative (*center*); 11-year postoperative (*right*). (*B*) Right oblique view. Preoperative (*left*); 2-week postoperative (*center*); 11-year postoperative (*right*).

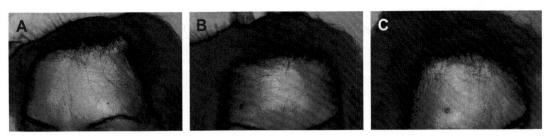

Fig. 14. Long-term scar camouflage 11 years after hairline advancement using the trichophytic incision and closure. (*A*) Left; (*B*) center; (*C*) right.

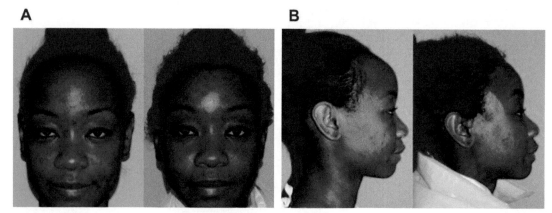

Fig. 15. Hairline advancement of 3.3 cm using a trichophytic incision. (*A*) Front view—preoperative (*left*) and postoperative (*right*). (*B*) Lateral view—preoperative (*left*) and postoperative (*right*).

initial insertion of a tissue expander with expansion of the scalp performed gradually over the following 4 to 10 weeks using similar methods as those described in the literature.[8] During the expansion period, patients have concealed their ever-enlarging scalps with adornments ranging from wigs to oversized hats. A second procedure, which, with the exception of removal of the expander, is exactly as that described earlier, takes place when desired expansion is achieved (**Fig. 12**). In the senior author's experience, this method has allowed for up to 10 cm of hairline advancement.

SUMMARY

With attention to detail and careful preoperative planning, the single-stage hairline-lowering procedure performed on a scalp with average laxity will allow for up to 2.5 cm of advancement with excellent long-term results (**Figs. 13** and **14**). Very lax scalps have allowed for up to 3.5 cm advancement with this one-stage approach (**Fig. 15**). This brief (1.5 hour) operation, which in the authors' experience has no more morbidity than an extensive FUT session, moves an average of 3000 follicular units at one time. The 2-stage procedure, despite having the disadvantages of prolonged, progressive deformity and the cost of an additional operation, is still efficient and cost-effective considering the fact that up to 12,000

follicular units can be advanced. Either procedure is generally well-tolerated with minimal morbidity, and the end result, whether achieved through a one-staged or 2-staged approach, has been met with excellent overall patient satisfaction.

REFERENCES

1. Kabaker SS, Yu KC. Ancillary surgical procedures: flaps. In: Unger W, Shapiro R, Unger M, et al, editors. Hair transplantation. 5th edition. London: Informa Healthcare; 2010. p. 496–503.
2. Marten TJ. Hairline lowering during foreheadplasty. Plast Reconstr Surg 1999;103(1):224–36.
3. Ramirez AL, Ende KH, Kabaker SS. Correction of the high female hairline. Arch Facial Plast Surg 2009;11: 84–90.
4. Mayer TG, Fleming RW. Aesthetic and reconstructive surgery of the scalp. St Louis (MO): Mosby-Year Book; 1992. p. 121–4.
5. Mayer TG, Fleming RW. Hairline aesthetics and styling in hair replacement surgery. Head Neck Surg 1985;7(4):286–302.
6. Kabaker S. Experiences with parieto-occipital flaps in hair transplantation. Laryngoscope 1978;538:73.
7. Kabaker SS. Juri flap procedure for the treatment of baldness: two-year experience. Arch Otolaryngol 1979;105(9):509–14.
8. Kabaker SS, Kridel RW, Krugman ME, et al. Tissue expansion in the treatment of alopecia. Arch Otolaryngol Head Neck Surg 1986;112(7):720–5.

Scalp Repair Using Tissue Expanders

E. Antonio Mangubat, MD

KEYWORDS

- Scalp defect • Tissue expanders • Hair restoration • Androgenetic alopecia

KEY POINTS

- The stretching of human skin via tissue expansion occurs as a result of biological and mechanical creep.
- Surgical planning is critical with tissue expansion to ensure that the repositioned scalp retains a natural hair direction.
- Overestimation of the required expansion is appropriate, and the largest commercially available expander for managing the patient's defect is usually required.
- Social factors like patient availability, distance from the surgeon, and pain tolerance determine how fast the expansion can be completed.
- Caution should prevail if the advancing flap proves incapable of resurfacing the entire scalp defect, because undue tension on the flap can increase the risk of flap necrosis.

INTRODUCTION

The most common cause of hair loss is androgenetic alopecia (AGA). Although not a scalp defect, understanding the cosmetic treatment of AGA greatly enhances our ability to treat severe hair loss deformities, allowing normal and natural-appearing results. Treating a large scalp scar that results in a different kind of scalp deformity often leads to dissatisfied patients and physicians, regardless of the success the procedure.

The various deformities and degree of deformity generally determine the treatment choice. The significant developments in hair restoration surgery (HRS) in the past 2 decades now yield natural and almost undetectable results. By using these cosmetic and reconstructive techniques, most scalp deformities can be treated effectively. It is important to understand the anatomy, physiology, and cosmetic treatments of AGA and that subject has been treated effectively by other investigators in this monograph.

This article concentrates on the treatment of large deformities of the scalp and hair by combining advanced techniques of scalp reduction and tissue expansion with contemporary hair transplantation.

HAIRLINE DESIGN

Perhaps the most deceptively difficult task in any scalp surgery is planning and executing a normal hairline with natural hair direction. Simple scalp coverage is unsatisfactory if the final result is unnatural. This situation is true of all scalp procedures, including hair transplants, scalp excisions, flap rotation, and movement of expanded scalp flaps and applies to all areas of the scalp. In general, frontal scalp hair points forward, parietal scalp hair points lateral and inferior, and occipital scalp hair is oriented posteriorly and inferiorly.

Addressing these subtleties is critical to avoid unnatural results. Even the untrained eye that does not understand the details of a natural hairline can detect an unnatural result.

ALOPECIA REDUCTION PROCEDURES

These techniques are acknowledged because some form of them is required in virtually all scalp

Disclosure: The author has no disclosures.
La Belle Vie Cosmetic Surgery and Hair Restoration, 16400 Southcenter Parkway, Suite 101, Tukwila, WA 98188, USA
E-mail address: tony@mangubat.com

Facial Plast Surg Clin N Am 21 (2013) 487–496
http://dx.doi.org/10.1016/j.fsc.2013.05.006
1064-7406/13/$ – see front matter © 2013 Elsevier Inc. All rights reserved.

repairs. Alopecia reduction (AR) allows the surgeon to eliminate unwanted scar. Originally, innovated for HRS in the 1970s, its popularity waned as hair transplantation techniques improved and our understanding of the natural history of hair loss became more refined, but the techniques remain valuable tools for scalp repair.

The first AR procedures were simple and involved rapid excision of bald scalp from the central area of hair loss. Limitations of AR were identified, including widening the bald area (also known as stretch-back),[1] slot deformity,[2] and visible scarring.

The extensive scalp lift (ESL) is one of the more interesting and effective ARs in that the dissection was carried out beyond the limits of the galea aponeurotica, marked by the nuchal line, extending it down to the nape of the hairline.[3] ESL permitted a greater reduction of bald scalp.

TISSUE EXPANDERS
Basic Principles

Tissue expansion is an extraordinary adjunct for repairing large skin defects. Before tissue expansion techniques, repair of large defects was crude and ineffective. The original work[4] on tissue expansion was not considered noteworthy and its significance remained unnoticed for almost 20 years, until a young surgeon showed its usefulness in breast reconstruction.[5] Its simplicity and popularity grew exponentially as an expander manufacturer became involved in producing a commercially viable product.

The technique involves gradual expansion of a balloon prosthesis implanted under the skin immediately adjacent to the defect. The expander is incrementally filled with sterile saline through a series of percutaneous injections into a self-sealing fill-port. As the balloon increases in size, the tissue compensates by stretching, increasing its length and mass through mechanisms known as mechanical creep (stretching the collagen fibers)[6] and biological creep (stimulating new tissue growth).[7] Mechanical creep is subject to shrinkage when the balloon is removed as the collagen fibers attempt to return to normal resting length. Biological creep, on the other hand, is not stretching in the traditional sense, because cellular activation increases the amount of tissue present. Both properties are critical to successful tissue expansion.

Surgical Planning

Surgical planning is critical to ensure that the hair-bearing scalp to be moved retains a natural direction. Midline scalp reductions were effective in removing bald scalp but resulted in an obviously unnatural result, known as the slot deformity (**Fig. 1**).

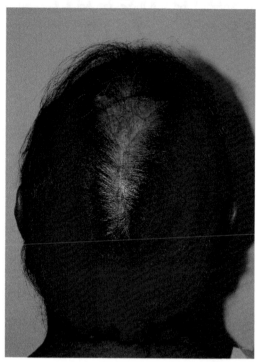

Fig. 1. Slot deformity resulting from midline scalp reduction. Note divergent hair directions, drawing attention to unnatural appearance.

The use of tissue expansion in cosmetic procedures is limited because of the significant deformity that the patient must temporarily endure during the final stages of the process (**Fig. 2**). Reconstructive patients, on the other hand, are more tolerant given the unsightly defects that they are trying to repair. The patient and family must be counseled to expect a cosmetic deformity, especially near the end of the expansion process.

The size, shape, and location of the expander(s) must be estimated preoperatively. Although there are many mathematical methods, none is exact. Overestimation of needed expansion is appropriate and I often choose the largest commercially available expander that fits the patient's anatomy. Ideally, the expander should have a base dimension roughly equal to the dimension of the defect, with the potential of a large vertical expansion dimension. Manufacturers publish tables of expander specifications, which eases the decision-making process.

Flap expansion in the vertical dimension produces greatest gain in flap length and thus provides for greatest coverage for larger defects. It is appropriate to choose an expander that possesses significant vertical rise. This strategy makes calculating the necessary expansion easy; when the distance over the expanded tissue is equal to 100% of the width of the defect, the expansion is theoretically

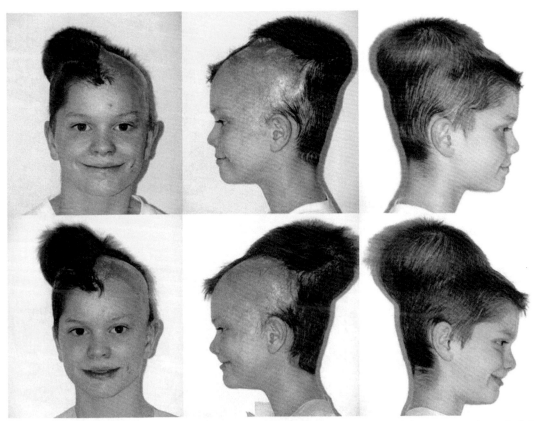

Fig. 2. Progressive tissue expansion in young burn victim with significant cosmetic deformity, near the end of the expansion process.

complete (**Fig. 3**). Because tissue tends to spring back, plan to overexpand to 120% to 130% of estimated length, because removing excess tissue is simpler and safer than attempting to undermine an expanded flap that falls short of complete coverage.

Ideally, the expander should be placed under the hair-bearing scalp parallel to the longest limb of the defect to provide the greatest coverage. This procedure is not always possible because the surgeon must plan for the hair direction in final repair to be natural. Otherwise, an abnormal result can occur. Consider the divergent hair direction of the old midline scalp reduction, in which complete coverage was achieved but the unnatural result was unsatisfactory.

It is often most efficient to match the shape of the expander shape to the shape of the defect. If the defect is long and curvilinear, choose a crescent-shaped expander to prepare a flap for advancement.

Expansion Process

Filling the expander is subject to variation. Social factors like patient availability, distance from the surgeon, and pain tolerance often determine how fast the expansion can be achieved. Expansion begins intraoperatively by filling the expander with 5% to 10% of the total expected fill volume. This procedure takes up dead space and tests the fill mechanism to identify any obstructions or leaks before wound closure. The expansion process then continues 2 to 3 weeks postoperatively. This interval allows the wound to gain tensile strength and the surgical pain to subside, making the first series of expansions more comfortable.

The goal is to expand as rapidly and as safely as possible, which allows faster treatment of the defect. If the patient is local and available, expansion can occur 2 to 3 times weekly. If the patient or a family member is medically trained, expansion can occur at their home with proper training. The most common end point of each expansion is pain; however, the surgeon must be constantly aware of tissue vascularity by monitoring adequate capillary refill. If skin blanching is slow or does not resolve, fluid should be removed. More technical methods of monitoring fill volumes have been described such as transcutaneous oximetry over the expanded flap and intraluminal pressure measurements; however, clinical observation is the mainstay in most cases.

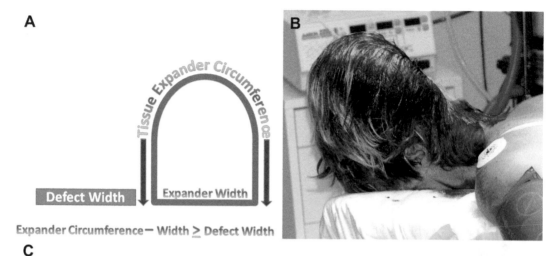

Fig. 3. (A) The width of the expanded flap is ideally equal to the width of the defect to be repaired. Vertical expansion provides flap length. The measured distance over the expanded flap minus the flap width yields the approximate distance of flap advancement. The actual yield is usually less than this measurement because of tissue contraction on removal of the expander, and thus an overexpansion is planned. (B) Patient with expanded flap in place. (C) Measurements of expanded flap.

Expander Removal/Flap Advancement

Once expansion is completed and the measured distance over the expanded flap is 120% to 130% of the width of the defect, the final flap advancement is executed. The initial incision in an advancement flap should be made immediately adjacent to the expander at the border of the defect. This strategy allows the expander to be removed immediately and the flap advancement tested to ensure that the complete defect can be excised.

Caution should prevail if the advancing flap proves incapable of resurfacing the entire scalp defect. Overextending an expanded flap places undue tension on the flap and increases the risk of flap necrosis; therefore, before excising the defect, the surgeon should attempt a trial advancement to visualize the area of coverage. If complete excision is not easily accomplished, it is advisable to leave some residual defect and excise only what can safely be removed. The same expander is then repositioned under the newly advanced flap for a second round of expansion, and the entire sequence of filling and flap advancement is repeated to safely complete the final excision.

CASE PRESENTATIONS

Case 1: Skin Cancer Resection and Radiation

A 45-year-old white woman was diagnosed with a fibrosarcoma of the posterior scalp at age 25 years. She underwent excision, skin grafting, and radiation, resulting in a large area of alopecia (**Fig. 4A–C**). She lived with this defect, being told that nothing more could be done. She underwent a 2 stage procedure with tissue expansion using a 1250-mL expander over an 8-month period (see **Fig. 4D–F**). This procedure provided adequate flap coverage to permit complete excision of the skin graft, and the radiation induced alopecia with the second procedure (see **Fig. 4G**). The width of the defect was 12 cm, the base width of the expander 10 cm, and the outer circumference of the expander 25 cm. Subtracting the outer circumference from the expander width gave a projected flap movement of 15 cm, thus enabling complete excision of the alopecia defect (see **Fig. 4H–L**).

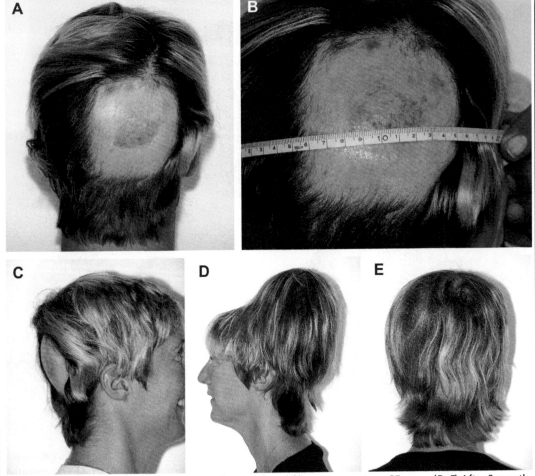

Fig. 4. (*A–C*) 45-year-old woman with excised and radiated fibrosarcoma at age 25 years. (*D–E*) After 9-month tissue expansion process.

(continued on next page)

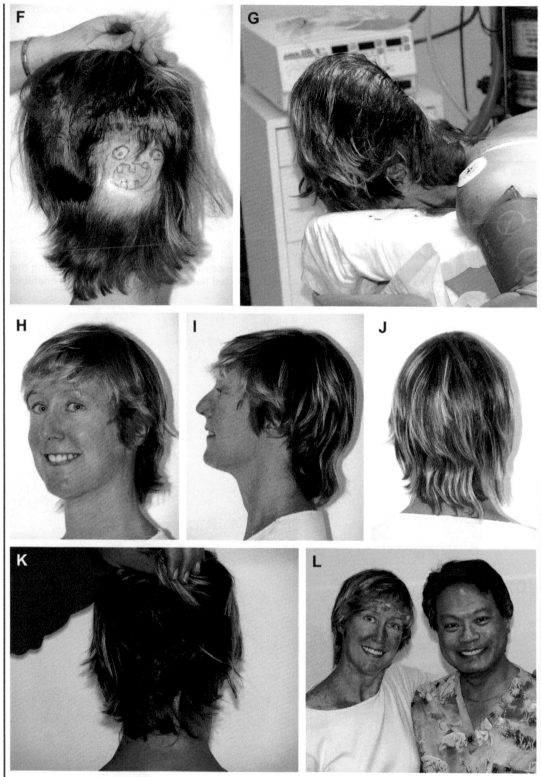

Fig. 4. (*F*) After 9-month tissue expansion process. (*G*) Perioperative prone position. (*H–K*) Postoperative photographs. (*L*) The author and patient 3 days postoperatively. Note minimal pain.

Case 2: Scalp Defect from Excision of Skin Neoplasm

A 7-year-old boy was referred for HRS after having a large giant congenital nevus (at significant risk for developing melanoma) excised as an infant (**Fig. 5A**). When he entered grade school, classmates began teasing him and he wished to have the defect repaired.

Treatment was undertaken during summer vacation, with a large tissue expander placed over the scalp vertex in such a position as to maximize movement of hair-bearing scalp. The expander was gradually inflated over a period of 2 months. Before the end of the summer vacation, expansion was sufficient that complete excision of the defect was possible (see **Fig. 5B, C**).

Note the hair direction was distorted but easily covered when his hair was longer (see **Fig. 5D**). The future potential for AGA was discussed with the family. If he were to develop male pattern hair loss during his young adult life, more HRS would be required. The situation may be more complicated as a result of the unusual hair distribution, as noted in his 3-year result (see **Fig. 5E**). However, his young life was free from childhood mockery, which could affect his social development.

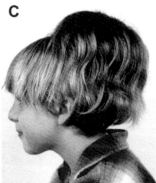
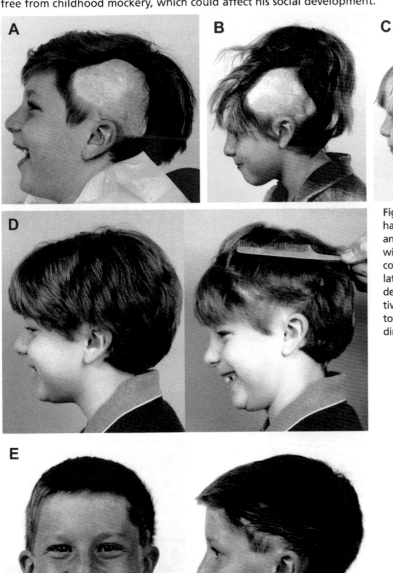
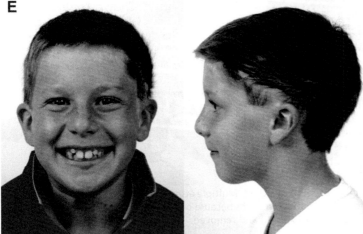

Fig. 5. (*A*) 8-year-old boy who had a giant nevus removed as an infant who was repaired with a skin graft. (*B, C*) The completed expansion 3 months later. (*D*) The closed scalp defect. (*E*) 3 years postoperatively. The results are satisfactory despite the aberrant hair direction.

Case 3: Large Burn Defect Presenting After Multiple Failed Treatment Attempts

Scalp burns are common causes of hair deformities (**Fig. 6**). If the burn is deep enough to destroy the hair follicles, scarring alopecia results regardless of burn depth. Burns are typically irregular, scarred, often large, and the resultant tissue is inelastic, making reconstruction difficult if not impossible using standard excisions. Tissue expansion is ideal for these difficult patients. However, tissue expansion is often prolonged because of the scar rigidity. Nevertheless, the expansion can be accomplished with minimal risk if patient compliance in follow-up is maintained.

A 35-year-old woman presented after having 5 previous procedures attempting to repair a grease burn that she suffered on her scalp as a child (see **Fig. 6A**). The procedures included 2 scalp reductions and 3 hair transplants using 4-mm punch grafts. She had to wear her hair long to camouflage the defect. The scar and surrounding tissue were thick and rigid, allowing little if any movement that would permit excising the 25-cm × 8-cm defect.

Treatment consisted of placing a large 1.3-L crescent-shaped expander in the occipital scalp directly adjacent to the defect. The extreme rigidity of the tissue required 9 months to complete the expansion process, about twice the duration required in an adult with a defect this size (see **Fig. 6B**). The process was prolonged because of pain resulting from the excessive tissue rigidity and extra expansion was planned for. The tissues were found to be rigid intraoperatively (see **Fig. 6C–E**). The result was particularly satisfying, in that with 2 simple procedures, the entire defect was closed (see **Fig. 6F, G**).

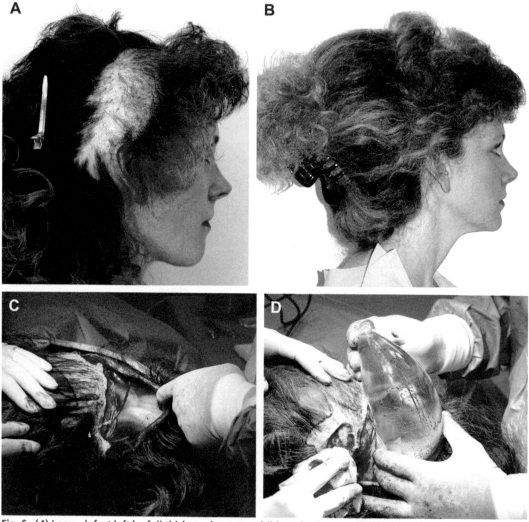

Fig. 6. (*A*) Large defect left by full thickness burn as a child. Multiple attempts at excision and hair transplants were not successful. (*B*) Expansion completed after 9 months because of rigid tissue. (*C*) Incision is made along the expanded flap border. (*D*) 1.3-L expander exposed and removed.

(continued on next page)

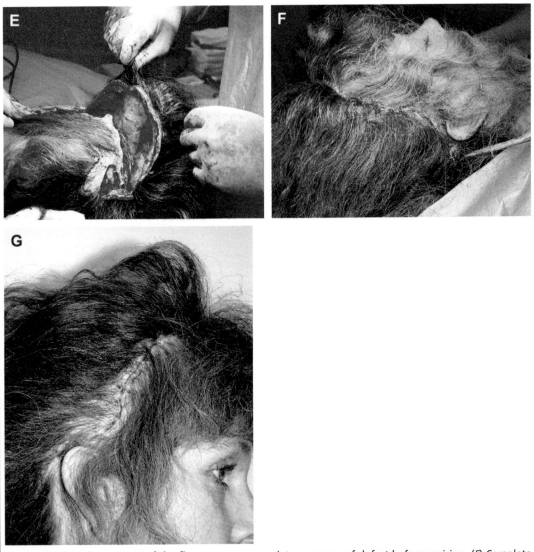

Fig. 6. (*E*) Trial advancement of the flap to ensure complete coverage of defect before excision. (*F*) Complete excision of large defect with immediate postoperative result. (*G*) Final result.

SUMMARY

To be able to treat the wide spectrum of hair deformities, the surgeon must possess a wide spectrum of skills in HRS, cosmetic surgery, and reconstructive surgery. Specific education and training in HRS are not a traditional part of formal surgical training, although much information is available through several national and international organizations. Being sensitive to the unique variables associated with HRS increases the chances of achieving a superior functional as well as cosmetic result when treating significant hair deformities. Tissue expansion offers a valuable ancillary resource for managing many challenging cases that are not amenable to correction using traditional cosmetic surgical hair restoration techniques.

REFERENCES

1. Nordstrom RE. "Stretch-back" in scalp reductions for male pattern baldness. Plast Reconstr Surg 1984;73(3):422–6.
2. Norwood OT, Shiell RC, Morrison ID. Complications of scalp reductions. J Dermatol Surg Oncol 1983; 9(10):828–35.
3. Brandy DA. The bilateral occipito-parietal flap. J Dermatol Surg Oncol 1986;12(10):1062–6.

4. Neumann CG. The expansion of an area of skin by progressive distention of a subcutaneous balloon: use of the method for securing skin for subtotal reconstruction of the ear. Plast Reconstr Surg (1946) 1957;19(2):124–30.

5. Radovan C. Reconstruction of the breast after mastectomy using a temporary expander. Plast Reconstr Surg 1982;69:195–206.

6. Mustoe TA, Bartell TH, Garner WL. Physical, biomechanical, histologic, and biochemical effects of rapid versus conventional tissue expansion. Plast Reconstr Surg 1989;83(4):687–91.

7. van Rappard JH, Sonneveld GJ, Borghouts JM. Histologic changes in soft tissues due to tissue expansion (in animal studies and humans). Facial Plast Surg 1988;5(4):280–6.

Scalp Micropigmentation
A Useful Treatment for Hair Loss

William R. Rassman, MD[a,*], Jae P. Pak, MD[a], Jino Kim, MD[b]

KEYWORDS

- Scalp micropigmentation • Medical tattoo • Balding or thinning hair

KEY POINTS

- SMP is a medical tattoo application for balding or thinning hair.
- SMP is a permanent concealer that reduces the color contrast between hair and scalp.
- SMP can be used for men or women with thinning hair.
- SMP can be used as an adjunct to hair transplantation.
- SMP can be used as a styling solution for a balding man who is willing to shave his scalp.
- SMP is an art form and requires a good understanding of the instability of the balding process.
- SMP can create extremely happy or unhappy patients so it is critical to fully implement informed consent.
- SMP is very effective for the treatment of scalp scars of almost any cause.

INTRODUCTION

A concealer is a product applied to the scalp to reduce the visual contrast between the color of the hair and the color of the skin. This procedure can be done by darkening the skin with powders, pastes, or paint-like substances, thickening the hair shafts with a keratin-like material or dying the hair to bring its color closer to the color of the scalp. Concealers are used by men and women with thinning hair or genetic patterned balding. The tattoo, when applied to the scalp, becomes a type of permanent concealer. The first recorded medical use for a tattoo as a concealer was published by Traquina[1] in 2001 but its use was crude and quite detectable. The refinement of the process, called scalp micropigmentation (SMP), requires that the tattoo pigment be placed in microdots of less than 1 mm in size and 1 mm apart, similar to the distance between follicular units evident on a shaved scalp.

SMP is like a stippled painting and it is an art form. The placement distance and the size of the pigment dots vary with the targeted goals of the surgeon (artist) and the patient. Although it is initially thought that the mathematical density of the dots for SMP should approximate the follicular unit density, in the authors' earlier experience,[2,3] we have since come to realize that the actual distribution of dots is not a purely mathematical constant tied to the follicular unit density of a particular patient. When used to address deformities of the hair and scalp, it is found that the pigment must be blended with the blemishes and scars found in the patients. What needs to be done is based on the "soft" requirements of the art form that best defines the dot size, density, and color of the pigment. The intensity of the dots and how they are worked on the scalp give shade and texture to the area being addressed. The requirement for each area of the scalp may vary based on many factors, including the following:

a. Presence of scars and/or hair
b. Smoothness of the scalp
c. Color of the skin and hair

[a] New Hair Institute, 5757 Wilshire Boulevard, Promenade #2, Los Angeles, CA 90036; [b] New Hair Institute, Gangnam Han-il B/D 7F, Yeoksam-dong 814-1, Korea
* Corresponding author.
E-mail address: wrassman@newhair.com

Facial Plast Surg Clin N Am 21 (2013) 497–503
http://dx.doi.org/10.1016/j.fsc.2013.05.010

APPLICATIONS AND INDICATIONS

Men and women have the option to control their hair length or to shave or buzz cut their hair. Creative hairstyling techniques have been adapted by many balding men and women to hide their thinning or balding problems. Shaving the scalp has been an acceptable styling option for balding men; however, when scars are present, the shaving options often disappear. In the 2011 International Society of Hair Restoration Surgery publication and presentation, SMP was presented for the treatment of many medical and surgically induced scalp problems, such as:

- Autoimmune diseases
- Genetic hair loss
- Surgical scarring from a variety of surgical procedures, including strip scarring from traditional hair transplant procedure
- Old punch graft donor sites
- Follicular unit extraction (FUE) scarring
- Craniotomy scarring
- Scars from scalp reduction surgery

The use of SMP has great value to augment a hair transplant in the many patients who do not have enough hair to undergo a hair transplant, whereby the hair supply does not meet the need for hair. SMP can also be an alternative to hair restoration surgery in some male patients who do not want to have a surgical procedure to treat their balding or the female patient who is thinning and may decide to use SMP as a permanent concealer. The best option for SMP in male patients who do not have enough hair for good coverage is to shave their head completely; however, the doctor may be able to design a strategy whereby SMP augments a hair transplant. When using SMP for this purpose, there must be some amount of hair present. If it is done when there is not enough density to obscure the dots, then the dots will easily be seen through the thin hair. The design criteria for using SMP as a background to thinning hair requires a unique strategy for each patient and varies with each problem being addressed.

THE SMP PROCESS

SMP is a highly sophisticated medical tattoo process whereby a dye is inserted into the skin using one or more needles. The needles require depth control to limit where the tattoo dye is placed. The dye can passively extend beyond the confines of the needle point where it is placed. SMP looks amazingly simple and in concept it is simple, but the techniques that were developed must be customized for each patient as the skin in each patient differs with regard to how the scalp reacts and holds on to the dye. There are many variables in performing SMP that makes this process more of an art form than a science. Bleeding of the pigment colors into the skin is the most common problem confronting the artist performing the SMP procedure because the dot sizes must be comparable to the diameter of a single hair or follicular unit at the completion of the process. The variables in the artist's control include the following:

- Size of the needles used
- Depth of needle penetration
- Duration of the penetration
- Puncture cycling of the needles if more than one is used
- Type of pigment used
- Incident angle of the needle entering the scalp

The SMP process is a labor-intensive process and could take multiple sessions and up to 20 hours of the surgeon's time to meet the patient's needs.

Once the SMP process is complete after the first session, the pigment is not stable and there is a tendency of the dots to fade or bleed (blend) into the surrounding skin, changing both the size and the color of the dot. The human body seems to attack the pigment such that the process often takes more than one procedure to produce a relatively stable result. A typical patient will come back for an additional treatment 2 to 3 times in a period of a month or so to refine the appearance of the pigment in the hope that the pigments that are placed are stable. Exposure to the sun can have an impact on the color and the size of the dots. It is important to explain to the patient that there may be a blue or green tint to the pigment. The greenish color of the black pigment is similar to how the red blood vessels appear green under the skin where the increased absorption of the red spectrum of light gives rise to a phenomenon explained by the trichomatic theory of color vision[2] (ie, if you absorb the red color, you will perceive a green hue).

Graying Hair Considerations in Micropigmentation

The provider performing this procedure must explain this to each and every patient in the disclosure of the informed consent that every patient must sign before undergoing the SMP process. The informed patient often asks about the graying of their hair as they get older because SMP is a permanent process, like any tattoo, and the concern is that if they develop gray hair, the pigment colors of the SMP process will be detectable. If they shave their scalp, this is not a problem, but if they allow their hair to grow out, then dying the hair may have to be considered if the color/contrast becomes a problem as the patient ages. Because of the high variability associated with the elements in performing the SMP process, many doctors and tattoo artists tend not to offer this service. Patient deformities created by inexperienced operators will, for the most part, be permanent. We tell our patients that, this is a permanent process, so they must be careful to select an experienced person to perform the procedure. The only option for a poor result may be the use of the laser to remove the pigments, but it may take many sessions to reverse the process adequately and the reversal is not guaranteed.

Micropigmentation Procedure

- The procedure is performed under local anesthesia—the procedure is painful without it. The authors use 0.5 Xylocaine and 0.25% Marcaine and the anesthesia often lasts through the entire 6-8 hour process.
- The hand piece the authors use has 3 needles in it that are cycled at a rate of 140 cycles per second (**Fig. 1**).
- A full head SMP takes between 5 to 7 hours.
- The dye insertion is often repeated 2 or 3 times because the dye is absorbed by the scalp in a patchy manner. Each subsequent procedure rectifies areas where the dye faded. In addition, the surgeon often underestimates the darkness of the color used and many patients ask for a darker color because they take more charge of what they want to look like.
- Second and third sessions are not unusual and each subsequent session often takes between 3 to 6 hours, depending on what is

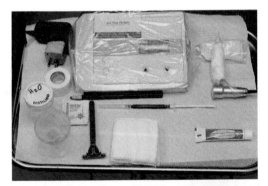

Fig. 1. Scalp micropigment kit. The kit includes handset with needles, control unit that regulates needle cycling, Vaseline, tape, razor, specialized ink, marking pen, electric shaver—all placed in a clean surgical field.

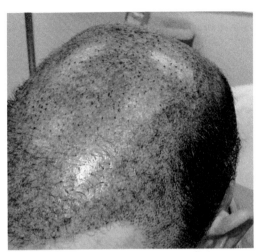

Fig. 2. A poorly done tattoo that eventually turned green. The tattoo dots were larger than the cross-section of a hair and the ink moved into the surrounding skin. The tattoo dots were only placed in areas of the head where balding existed at that time it was done and the tattoos became isolated in a patch-like quilt pattern.

needed to satisfy the patient. The timespan between sessions can be relatively short (about 1 week), but often the patients are seen a few months after the last procedure is done for touchups.

Pigment Bleeding in Scalp Micropigmentation

The occurrence of bleeding pigments from one dot to another is not uncommon. This process is most often caused by the patient who pushes us to do it again and again, or because the surgeon does not adequately control the depth or the length of time the needles are in the skin (**Fig. 2**). The need to have a patient who is willing to follow the strategy that is given is critical to preventing pigment bleeding. Pigment bleeding may be controlled with careful depth control and the use of small dots; however, the authors have seen pigment bleeding that has been significant in a small very rare subset of cases. When that happens, the use of a laser may be the only option available.

Good patient education and communication are critical. Many patients have developed a simple view of what they need and often try to direct the process. There is a continuing dialogue with many patients, finding a middle ground between what they want and what is thought will work for them can be challenging.

RESULTS

Examples of various SMP applications are presented:

SHAVED HEAD: If the entire head is shaved, SMP can be a styling option or a treatment modality for men with genetic androgenic alopecia. This is a purely cosmetic application (**Figs. 3** and **4**).

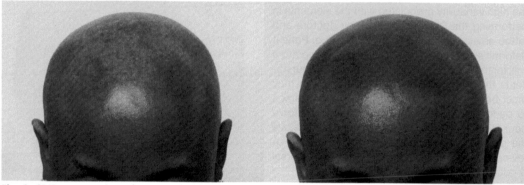

Fig. 3. SMP on genetic androgenic alopecia (before/after) on patient with skin mottling possibly from sun damage.

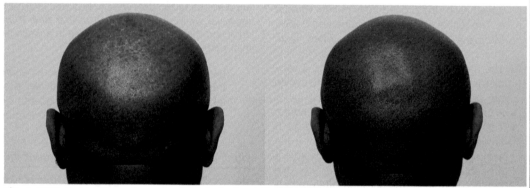

Fig. 4. SMP on genetic androgenic alopecia (before/after) in dark skinned man.

ENHANCING THE THINNING HEAD OF HAIR: If the hair is left at an adequate length and there is enough hair present, SMP can be used as a permanent concealer to soften the contrast between the hair and skin color giving the appearance of a fuller head of hair. This is a very valuable option for individuals who have a depleted donor supply and who can simply not get the final results they need (**Figs. 5** and **6**).

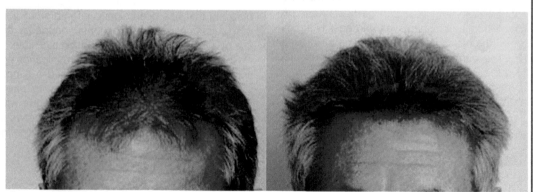

Fig. 5. SMP on thinning hair (before/after).

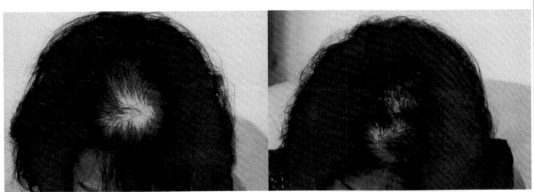

Fig. 6. SMP on thinning hair (before/after). Note that the frontal centimeter was not pigmented.

TREATMENT OF VARIOUS SCARRING ALOPECIAS: In conditions such as alopecia areata, alopecia totalis, where hair transplant is not an option, SMP can blend in the bald patches with the surrounding hair. If the patches of hair loss are extensive in the male, this is an option as long as the patient is willing to shave their scalp to create the even appearance (**Figs. 7** and **8**).

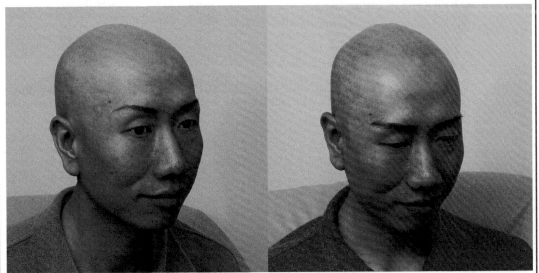

Fig. 7. SMP on patient with Alopecia Totalis (before/after). The eyebrows reflect a hair system application.

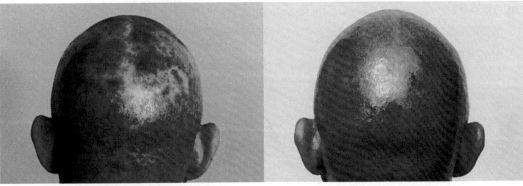

Fig. 8. SMP on scarring alopecia (before/after).

CAMOUFLAGING THE HAIR AND SKIN DEFORMITIES ASSOCIATED WITH OLDER, OUTDATED HAIR TRANSPLANT PROCEDURES (plugs, scalp reductions) are shown here and include the older punch graft scars, widened strip scars, FUE scars, and irregular cobble-stoning scar deformities of the scalp. SMP can greatly reduce the contrast and unsightly appearance of the scars where it may be undetectable by a casual observer (**Figs. 9–12**).

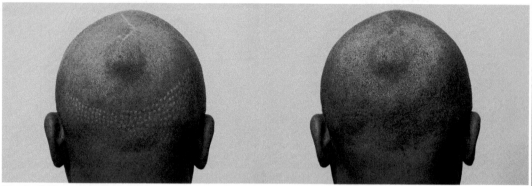

Fig. 9. SMP on old punch graft scars and a scalp reduction scar (before/after).

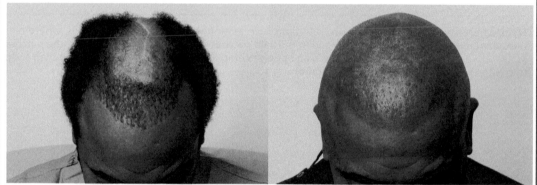

Fig. 10. SMP on old punch graft scars and a scalp reduction scar (before/after). Fillers can be used to treat the divots on the skin surface.

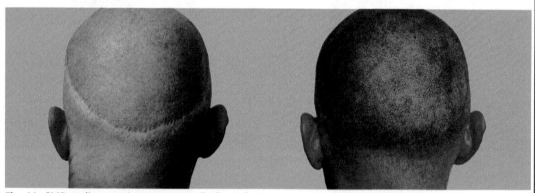

Fig. 11. SMP on linear strip surgery scar (before/after).

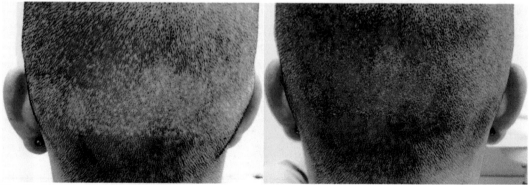

Fig. 12. SMP on FUE scars (before/after).

SUMMARY

Tattooing of the scalp is not new. This technique has been attempted by tattoo artists for years. It is a niche segment of the permanent makeup industry in Asia, Europe, and the United States. In general, scalp tattooing is shunned by most physicians and potential patients because the results are highly variable. The SMP technique takes considerable time to learn. This process is a great adjunct for the hair restoration surgeon as sooner or later many patients will run out of donor hair or the funds to complete the process, once started. The limitations of the technique must be understood by the surgeon as the appropriate potential candidates are chosen.

REFERENCES

1. Traquina AC. Micropigmentation as an adjuvant in cosmetic surgery of the scalp. Dermatol Surg 2001; 27(2):123–8.
2. Pak JP, Rassman WR, Kim J. Scalp micropigmentation (SMP): novel applications in hair loss. Hair Transplant Forum 2011;21(6).
3. Kienle A, Lilge L, Vitkin IA, et al. Why do veins appear blue? A new look at an old question. Appl Opt 1996; 35(7):1151.

Complications in Hair-Restoration Surgery

Raymond J. Konior, MD[a,b,*]

KEYWORDS

- Complication • Shock-loss • Scalp necrosis • Plugs • Donor-site scar • Unnatural hairline

KEY POINTS

- Complications associated with surgical hair restoration are usually preventable and most often arise as a consequence of poor planning or faulty surgical technique.
- Preoperative education and active patient participation are vital components for a successful, problem-free restoration of hair.
- Young patients are most likely to experience a planning error because of their frequent desire for aggressive restoration schemes and the unpredictability of progressive hair loss.
- A scar-related complication is one of the most common problems encountered at the donor site.
- A thorough preoperative screening program is mandatory to exclude patients with unattainable goals and unrealistic expectations.

INTRODUCTION

Serious complications arising from surgical hair restoration (SHR) are relatively uncommon following well-performed and well-planned surgery. Hair transplant patients are much more likely to experience temporary inconveniences such as:

1. Excessive pain
2. Pronounced edema
3. Temporary thinning of hair within the surgical site
4. Prolonged crust formation over the grafts or incision line
5. Short-term hypoesthesia within the graft or donor-site regions

Complications that follow SHR can be placed into 1 or more of the following categories:

1. Standard surgical risks
2. Physician planning errors
3. Physician technical errors
4. Patient compliance factors
5. Patient physiology factors
6. Miscellaneous causes

Surgical complications can often be secondarily categorized as those which occur in the recipient site and those which occur in the donor site.

Risk follows all forms of surgical intervention. Complications can occur unexpectedly despite even the most optimal conditions relating to patient health, patient preparation and education, surgical technique, and operative plan. Fortunately, the commonly recognized surgical risks of infection and bleeding are extremely uncommon for patients undergoing SHR, as the scalp is privileged with an extraordinary circulation that provides relative resistance to such issues. Problems associated with SHR are much more likely to arise from elements that are directly controlled by the surgeon or by the patient. Mistakes such

Disclosure Statement: The author has nothing to disclose and has no conflicts of interest with respect to the content of this article.
[a] Department of Otolaryngology – Head and Neck Surgery, Loyola University Medical Center, 2160 South First Avenue, Maywood, IL 60153, USA; [b] Chicago Hair Institute, 1S280 Summit Suite C-4, Oakbrook Terrace, IL 60181, USA
* Chicago Hair Institute, 1S280 Summit Suite C-4, Oakbrook Terrace, IL 60181.
E-mail address: drkonior@sbcglobal.net

Facial Plast Surg Clin N Am 21 (2013) 505–520
http://dx.doi.org/10.1016/j.fsc.2013.05.012

as placing a hairline too low or inserting a graft upside-down are fully controlled by the surgeon, and therefore completely preventable. Strategic planning and implementation errors typically result from inexperience.

Patient-related factors and patient participation can also influence the occurrence of postoperative problems. Preoperative education and training as to the importance of medication schedules, scalp hygiene protocols, activity restrictions, and dietary recommendations are mandatory to assure that the patient will not put himself or herself at greater risk for a postoperative complication. Despite rigorous education and diligent compliance, however, the patient may still be at risk for a complication related to an unexpected physiologic healing disorder.

Other potential causes for SHR complications include patient dissatisfaction associated with body dysmorphic disorder and the unexpected loss of donor hair that can rarely occur many years far removed from the restoration procedure.

GENERAL COMPLICATIONS
Bleeding

Bleeding following hair transplantation can occur in both the recipient and donor areas. Preoperative evaluation should screen for history of bleeding diathesis and for intake of aspirin, nonsteroidal anti-inflammatory agents, vitamin E, alcohol, anabolic steroids, or other anticoagulative agents. Intraoperative recipient-site bleeding is not uncommon and can usually be minimized by injection with epinephrine-containing solutions.[1] Significant bleeding in the donor region can be encountered with strip harvesting or punch extraction following inadvertent vascular transection in the supragaleal plexus. Suture ligation best controls hemorrhage from large vessels. Coagulation is effective for sealing small vessels located in the deep tissue bed, but should be avoided for dermal bleeding whereby follicles risk thermal injury. Dermal oozing is best controlled with epinephrine-containing solutions and with meticulous wound closure that firmly approximates the opposing subcutaneous edges. Patients are instructed to control postoperative oozing from either the recipient or donor sites with 10 to 15 minutes of continuous pressure. Persistent bleeding from either region requires professional evaluation.

Infection

Although the incidence of infection following hair transplantation is low, localized infections can occur in both the recipient- and donor-site regions. Serious infections occur in less than 1% of cases and are usually associated with poor hygiene, excessive crust formation, or a preexisting medical risk factor.[2] Prompt detection is vital for containing the problem and assuring a rapid recovery.

Donor-site infections may be more prevalent following a high-tension closure secondary to the circulatory compromise that accompanies this situation. Pronounced crust formation favors localized bacterial proliferation, which can increase the risk of infection. Recipient-site infections often present with papulopustules localized to the affected area, whereas donor-site infections commonly show excessive crust formation, inflammation, and light purulent discharge from individual suture or staple perforation points. Early donor-site problems often respond positively to staple and suture removal. Low-grade infections in either zone tend to improve quickly with excellent wound care that encourages the removal of overlying crusts. Moist compresses and frequent shampooing are recommended to soften and dislodge adherent crusts within the recipient site and along the donor incision line. Topical antibiotic ointment is applied 3 to 4 times daily over any involved area to contain inflammation and prevent additional crust formation.

Occasionally a localized area in the graft site or along the incision line will demonstrate fluctuance, erythema, and tenderness suggestive of abscess formation. Localized purulent fluid collections require drainage and wound care with moist gauze packs. Fluid samples should be submitted for culture and sensitivity testing to guide antimicrobial management. Although topical antibiotic ointments may suffice for managing small, well-localized inflammatory reactions, diffuse infections with surrounding erythema, edema, or tenderness generally require systemic broad-spectrum antibiotics with ideal coverage determined by final culture report. Open wounds are maintained using a moist dressing protocol and are allowed to heal via secondary intention. Secondary scar revisions can be performed at a later date on complete resolution of the inflammatory process.

Edema

Hairline restoration inevitably generates some soft-tissue edema within the forehead and surrounding areas. Left unmanaged, forehead edema can spread to the periorbital region, which occasionally may force the eyelids to close for 1 or more days. Some patients correlate demonstrable edema with a negative experience. Pharmacologic and nonpharmacologic interventions help to minimize this problem and enhance the overall patient experience.

Forehead edema results from the cumulative anesthetic and tumescent fluid loads injected into the recipient site and from the venous and lymphatic congestion that accompanies incising the recipient site. Patients undergoing a dense-pack or a megasession procedure are especially predisposed because of the compromised venous and lymphatic flow that is associated with these transplant methods. Peak facial edema commonly occurs 2 to 4 days postoperatively. Patients are encouraged to rest, maintain a 45° head elevation, perform frequent ice-pack massage over the fore-head region, and maintain a low sodium diet. Massaging the lower forehead above the brows with a central to lateral motion diverts fluid away from the periorbital region toward the temple, which then can migrate inferiorly into the less aesthetically sensitive cheek region. Systemic corticosteroids are a useful adjunct for managing postoperative swelling.[3] A 6-day tapering dose of methylprednisolone is one option to help speed resolution of clinically disturbing periorbital and forehead edema.

DONOR-SITE COMPLICATIONS

Table 1 summarizes donor-site complications.

Wide Scars

Unpredictable physiologic healing variations risk the chance of a wide donor scar for some patients despite excellent surgical technique. Most patients, however, heal with narrow scars that are easy to camouflage when subjected to a technically superior donor strip harvest. Operative strategies that encourage optimal healing include:

1. Minimizing incision-line tension, especially in the region above the mastoid process where a higher intrinsic tension predisposes many patients to wide scars
2. Avoiding follicular transection by performing meticulous incisions that traverse a precise path between each follicular unit along the entire length of the donor strip
3. Utilization of multilayered closure techniques that limit superficial tension via secure approximation of the deep fascia
4. Avoiding low donor incisions near the nape of the neck where scar stretching is more prevalent[4]

Patient-related influences can also affect donor-scar width, especially during the early healing phase when scars possess limited tensile strength. Wound strength may remain compromised for weeks to months following suture removal until completion of the scar maturation process. Patients are often eager to resume normal activities immediately after suture removal, at which time the increased donor-site tension that accompanies neck flexion can widen a vulnerable scar (**Fig. 1**). Patient education should emphasize the adverse consequences associated with tension-inducing forces along the donor-site incision line. Neck-flexion restrictions are recommended for 4 to 6 weeks or until the scar reveals evidence of complete maturation. Ironically, patients with hyperelastic skin, whose donor sites routinely close with minimal effort, occasionally heal with a scar much wider than expected, possibly secondary to intrinsic hyperelastic scar formation.

Table 1 Donor-site and recipient-site complications in hair-restoration surgery	
Donor Site	**Recipient Site**
Wide scars	Hairline location or shape error
Cross-hatch scars	Prediction of male pattern baldness progression error
Keloid scars	Graft type error
Multiple scars	Graft placement error
Visible scars	Hypopigmentation
Donor-site depletion	Hair color mismatch
Wound dehiscence	Chronic folliculitis
Necrosis	Necrosis
Effluvium (shock-loss)	Effluvium (shock-loss)
Hypoesthesia	Ingrown hairs
Neuralgia and neuromas	Cysts
Hematoma	Low graft yield

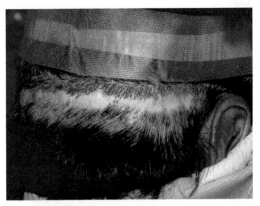

Fig. 1. Wide donor scar that resulted from a combination of faulty surgical technique and premature strenuous physical activity.

Unsightly wide scars that result from technical mishap or poor patient compliance may benefit from scar revision. Preoperative scalp massage to promote local scalp laxity and prolonged neck-flexion restrictions may increase the odds of a successful repair. Unfortunately, some wide scars are destined to recur despite even the best scar revision. Patients with recurrent widening despite proficient surgical technique may be dependent on topical concealers, micropigmentation, or follicular-unit extraction (FUE) to provide effective camouflage.

Cross-Hatch Scars

Unsightly cross-hatch donor-site scars are possible with both suture and staple wound closures. A tight closure and pronounced edema can create a strangulation effect on the skin surface arising from snug overlying sutures or staples. A critical pressure force will cause a suture loop or staple crown to cut through the skin with a resulting cross-hatch scar pattern that runs perpendicular to the donor incision line (**Fig. 2**). Follicular devitalization ensues beneath each cross-hatch scar to further exacerbate the consequences of this complication. Cross-hatching seems to be less prevalent with staples because the staple crown rests 1 to 2 mm above the donor skin, thereby creating a small buffer zone in which the skin can swell before encountering any significant pressure effect. Preventive measures begin with minimizing incision-line tension through the use of conservative strip widths and layered wound-closure techniques. A thorough approximation of the deep fascia along the entire length of the donor incision line helps reduce local tension so that epidermal sutures and staples can be positioned without strangulating forces. Patients are encouraged to use frequent postoperative icing to minimize incision-line edema, and to limit neck flexion until sutures have been removed.

Keloid and Hypertrophic Scars

Donor-site keloid and hypertrophic scar formation occurs infrequently in patients without prior history of such scarring. Patients with a documented keloid tendency are best discouraged from undergoing elective scalp surgery (**Fig. 3**). High-risk patients who wish to pursue the restorative process can be screened using a test session consisting of a very limited donor harvest and subsequent graft placement into a well-camouflaged fringe area that would remain undetectable in the event of adverse healing. Proliferative scars can be managed with intralesional injections using triamcinolone acetonide, 10 to 40 mg/mL every 2 to 4 weeks, until softening occurs.

Multiple Scars

The older strategy of excising donor strips with multiple scars has fallen into disfavor. Patients often have greater difficulty camouflaging multiple donor-site scars, especially with shorter hair styles.

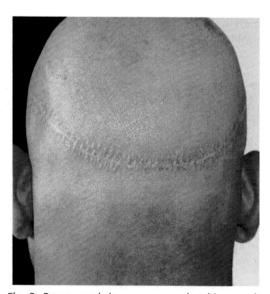

Fig. 2. Pronounced donor scar cross-hatching resulting from a tight suture closure.

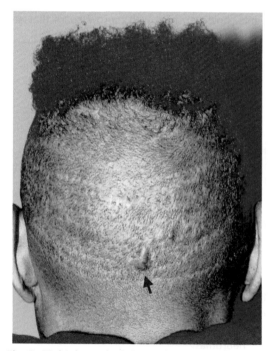

Fig. 3. Multiple stacked donor-site scars with an isolated central occipital keloid scar (*arrow*).

Multiple scars scattered throughout the donor area have an adverse effect on local scalp circulation. Circulatory compromise is further exaggerated when only a narrow bridge of donor scalp is preserved between adjacent incisions so as to increase the risk of telogen, scar widening, and permanent hair loss (**Fig. 4**). The multiscar harvesting approach is inefficient with respect to the use of available follicular stores because more donor hair must be preserved to camouflage several scars than would be needed to hide a single scar. An ideal donor-site management plan for secondary and tertiary strip harvest procedures favors retention of a single scar line, accomplished by positioning a prior scar within the new donor strip or by placing it along the upper or lower edge of the newly excised strip. This strategy maintains a single scar within the dense central donor region, thereby optimizing graft quality and reducing postoperative styling restrictions. The single-scar approach minimizes local circulatory compromise and maximizes long-term graft availability.

Visible Scars

Visible scarring within the donor region is one of the most common complications encountered in SHR. The detectability of donor-site scars is influenced by the absolute scar mass (ie, the overall number and width of scars) and the ability of the remaining donor hair population to hide the scars (**Fig. 5**). For some patients the visibility of even a single, relatively narrow scar can result in tremendous anxiety and frustration.

Surgeons who attempt to maximize graft yields through the use of aggressive donor harvesting approaches increase the risk of a long-term visible scar dilemma. Methods that increase this risk include:

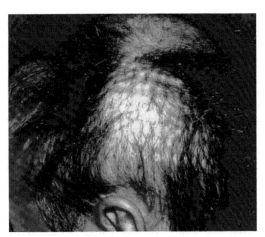

Fig. 5. Visible donor-site scarring resulting from an extremely aggressive graft-harvesting plan. The final scar mass overwhelms the native hair population so that effective camouflage is impossible.

1. Use of multiple donor incision lines scattered throughout the donor region
2. Strip excisions that are placed in the inferior donor region where the prevalence of scar stretching is increased
3. High-density FUE graft depletion
4. When strip or FUE harvests venture superiorly into donor-site fringe zones that possess a risk for future thinning

This last point assumes greater significance for young men in whom the risk of unpredictable fringe erosion is especially high. Unexpected downward migration of the donor fringe arising from progression of the balding process has the potential to expose poorly planned superior incision or extraction sites. An increasing scar mass from aggressive and repetitive donor harvests can result in "see-through" hair, which exposes donor scars even when the remaining hair is grown long. The risk of see-through hair is increased at the donor rim and between closely stacked incision lines, where follicular depletion from vascular compromise and interscar stretching further exaggerates the see-through effect. Correction of visible scarring arising secondary to a see-through effect is difficult in light of the implicit follicular depletion that accompanies this problem. Donor scar grafting with body or beard hair and cosmetic tattooing are potential treatment options.[5]

Donor-Site Depletion

Donor-site depletion is an end-stage condition whereby scalp follicles are no longer available for harvest. This complication can be devastating for those patients who are in need of recipient-site

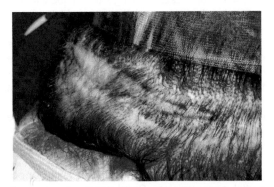

Fig. 4. A pair of wide donor scars impinge on each other in the central occipital region. Compromised follicular viability and stretching along the interposed skin bridge created an extremely wide alopecic zone.

repair or who simply have an incomplete restoration. End-stage depletion most often arises from a combination of poor surgical planning and substandard surgical techniques. Patients in this group commonly present with multiple problems including low graft yields, unnatural hairlines, inefficient graft distribution, and diffuse donor-site scarring that often demonstrates a see-through appearance. FUE of body and beard follicles[6] and scalp micropigmentation offer hope for improving the appearance of both the donor and recipient sites in these patients.

Wound Dehiscence

Donor-site wound dehiscence is extremely uncommon, as scalp incisions tend to heal quickly because of favorable local circulation patterns. Most surgeons remove sutures 8 to 14 days following surgery, at which time the tensile strength along the donor incision line is adequate to maintain approximation of the wound edges. Circulatory compromise, however, can delay healing and increase the risk of suture-line dehiscence. Predisposing factors such as diabetes, a high-tension closure, coexisting suture-line infection, premature removal of sutures, and excessive early physical activity place the patient at greater risk for unexpected donor-site dehiscence.[7] This complication is best avoided by using a layered wound closure to reduce incision-line tension, minimizing local incision-line inflammation with meticulous postoperative wound care, avoiding early removal of sutures, and limiting any physical exertion that places a distracting force on the incision line for at least 1 week following suture removal.

Necrosis

Donor-site necrosis occurs most commonly from a technical error that places excessive tension along the donor incision line. Inordinate tension predisposes to a localized microcirculatory collapse. Donor-site necrosis is a serious complication that destroys soft tissue and permanently damages follicles within the affected area (**Fig. 6**). Patients with a history of prior scalp reduction or previous strip harvesting may have elevated intrinsic tension within their donor area, placing them at even greater risk. The possibility for necrosis is increased with preexisting conditions such as diabetes mellitus, smoking, donor-site scarring, and intraoperative mishaps such as inadvertent transection of the occipital artery.

Necrosis is best avoided by preventing excessive tension anywhere along the donor incision line. The area superior to the mastoid process is particularly susceptible to a tension-related

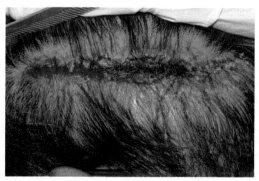

Fig. 6. Donor-site necrosis resulting from a high-tension suture closure. Eschar is identified over the necrotic site in this 2-week postoperative photo. Early postoperative effluvium surrounds the devitalized incision site.

problem, as it often demonstrates limited laxity secondary to rigid deep scalp attachments. Caution must also be exerted with wide strips that often accompany megasession donor harvests, as these invariably have the potential to generate high donor tension. Patients who demonstrate limited elasticity can often improve scalp laxity with several weeks of preoperative daily scalp massage.

Experience is perhaps the most valuable resource for determining acceptable tension levels during the donor harvest. However, even an experienced surgeon may overestimate a tolerable strip width and face the challenge of a tight closure. Proper management of this situation begins by avoiding any forced wound closure and using a multilayered closure to approximate only those areas along the incision line with favorable tension dynamics. Any high-tension zone is left open to be managed with moist dressings and secondary-intention healing.[8] Once fully healed the patient is instructed on scalp massage techniques to enhance local scalp elasticity, after which a controlled scar revision can be performed.

Once established, donor-site necrosis can be managed using antibiotic ointments to provide moist occlusion to the devitalized area. Conservative debridement of loose peripheral necrotic crust is performed on a regular basis to maintain a clean healing environment. Necrotic wounds often take weeks to months to heal, and typically conclude with inelastic cicatricial scar formation. The patient is encouraged to perform scalp massage for several weeks to improve local scalp laxity for potential scar revision. Serial excisions or tissue expansion may be required for large scars and when high intrinsic tension levels dominate the donor site.

Donor-Site Effluvium (Shock-Loss)

Minor occurrences of donor-site effluvium are not uncommon. Thinning usually remains confined to a region located immediately above and below the harvest incision line. Often referred to as shock-loss, peri-incisional thinning is almost always temporary, with full recovery occurring about 3 to 4 months following surgery. Physiologic alterations in the native follicle population arising secondary to regional edema, inflammation, and localized vascular compromise along the suture line are probable contributing factors. Patients are encouraged to control edema with frequent incision-line cooling, and are also instructed on maintaining excellent donor hygiene with daily cleaning and antibiotic ointment applications to control suture-related inflammation. Preexisting donor-site scars and technical miscalculations that generate excessive donor-site tension or that inadvertently transect major vascular supply vessels increase the chance of a more profound effluvium event. Fortunately, a full recovery is still the norm even for those with dramatic shock-loss (**Fig. 7**). Topical minoxidil is commonly recommended to speed follicular recovery within the shocked zone.[9]

Neuralgias, Neuromas, and Hypoesthesia

Partial or complete nerve transection of the greater occipital, lesser occipital or auriculotemporal nerves may follow carelessly performed deep donor-site incisions. Hypoesthesia localized to the innervation zone can result from accidental nerve transection. Aberrant neural healing can cause persistent scalp hyperesthesia or regional discomfort. A faulty healing response may also generate a neuroma: a tender, palpable nodule that develops from fibrous tissue proliferation surrounding the injured nerve. One can attempt to treat neuropathic pain or hypersensitivity arising from an injured nerve with regional infiltrations of local anesthetics and corticosteroids. Monthly injections using a mixture of triamcinolone acetonide, 10 mg/mL, diluted 2:1 with 2% lidocaine, has been advocated for this problem.[10] Extreme hyperesthesia or discomfort that resists infiltrative therapy may require referral to a neurologist for possible pharmacologic management. Persistent pain or sensitivity arising from a palpable neuroma may require surgical intervention to remove the pathologic mass.

Hematoma

Donor-site hematomas are rare and are usually associated with inadvertent transection of a major vascular branch such as the occipital or superficial temporal arteries. Cutting too deep during strip harvesting can lacerate these vessels and, when unrecognized, may result in a donor-site hematoma. Hematomas are best avoided by limiting donor-site incision depth and carefully exploring the wound bed for evidence of vascular damage. Major vessel transections require careful suture ligation for effective control. A multilayered closure technique is preferred to eliminate any dead space that could potentially harbor a fluid collection. An active donor-site hematoma will often produce pain, swelling, and localized ecchymosis. Once established, this complication is best corrected by wound exploration, suture ligation, or cauterization of actively bleeding vessels, and layered wound closure. Failure to promptly address this problem within 24 hours may increase the risk of donor-site necrosis and permanent hair loss.[11]

RECIPIENT-SITE COMPLICATIONS

Table 1 summarizes recipient-site complications.

Hairline Location and Shape Errors

Hairline location and shape errors occur most often in young men who often prefer relatively

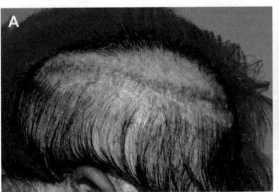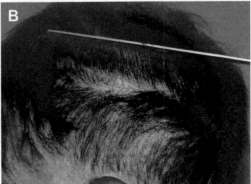

Fig. 7. Donor-site shock-loss. (*A*) Dramatic donor-site effluvium in a patient with a history of 3 prior strip procedures. (*B*) Full recovery of donor-site effluvium is apparent in this 6-month postoperative photo.

low and straight hairlines. Such hairlines may appear acceptable if the balding process remains stable. However, the adverse aesthetic consequences of opting for such a hairline plan may only emerge years later if progressive balding leads to temporal hairline recession and significant balding posterior to the previously set hairline (**Fig. 8**). Hairline design and location are determined by many factors including patient goals, available donor supply, and the potential for future hair loss. In general, higher hairlines that follow a gentle upward path from the central hairline to the lateral frontotemporal recession tend to maintain a more natural appearance over time, despite aging and the ongoing progression of pattern hair loss. Drastic maneuvers are often required to correct a cosmetically undesirable low hairline.[12] Forehead lifting with or without tissue expansion is one option for raising and reshaping a low hairline. The forehead skin is first elevated via a pretricheal incision and then advanced superiorly to allow removal of the unattractive, inferiorly positioned hairline grafts. A trichophytic closure can be performed to help optimize healing along the frontal hairline incision. Staged hairline restoration or frontal scar refinement can be planned several months later on normalization of vascular flow within the frontal scalp region.

Prediction of Male Pattern Baldness Progression Error

A long-term planning mistake is most likely to occur in young patients because of the difficulty associated with accurately predicting the final extent of hair loss, a process that may take decades to declare.[13] Early-onset hair loss,

especially during adolescence, may be a predictor for future evolution to a high-grade pattern. Young patients who can advance to class 6 and class 7 patterns are especially problematic, as these individuals often present with lofty goals that favor a low hairline, high density, and full scalp coverage. Aggressive restoration plans that attempt to satisfy these goals have the potential to create cosmetically disfiguring graft distributions (**Fig. 9**) and to deplete the donor graft supply from any ongoing pursuit to keep pace with the progressive balding process. For these reasons many surgeons advocate limiting or avoiding surgical restoration for patients younger than 24 to 26 years.

Graft Type Error

Over the years hair restoration has progressed from a procedure that involved a small number of large grafts (plugs) to one that consists of a large number of small grafts (follicular units). The cosmetic deficiencies of large plug techniques are readily apparent. The primary goals of restoration focus on objectives relating to density and naturalness. Naturalness is best assured by the careful placement of meticulously dissected, individual follicular units. Some physicians, however, continue to advocate the use of larger minigrafts or double-unit grafts as a means of enhancing density. Although these grafts tend to produce acceptable results with low-contrast hair-skin color combinations, and fine or textured hair, they have a greater potential for creating aesthetic problems. Double-unit grafts, single-unit grafts, and even single hair grafts have the potential to produce an unnatural look when used inappropriately. The anterior frontal hairline is most prone

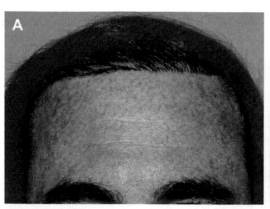 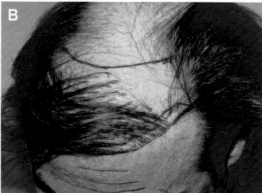

Fig. 8. (*A*) A very straight and low hairline was placed on this 47-year-old patient 22 years earlier at 25 years of age. The patient experienced only limited frontal recession at that time and was encouraged to pursue a low hairline design. (*B*) Oblique view reveals marked progression of hair loss that occurred over 22 years following the initial restoration. The low hairline appears unbalanced, and he does not have sufficient donor supply for a complete restoration.

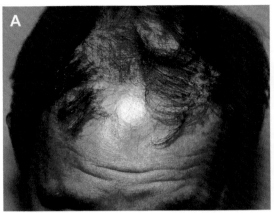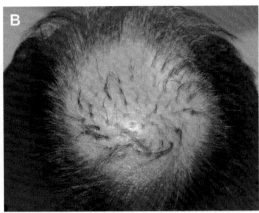

Fig. 9. Prediction of male pattern baldness progression error. (*A*) The patient received an isolated frontotemporal recession transplant in his early twenties. Twenty-year progression of hair loss has left him with an unnatural "horn deformity." (*B*) The patient underwent plug session for early crown thinning during his early twenties. Two decades of progressive thinning have left an unnatural island of plugs surrounded by a halo of bald skin.

to a detectable error of graft choice, as this is usually the most revealing zone of the restoration process. Patients with thick skin, high-caliber hair, and a contrasting dark hair–light skin combination are especially susceptible to graft detectability (**Fig. 10**). These high-risk patients should be approached cautiously, particularly at the frontal hairline, where carefully dissected, small-caliber single-hair grafts should be inserted along the leading edge of the frontal hairline to assure a completely undetectable appearance.

Graft Placement Error

Graft placement complications commonly fall into 1 of 3 categories:

1. Graft direction error (ie, wrong angle or incorrect right/left orientation)
2. Graft height error (ie, too high or too low)
3. Graft rotational error

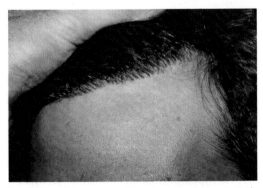

Fig. 10. Graft type error. Multihair grafts used at the leading edge of the frontal hairline look bulky and unnatural.

Errors relating to graft placement are completely dependent on the technical expertise of the surgical team.

Directional errors originate during preparation of the recipient sites, at which time the graft trajectory is predetermined by the path created from the blade cut into the scalp. Failure to follow the normal or intended directional flow of hair can have adverse cosmetic consequences, the significance of which may be exaggerated by contrasting and high-caliber hair. Right/left directional discrepancies can create styling problems, such as difficulty establishing a natural part or hair that does not flow evenly over the recipient site. Angle-related errors are common among novice surgeons, as the natural tendency is to create an opening less acute than the natural hair-exit angle. Graft insertion perpendicular to the scalp surface often looks unnatural and emphasizes hairline transparency because of inefficient recipient-site coverage dynamics (**Fig. 11**).

Rotational and height errors are controlled by the graft placement team. Grafts placed too high result in a cobblestone appearance, the significance of which can be exaggerated by larger and poorly trimmed grafts. Grafts inserted too low tend to form unattractive pits. The contractile forces of healing will typically compress multihair grafts so as to further accentuate the unnaturalness of the surface contour irregularities that accompany cobblestone and pit formation (**Fig. 12**). Extreme pitting along the frontal hairline may require FUE extraction to remove problematic grafts. Graft rotational errors originate from the hair shaft's natural curl, a physical characteristic that imparts some element of curvature to even fine, straight hair. Aesthetic imperfections associated with this

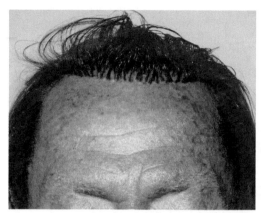

Fig. 11. Graft direction error. Improperly angled grafts placed perpendicular to the frontal scalp create an unnatural vertical wall of hair.

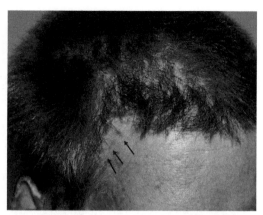

Fig. 13. Graft rotation error. Grafts were placed with the hair shaft "curl" rotated anteriorly (*arrows*), which causes transplanted hair at the temporal hairline to grow toward the forehead rather than in the natural posterior direction toward the temporal hair.

technical error are most prevalent at the anterior temporal hairline. Hair in this area characteristically possesses an acute angulation and a backward direction. Failure to meticulously control the rotational component of graft placement so as to orient the curl backward toward the temporal hair can result in an unnatural appearance along the temporal hairline where hairs haphazardly grow forward, upward, or with some other unfavorable orientation (**Fig. 13**).

Hypopigmentation

Hypopigmentation can occur in either the donor or recipient areas. Donor-site hypopigmentation is a definite risk of aggressive FUE graft harvests (**Fig. 14**). The risk for this problem increases with larger incisions and for those with a genetic predisposition to hypopigmentation. Clinically disturbing donor-site hypopigmentation that cannot be concealed by native donor hair may benefit from camouflage using body hair transplants, micropigmentation, or topical concealers. Recipient-site hypopigmentation is more prevalent with larger incisions, and can be especially problematic when low graft yields fail to produce sufficient hair for adequately camouflaging the scalp. Hypopigmentation in the recipient site is minimized by meticulously sizing each follicular-unit graft to its respective opening so as to avoid unnecessarily long recipient openings.

Hair Color Mismatch

The transformation of youthful hair pigment to that of graying is common with advancing age, but the distribution pattern of gray hair on a mature scalp

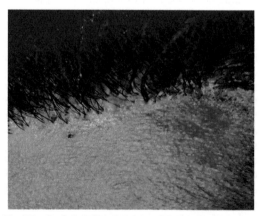

Fig. 12. Graft height error. Careless graft placement resulted in a combination of cobblestoning (too high) and pitting (too low).

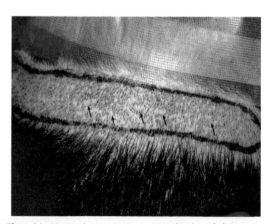

Fig. 14. Hypopigmentation. Hundreds of hypopigmented punctate scars (*arrows*) from a prior follicular-unit extraction procedure are scattered throughout the previous extraction site.

can be highly variable. Some patients demonstrate a homogeneous distribution of gray hair throughout the scalp such that donor harvesting will remove a hair population with color characteristics comparable to those of hair in the recipient site and along the adjacent temporal scalp. However, some patients demonstrate a strong bias for advanced graying or white hair transformation primarily at the anterior temporal scalp and temporal point regions while maintaining a much higher percentage of normal-colored hairs within the occipital donor area. Failure to recognize a regional color discrepancy can result in the creation of an unnatural color contrast problem whereby a stark, dark frontal hairline suddenly abuts against a white temporal hairline (**Fig. 15**). Significant color discrepancies must be recognized during the planning phase so that the donor harvest includes follicles from the distinctly different temple regions. Hair harvested from this area should be separated during the dissection process and strategically integrated among hairline grafts adjacent to the temporal hairline. Careful graft integration in this zone will allow for a natural color blend at the frontotemporal interface.

Chronic Folliculitis

Chronic folliculitis is an uncommon complication of SHR.[14] Culture and sensitivity examination is recommended for affected patients, but results are typically nondiagnostic. Predisposing factors such as poor hygiene or a preexisting dermatologic disorder should be investigated for a possible etiologic source. Similar to chronic acne vulgaris, patients may demonstrate resistance to treatment. Management is usually initiated with a vigorous scalp

hygiene regimen that can include daily cleansing with chlorhexidine gluconate or povidone-iodine shampoos. Topical antibiotic creams or ointments are applied over active lesions, with low-dose systemic oral antibiotics being reserved for more diffuse and resistant cases. Refractory cases may require modified antibiotic regimens for the control of recipient-site inflammation. An aggressive management plan is suggested, as chronic folliculitis has the potential to permanently destroy transplanted follicles via the induction of cicatricial scarring (**Fig. 16**).

Ingrown Hair

The appearance of 1 or more ingrown hairs is a common occurrence following hair transplantation. This problem is usually a limited one, with minor inflammatory reactions typically appearing 8 to 12 weeks after the transplant procedure on completion of the obligatory posttransplant follicular dormancy phase. Occasionally ingrown hairs present as a more significant problem, with a high percentage of the graft population being affected by large inflammatory eruptions. Problematic eruptions can last for months until all of the transplanted hairs have emerged from their subcutaneous implantation site. There appears to be an increased predisposition to ingrown hair inflammatory reactions in patients with large-caliber hair, thicker skin, and increased sebaceous gland activity. Treatment focuses on containing the inflammatory reaction and facilitating emergence of the trapped hair. Low-grade eruptions often resolve quickly with vigorous shampooing regimens that encourage exfoliation of the

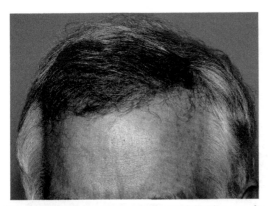

Fig. 15. Hair color mismatch. Frontal hairline grafts that were harvested exclusively from the occipital region have a significantly darker color than the white temple hair. Blending some donor hair from the temple into the frontal restoration could have provided for less color contrast between the 2 regions.

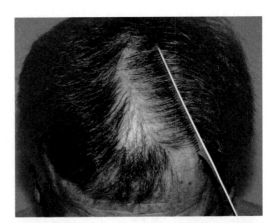

Fig. 16. Chronic folliculitis of unknown etiology developed 3 years following a successful frontal restoration. Lingering inflammation resistant to medical management for more than 1 year resulted in cicatricial alopecia and significant density reduction throughout the previously thick transplant site.

overlying skin. More profound reactions can benefit from moist, warm compresses 3 to 4 times a day, shampooing with chlorhexidine gluconate or povidone-iodine once or twice a day, and applying a topical antibiotic cream to individual inflammatory sites. Persistent or widespread eruptions may require low-dose systemic antibiotics to suppress inflammation until complete emergence of all transplanted hairs.

Cysts

Epidermal cysts originate from graft placement errors when a graft is buried beneath the recipient-site epidermal opening or when a graft is inadvertently "piggy-backed" over a previously placed graft.[15] Cysts in the donor site are also a potential risk with FUE, particularly following the use of a dull punch, which has the potential to push a graft deep into the donor extraction site. These technical mishaps are more common in the presence of excessive bleeding, with an inexperienced placement team, or when failing to use adequate magnification to facilitate visualization of the surgical field. An epidermal cyst often presents as a tender, palpable nodule with or without surrounding erythema. Rapid resolution generally follows incision and drainage of entrapped sebaceous debris, remnant hairs, and malpositioned follicles. Localized inflammation is managed with warm moist compresses 2 to 3 times a day and application of a topical antibiotic over the affected site. Diffuse infection may necessitate the use of systemic broad-spectrum antibiotics.

Low Graft Yield

A high graft yield of greater than 90% is both desirable and possible with follicular-unit restoration.[16]

A low graft survival rate is a complication influenced by physician-related and patient-related factors. Follicular injury that accompanies careless graft harvesting, graft preparation, or graft insertion can adversely affect graft survival. Graft desiccation is perhaps one of the most common preventable errors that predisposes to a low yield as the minuscule grafts typically remain vulnerable to exposure for long periods of time during the various phases of extraction, dissection, and insertion. Vascular compromise associated with conditions such as diabetes and preexisting scarring from prior trauma, previous hair restoration, or cicatricial alopecia can negatively affect graft yield. Extremely dense packing and large recipient-site incisions are other associated causes (**Fig. 17**). Patient-related factors that contribute to low graft yield include direct manipulation of the graft bed, for example with scratching, massaging, or aggressive shampooing. Although smoking has been indicted as a contributing factor, many smokers have demonstrated excellent graft yields. In general, superb technical implementation and diligent self-care by the patient helps to assure excellent graft survival rates.

Effluvium (Shock-Loss)

Recipient-site effluvium, commonly referred to as shock-loss, occurs to some degree in most patients who continue to have preexisting hair within the transplant zone. Anagen effluvium, telogen effluvium, or some combination of the two is responsible for the shedding of native hair, which typically begins 2 to 6 weeks following surgery. Female patients and those with advanced miniaturization seem to be at higher risk for recipient-site effluvium (**Fig. 18**). Most often shock-loss is

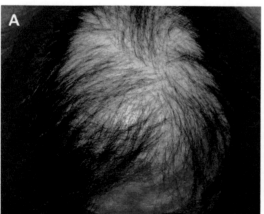
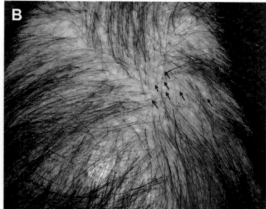

Fig. 17. Low graft yield. (*A*) Patient with very low yield following what was reported to be a 3000-graft session. (*B*) Close-up view of the transplant site reveals numerous hypopigmented scars (*arrows*) indicating previously placed grafts that failed to grow.

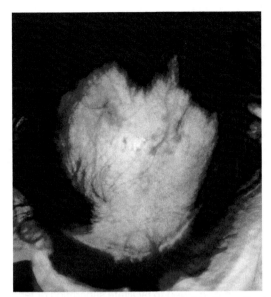

Fig. 18. Recipient-site effluvium. A female patient demonstrates profound recipient-site effluvium 3 weeks following a scalp advancement procedure.

strategies that limit graft incision size, minimize the use of epinephrine infiltration, avoid dense packing, and meticulously control opening direction so as to avoid native recipient-site follicles. Postoperative care regimens should aggressively manage recipient-site edema and inflammation. Topical minoxidil has been advocated to reduce the risk of effluvium as well as to speed the recovery of the dormant follicle population.[17] Cosmetically effluvium may benefit from topical fiber, spray, powder cake, or lotion camouflage agents.

Recipient-Site Necrosis

The frontal hairline and midscalp regions are well vascularized via a relatively robust centripetal blood supply. Recipient-site necrosis is a rare complication arising from a catastrophic vascular compromise that overwhelms local circulation within the transplant zone (**Fig. 19**). The intraoperative appearance of localized cyanosis in the central graft zone should alert the surgeon to the possibility of an impending vascular collapse. Persistent duskiness is an ominous sign that should signal immediate cessation of any additional incision or injection with epinephrine-containing solutions. Over the ensuing days a critically compromised area will typically darken further and develop a tightly adherent superficial crust overlying the damaged soft tissue bed.

Recipient-site necrosis is a consequence of vascular compromise. Predisposing influences such as diabetes mellitus, smoking, atrophic skin damage, preexisting recipient-site scarring, or prior scalp surgery may increase the risk of a necrotic event. Prevention begins with preservation of the scalp's vascular supply during the donor-area graft harvesting procedure. Technical

temporary, but a permanent reduction in the native hair population may occur, especially in those hairs that are near the end of their natural life cycle. The effluvium process advances the hair cycle with the result that genetically predisposed hairs destined to short-term loss will not recover. Recovery from recipient-site effluvium generally begins about 3 months postoperatively, when the transplanted follicles initiate their new growth cycle. Direct follicular injury, regional vascular compromise, recipient-site inflammation, and perifollicular edema increase the risk of this complication. These influences may be curtailed with technical

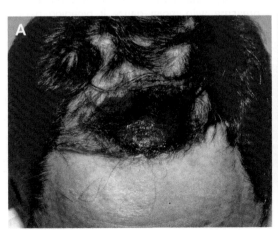

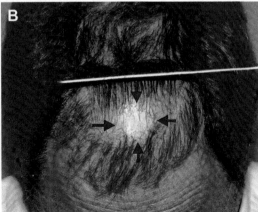

Fig. 19. Recipient-site necrosis. (A) Two-week postoperative photo shows dry crust densely adherent to underlying frontal graft zone. (B) Two-year postoperative photo demonstrates cicatricial alopecia (*arrows*) localized to the prior necrosis zone.

factors associated with recipient-site graft placement strongly influence the potential for necrosis. Large openings, megasessions, dense packing, epinephrine solutions injected directly into the recipient site, and deep recipient incisions are possible contributing factors.

Patience is required, as a necrotic event may take weeks or months to heal. Early crust formation is best managed conservatively with moist dressings and topical antibiotics to minimize local bacterial loads and to facilitate separation of the overlying crust. A clean eschar functions as a biological dressing for the underlying wound bed, and is best managed with conservative debridement as the peripheral edges begin to separate from the scar bed below.[18] End-stage healing is marked by the emergence of cicatricial scarring. The fibrotic scar tissue observed at this stage can reveal varying degrees of atrophy and has a predictably tenuous vascularity. Camouflage may be possible with a cautious grafting strategy that uses staged, low-density graft sessions. This approach increases the odds for graft survival while reducing the risk of a secondary vascular insult within the compromised scar bed. Tissue expansion may be required to reconstruct large areas of devitalized tissue.

PATIENT-RELATED COMPLICATIONS

Patient-related complications are listed in **Box 1**.

Excessive Crusting

Grafts typically develop localized crusts over the insertion sites within 24 hours of surgical implantation. Small crusts usually shed within 7 to 10 days while large crusts can last for 2 weeks or more. Crust formation normally does not create any long-term healing problems, but excessive crust formation can impose a cosmetic burden and may incite undesirable inflammation within the recipient site. Crust formation is best minimized with a diligent moisture-based hygiene protocol that begins immediately on completion of the procedure, at which time the recipient area is

---

| **Box 1** |
| **Patient-based complications** |

- Excessive crusting
- Displaced grafts
- Excessive edema
- Wide scars
- Low graft yield

---

thoroughly sprayed with sterile saline solution to remove any residual blood and serum from all graft insertion sites. An early postoperative visit within 24 to 48 hours of surgery is encouraged so that staff may inspect the recipient site under magnification and to remove dried serum and blood deposits with vigorous saline sprays. Patients are advised to continue spraying frequent saline mists over the graft zone and to gently shampoo the recipient site on a daily basis until all crusts have shed. Thorough patient education as to proper spraying and shampooing methods is crucial, as some patients avoid the necessary moisturizing activities for fear of dislodging their grafts. Neglecting to maintain proper hydration can lead to dense and profuse crusting that has the potential to inflame the recipient site and possibly compromise graft growth (**Fig. 20**). Moist compresses, scalp soaks, and topical ointments or gels can be used as needed to facilitate separation of tenaciously adherent crusts.

Displaced Grafts

Patient education and compliance with postoperative instructions are vital for prevention of early postoperative graft dislodgment. Freshly placed grafts remain stable in their insertion sites only by the force of the surrounding recipient-site tissue bed and by adherence from the overlying crust. Normal wound healing requires at least 3 to 4 days to establish any significant stability between the graft and the scalp. Patients place themselves at risk during this vulnerable period with any activity that involves rubbing, combing, brushing, or striking the recipient site with a blunt or sharp force. An acutely dislodged graft will often be accompanied by a sudden stream of profuse bleeding. Patients are advised to apply a gentle pressure with moist gauze if bleeding persists beyond a short time. Displaced grafts should be placed in a clean, moist cloth, preferably using saline solution if possible. Well-hydrated grafts can be reinserted on return to the physician's office. Unfortunately, patients often return with desiccated grafts that lack viability. In this case, a small donor harvest may be required to fill an empty zone from where the displacement occurred (**Fig. 21**).

Excessive Edema, Wide Scars, Low Graft Yield

The key components in minimizing patient-related complications include:

1. A comprehensive patient education program that contains clear written instructions
2. Regular staff encouragement for patient compliance with postoperative care requirements

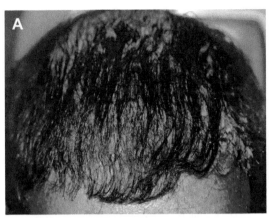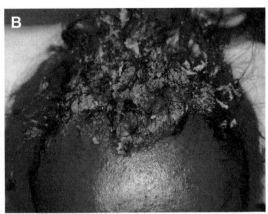

Fig. 20. Postoperative crusting. (*A*) The patient failed to wash the frontal graft zone for 1 year, fearing that he would damage grafts. (*B*) Separation of adherent, greasy, sebaceous debris reveals minimal graft survival in what was reported to be a 2000-graft session.

3. Frequent patient follow-up to ensure proper self-care

Inadequate postoperative care by the patient can increase the risk of cosmetically debilitating edema, wide donor-site scars, low graft yield, and a variety of other potential problems.

MISCELLANEOUS COMPLICATIONS
Unexpected Progression of Hair Loss

The incidence of senile alopecia increases with advancing age, especially after the age of 70 years. The emergence of senile alopecia in a patient with androgenic alopecia whose hairline had previously been restored can result in unpredictable thinning within the transplanted zone that may surprise even the most seasoned surgeon.[19] Young patients with evidence of donor-area miniaturization are perhaps most vulnerable to an unpredictable

long-term hair loss. Unexpected progressions may take decades to emerge, a fact that should instill caution with respect to surgical planning for young patients and anyone with evidence of significant donor-region miniaturization (**Fig. 22**).

Failure to Achieve Patient Expectations

Sooner or later, most surgeons will encounter an unhappy patient who reveals a result judged to be good or excellent by the surgeon, staff, and peers. This frustrating scenario is best avoided by rigorous preoperative patient screening, which begins with a comprehensive preoperative portrayal of what can be expected in terms of density, coverage, styling requirements, and any potential risks associated with the restoration process.

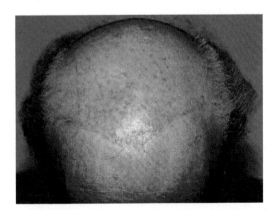

Fig. 22. Unexpected progression of hair loss. Frontal hairline of a patient who 30 years earlier underwent what was reported as a successful hair transplant that held stable for more than 20 years. He reported progressive loss of his graft hair over a 10-year period that was associated with comparable donor-site thinning, presumably arising secondary to the emergence of senile alopecia.

Fig. 21. Dislodged grafts. The patient hit his head on a kitchen cabinet within 30 minutes of returning home after a 3500-graft session. Dislodged grafts appear desiccated and devitalized.

Individuals with undue anxiety, unrealistic goals, or unreasonable expectations are approached with caution.[20] Openly hostile patients with unwarranted complaints regarding prior procedures from another physician may be especially hard to please. When faced with this problem, the physician should consider additional surgery only if a detailed discussion with the patient confirms his or her full comprehension of the situation and that an acceptable outcome will likely follow. Patients who continue to maintain unrealistic goals and expectations should be discouraged from pursuing surgery until they are willing to accept the realities of what can be accomplished. The treating physician should always remain positive, supportive, and available for future discussion, so as to never alienate or anger a problematic patient.

SUMMARY

Complications following hair transplantation occur infrequently with proper patient selection, a strategic operative plan, and careful execution of the restorative procedure. Patients are screened for having realistic goals and a pattern that is amenable to aesthetic restoration. A sound treatment plan must factor in the potential for long-term progression of hair loss as regards its influence on the stability of the proposed restorative scheme. Excellent technique strives to create perfectly natural-looking hair that balances the density and coverage goals agreed on by both patient and surgeon. Compromising any of these key elements can precipitously increase the risk of complications and patient dissatisfaction.

When to Refer

1. Patients with unrealistic goals or expectations
2. Patients with complicated donor-site scarring
3. Patients with visible donor-site scars or a depleted donor area
4. Patients with an unexplained history of a low graft yield
5. Patients who are openly hostile toward a prior physician
6. Patients who require technically challenging hairline relocation

REFERENCES

1. Coleman WP III, Klein JA. Use of tumescent technique for scalp surgery and dermabrasion, and soft tissue reconstruction. J Dermatol Surg Oncol 1992;18:130–5.
2. Farjo N. Infection control and policy development in hair restoration. Hair Transplant Forum Int 2008; 18(4):141–4.
3. Nordstrom RE, Nordstrom RM. The effect of corticosteroids on postoperative edema. In: Unger WP, Nordstrom RE, editors. Hair transplantation. 2nd edition. New York: Marcel Dekker; 1988. p. 391–4.
4. Knudsen RG. The donor area. Facial Plast Surg Clin North Am 2004;12(2):233–40.
5. Pak JP, Rassman WR. Scalp micropigmentation (SMP): novel applications in hair loss. Hair Transplant Forum Int 2011;21(6):181–7.
6. Cole J. Body to scalp. In: Unger WP, Shapiro R, Unger R, et al, editors. Hair transplantation. 5th edition. London: Informa Healthcare; 2010. p. 304–6.
7. Kulaylat MN, Dayton MT. Surgical complications. In: Townsend CM, Beauchamp RD, Evers BM, et al, editors. Sabiston textbook of surgery. 18th edition. Philadelphia: Elsevier Saunders; 2008. p. 1589–623.
8. Mangubut EA. Donor area vascular damage and sequelae. In: Unger WP, Shapiro R, Unger R, et al, editors. Hair transplantation. 5th edition. London: Informa Healthcare; 2010. p. 270–1.
9. Parsley WM, Waldman MA. Management of the postoperative period. In: Unger WP, Shapiro R, Unger R, et al, editors. Hair transplantation. 5th edition. London: Informa Healthcare; 2010. p. 416–9.
10. Knudsen RG. Unger. Donor area complications. In: Unger WP, Shapiro R, Unger R, et al, editors. Hair transplantation. 5th edition. London: Informa Healthcare; 2010. p. 419–22.
11. Stough DB, Randall JK, Schauder CS. Complications in hair replacement surgery. Facial Plast Surg Clin North Am 1994;2(2):219–29.
12. Epstein JS. Different options in revision surgical hair restoration. Hair Transplant Forum Int 2010;20(3): 73–9.
13. Marritt E, Konior RJ. Patient selection, candidacy, and treatment plan for hair replacement surgery. Facial Plast Surg Clin North Am 1994; 2(2):111–37.
14. Unger WP. Complications of hair transplantation. In: Unger WP, editor. Hair transplantation. 3rd edition. New York: Marcel Dekker; 1995. p. 363–74.
15. Beehner ML. Cyst formation post-transplant. Hair Transplant Forum Int 2007;17(1):30.
16. Tsilosani A. One hundred follicular units transplanted into 1 cm2 can achieve a survival rate greater than 90%. Hair Transplant Forum Int 2009;19(1):1–7.
17. True RH, Dorin RJ. A protocol to prevent shock loss. Hair Transplant Forum Int 2005;15(6):197.
18. Nusbaum BP, Nusbaum AG. Recipient area complications. In: Unger WP, Shapiro R, Unger R, et al, editors. Hair transplantation. 5th edition. London: Informa Healthcare; 2010. p. 422–4.
19. Rassman W. Case of long-term graft failure. Hair Transplant Forum Int 2002;12(5):186.
20. Knudsen R. The pursuit of perfection. Hair Transplant Forum Int 2009;9(2):45–6.

Future Horizons in Hair Restoration

Bryan T. Marshall, PhD[a], Chris A. Ingraham, PhD[a],
Xunwei Wu, PhD[a], Ken Washenik, MD, PhD[a,b,c,*]

KEYWORDS

- Cell therapy • Trichogenicity • Regenerative medicine • Dermal papilla • Hair follicle
- Induced pluripotent stem cells (iPS) • Hair transplantation

KEY POINTS

- Hair follicles can be regenerated from cultured cells.
- Culture conditions impact the trichogenic property of cells.
- The delivery method impacts the potential for a cell-based therapy to produce follicle outgrowth.
- Advances in cell biology provide the possibility of follicle regeneration from additional cell sources.

INTRODUCTION

The most common form of hair loss is androgenetic alopecia (AGA). Those affected by AGA display an increased sensitivity to androgens, which leads to reduced follicular diameter. Orientreich[1] was the first to show that transplanted hair follicles retain the characteristics of their original location (namely androgen resistance when placed into an androgen-sensitive area). This concept is termed donor dominance. The growth pattern dominance of the follicular origin over recipient site placement has enabled surgical hair transplantation to be one of the most effective treatments to date. Despite the effectiveness of modern hair transplantation, there are challenges associated with this method such as the limitation of donor hair follicles. Currently, medical treatments attempting to bypass the need for additional donor follicles include minoxidil, a potassium channel agonist, and finasteride, an inhibitor of 5 alpha- reductase.[2] These drug therapies require continual use and can be associated several adverse effects. More recently, hair loss therapies based on the cellular components of hair follicles and the growth factors that drive the behavior of those cells have become foci of research efforts. Autologous cell-based therapies offer a unique solution requiring the potential of single treatment and the possibility of no significant systemic adverse effects. Several advances have been made in the fields of stem cell biology and regenerative medicine in the last decade. These advances have laid the foundation to develop new strategies to treat hair loss. The possibility now exists to harvest a small number of hair follicles from the occipital area of the patient, expand the trichogenic, or hair follicle growth-inducing, cell population from this tissue, and transfer these cells back to the patient as a regenerative treatment. Aderans Research Institute Incorporated (ARI, Marietta, GA) and Replicel Life Sciences Incorporated (Vancouver, Canada) are currently conducting separate clinical trials with cell-based solutions for alopecia. Similar clinical trials have also been undertaken by Intercytex, Incorporated. Additionally, Histogen Incorporated (San Diego, CA) and Follica Incorporated (Cambridge, MA) are both conducting phase 1 clinical trials exploring the use of

Disclosures: The authors have a royalty agreement with the Aderans Research Institute should future revenue result from the sale of this technology.
[a] Aderans Research Institute, 2211 Newmarket Parkway, Suite 142, Marietta, GA 30067, USA; [b] Bosley, 9100 Wilshire Boulevard, East Tower Penthouse, Beverly Hills, CA 90212, USA; [c] Department of Dermatology, New York University School of Medicine, 550 First Avenue, New York, NY 10016, USA
* Corresponding author. Bosley, 9100 Wilshire Boulevard, East Tower Penthouse, Beverly Hills, CA 90212.
E-mail address: washenik@bosley.com

molecular growth factors aimed at the reinvigoration of dormant follicles. These small molecules are known agonists of follicular formation and growth pathways (eg, Wingless-related integration site [WNT], Sonic hedgehog [SHH], and fibroblast growth factors [FGF]).

Unlike most organs, hair follicles do not reach homeostasis once they mature. Instead there is a continuous cycle of growth, regression, shedding, and regeneration throughout life.[3] This inherent ability of hair follicle cycling lends credence to the idea of regenerative cell populations existing in the hair follicle itself. Several groups have demonstrated regeneration of hair follicles using cells dissected from the dermal papilla and dermal sheath of the hair follicle,[4–10] as well as follicular epidermal cells to form all lineages of the hair follicle[11,12] in animal models. This article addresses the history of hair follicle regeneration from follicular fragments and dissociated cells. The challenges of trichogenic in vitro culture and subsequent delivery into the patient are discussed, as well as cosmetic acceptance, recent achievements on regeneration of human hair follicles, and new potential cell sources (skin derived precursor cells [SKPs], Induced pluripotent stem cells [iPS]) for hair regeneration.

REGENERATION OF THE HAIR FOLLICLE FROM DISSECTED FRAGMENTS

One solution to increase the number of possible donor follicles is to divide up the hair follicle into dissected fragments in the hope that upon transplantation each fragment would develop into a complete follicle. While horizontal division of the hair follicles[13] has resulted in a complete hair follicle from the upper two-thirds, the lower one-third was not able to produce a follicle. A second study using transverse division[14] produced hair follicles from only one of the upper implants. The studies of these approaches were limited in size.

Another approach, using microdissected follicular dermal papillae (DP) or connective tissue sheaths (CTS),[4–10] was able to regenerate follicles upon insertion into afollicular skin. In people, the transplantation of male scalp dermal sheath (DS) fragments into female forearm skin resulted in follicular growth with male dermal lineage.[15]

The major caveat to these methods is the poor efficiency of regeneration (ie, they did not result in increase in the resultant number of hairs compared with the number of follicles used). The numbers of hairs were not increased, because at least 1 DP, DS, or CTS is required to form a new hair follicle. Hence, the major contribution of this research was the realization that cells within dissected

follicular fragments are able to reorganize and induce new hair follicles or follicular growth. These experiments prompted additional research investigating the cells derived from these follicular fragments and the development of in vitro culture methods directed at trichogenic cell proliferation and maintenance of their inductive capabilities.

REGENERATION OF THE HAIR FOLLICLE FROM DISSOCIATED CELLS

A second approach, designed to create more hair follicles from the same number of donor follicles, consists of dissociated cell culture. Regeneration using dissociated cells has been tested in various models, mostly involving embryonic and neonatal mouse cells. The chamber assay[16,17] uses dissociated mouse neonatal dermal (MND) and mouse neonatal epidermal (MNE) cells combined (to a total of 10 million cells) and delivered into a silicon chamber already grafted onto the back of an immunocompromised (nu/nu) mouse. After 1 week, the chamber is removed to ultimately yield tufts of mouse hair on the back of the host mouse after 1 month, thereby indicating the trichogenic potential of the cells (**Fig. 1**). Zheng and colleagues[18] reported on the patch assay in 2005, which consists of a mixture of MND and MNE injected into the dermis of nu/nu mouse dorsal skin to generate hair after 10 to 14 days. Upwards of 10 samples were injected into a single mouse, with each injection using only 2 million total cells. Variations included placement of the cells into a kidney capsule or into a trachea.[12,19,20] In 2008, Qiao and colleagues[21] used a flap assay (a modification of the chamber assay) involving the use of a skin flap.

Recently, Lee and colleagues[22] combined aspects of the chamber assay and trichogenic patch assay to create a reconstituted hair assay in a nu/nu mouse model. Hair was formed using

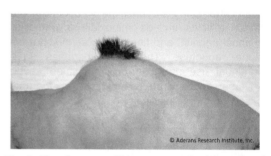

Fig. 1. Chamber assay. Mouse neonatal epidermal and dermal cells were isolated and delivered (at a concentration of 10×10^6) into a silicon chamber implanted in the dorsal region of a nu/nu mouse to generate a tuft of hair (1 week = chamber removed, 4 weeks = assay completed). (*Courtesy of* Aderans Research Institute Inc., Marietta, GA; with permission.)

dissociated cells placed under a membrane over a wound created on the dorsal side of the mouse. The technique is simpler and more efficient than the chamber assay and, although less efficient than the trichogenic patch, this method results in hair follicles observable from the surface of the skin. The graft can be made with flexibility into different shapes and sizes depending on cosmetic needs.

Hair follicles regenerated using dissociated cells in the patch assay[18] contain pigmented shafts complete with sebaceous glands and are characteristic of the donor (**Fig. 2**). The newly generated follicles cycle normally through anagen, catagen, and telogen. Generation of hair follicles in the patch assay as well as the chamber assay continues through multiple cycles when they are allowed to egress to the surface of the skin.

TRICHOGENIC MAINTENANCE OF DISSOCIATED CELLS

Initial studies took advantage of the intrinsic trichogenicity of cells isolated from dissociated tissue. Most successful in vivo hair reconstitutions from dissociated cells are from freshly isolated cells not cultured, expanded cells. Therefore, it is crucial to maintain inductive activity of cells in vitro as the cell number is expanded.

Rat vibrissa dermal papilla cells were first cultured in 1981 by Jahoda and Oliver[23] and later by Messenger in 1984.[24] Although DP and DS

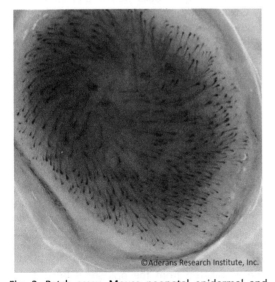

Fig. 2. Patch assay. Mouse neonatal epidermal and dermal cells were isolated and delivered (at a concentration of 2×10^6) into the dermis of the dorsal region of a nu/nu mouse to generate a cyst of hair in the mouse dermis (10–14 days = assay completed). (*Courtesy of* Aderans Research Institute Inc., Marietta, GA; with permission.)

cells can generate new hair follicles when implanted,[8,25–27] they lose their trichogenic potential rapidly following in vitro culture. Maintenance of trichogenicity in vitro has concentrated on culture medium supplementation[28] and the retention of a follicular DP gene expression profile.[29]

The addition of Wnt3a protein to culture media extended the inductivity of dermal cells in vitro.[30] Adding bone morphogenetic protein (BMP) to cultured mouse DP prolonged in vitro DP-specific marker expression and trichogenicity.[31] Osada and colleagues[32] discovered that basic fibroblast growth factor (FGF2) is critical to mouse vibrissae maintenance in vitro.

An interesting characteristic of early DP culture is that the cells primarily grow in aggregates immediately following isolation from tissue.[23,24,33] This phenomenon is lost throughout culture and may suggest a link between aggregation and trichogenic activity. Cultured mouse vibrissae DP cells lost their aggregation and trichogenicity over time in culture but recovered their trichogenicity, as well as DP-specific marker expression, following aggregation to spheres.[32]

In the mouse model, the relationship between follicular dermal cells and aggregation was further exploited by Fernandes and colleagues.[34] Miller's group demonstrated that a highly multipotent cell type, termed SKPs, are derived from the follicular portion of mouse dorsal skin. These cells self-select under appropriate culture conditions to form spheres. The cells that make up the spheres trace their origin to the follicular DP and DS and also express DP-specific markers SOX2, nestin, fibronectin, and vimentin. SKP cells can be passaged multiple times and are able to form new hair follicles in the patch assay as well as homing to and incorporating into existing follicles in a wound assay.

Work by Shimizu and colleagues[35] investigated the impact of aggregative culture on lung fibroblasts. The group discovered that aggregation upregulated LEF1, a transcription factor associated with the WNT pathway, a known follicular pathway. More striking was that long-term aggregative culture resulted in lung fibroblasts inducing hair formation in the patch assay, demonstrating the plasticity of cultured fibroblasts induced by their culture conditions.

Kang and colleagues[36] used aggregative culture techniques (spheroid culture) to restore the inductive ability of human DP cells. In these experiments, late-passage DP cells (P10) regained their inductive ability when cultured and assayed as spheroids. Clearly the microenvironment created by a 3-dimensional culture helps to maintain and induce trichogenic properties in dermal cells.

The majority of the work investigating cell based follicular neogenesis has focused on retaining or enhancing the trichogenicity of the dermal follicular progenitor cells. Much progress has been made to maintain dermal follicular progenitor cell trichogenicity; however, very little attention has been paid to the epidermal cells. Recently, Atit's group[37] clearly showed that the original signal resulting in hair follicle morphogenesis is initiated by the epidermal cells; therefore, it will be crucial to study the role of epidermal cells in follicle neogenesis and develop appropriate assays to evaluate the trichogenicity of epidermal cells. Recently, ARI improved the epidermal culture conditions of mouse neonatal cells. The improved culture condition resulted in an epidermal cell that was able to form an epidermal basal layer when injected in vivo. With this enhanced epidermal cell preparation, ARI was able to create a mouse follicle using cultured mouse-derived epidermal and dermal cells for the first time (Xunwei Wu, unpublished data, 2012).

REGENERATION OF HUMAN HAIR FOLLICLES IN VIVO

The hair reconstitution assays mentioned work very well with mouse cells; however, it has been a long-time challenge to regenerate human hair follicles in vivo. Recently, a big breakthrough was made by Li and colleagues,[38] who created human follicles from cultured dermal and epidermal cells in a nu/nu mouse model. In their initial work, TSC2 null fibroblasts were combined with foreskin keratinocytes in a skin construct model. Once a nascent epidermal basal layer was formed in vitro, the skin construct was grafted on the back of a nu/nu mouse. The continued development of the skin resulted in the formation of hair follicles and sebaceous glands. The initial work was repeated using DP-derived fibroblasts in place of the TSC2 null fibroblasts. This work represents the first published account of the formation of human hair from cultured cells. In a separate system, Higgins and colleagues[39] reported the formation of human hair using DP cells cultured as spheroids and combined with the epidermis of an excised human foreskin in a sandwich assay. For the first time, cultured human cells were used to form a completely human hair follicle. The expansion of these techniques provides a potentially unlimited supply of hair for the treatment of alopecia. ARI recently successfully generated human hair follicles by grafting dissociated and cultured expanded cells (manuscript in preparation). Taken together, it is expected that more mouse models with reconstituted human hair follicles regenerated will be seen in the near future. This will improve therapeutic product development for treating hair loss.

ALTERNATIVE CELLULAR SOURCES

A revolutionary breakthrough in the field of cell biology was the discovery of induced pluripotent stem cells (iPSCs). The work by Takahashi and colleagues[40] described the ability of 4 transcription factors (SOX2, OCT4, c-MYC, and KLF-4) to reprogram differentiated fibroblasts into an embryonic stem cell state. From these cells, the creation of every lineage is possible. Bilousova and colleagues[41] have exploited this process to produce a multipotent keratinocyte lineage from mouse iPSCs. Retinoic acid, BMP4, and a collagen IV substrate were used to push the fate of the iPSCs to a keratinocyte lineage. The keratinocytes produced by this method demonstrated the ability to form skin and all of its appendages including the hair follicle. Itoh and colleagues[42] used similar methods to generate human keratinocytes from iPSCs and produced 3-dimensional skin equivalents. In this human model, appendages were not produced, but the foundation of reprogramming iPSCs into keratinocytes was established. iPSCs represent an unlimited supply of cells for each patient. The potential will be unlocked as research groups develop methods to differentiate iPSCs into follicular progenitor cells.

The plasticity of cells was further established by Bonfanti and colleagues[43] who demonstrated microenvironmental reprogramming of thymic epithelial cells to skin multipotent cells. Cultured thymic epidermal cells were transformed into epidermal multipotent hair follicles when exposed to an inductive skin microenvironment. These experiments demonstrate that, with the right environment, cells from multiple sources could be used to develop cell-based therapy for alopecia.

FOLLICULAR NEOGENESIS

Hair follicle formation from dissociated cells progresses through similar morphologic stages and uses the same molecular pathways observed during follicular morphogenesis. The seminal work describing the morphogenesis in the human scalp was done by Karen Holbrook.[44] Follicular formation is initiated from the epidermal basal layer. The first morphologic evidence is the formation of the epidermal placode, which is followed by the dermal condensation, peg formation, and follicle formation. The molecular mechanisms underlying the reciprocal signaling between the dermal and epidermal cells are described in detail in the review by Millar.[45] In this work, WNT, Notch, BMP, and SHH pathways were identified as critical. These pathways and associated molecules have been used by multiple groups to maintain and induce trichogenicity in cultured cells.[30,31]

Zheng and colleagues[18] described the conservation of the morphogenesis process using dissociated dermal and epidermal cells. In this process, the injected epidermal cells formed an initial cyst. The outermost layer of the cyst provided the epidermal basal layer from which the injected dermal cells initiated follicles. The follicle morphogenesis progressed from placode, to peg to follicle, and when the cells were implanted in close proximity to the host epidermis, the cyst fused with the host skin, resulting in emergent hair follicles (**Fig. 3**).

In a different scenario, the host epithelium provides the epidermal cell source. McElwee and colleagues[8] injected cultured vibrissae dermal sheath cells into the ear of SCID (Severe Combined Immunodeficiency) mice. This treatment resulted in vibrissae-like follicles emerging from the mouse ear. Two mechanisms were proposed: the injected dermal cells induced follicle neogenesis with the host epithelium, or the injected dermal cells

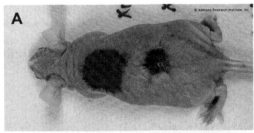

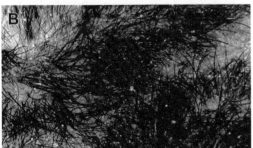

Fig. 3. Reconstituted hair assay. Mouse neonatal epidermal and dermal cells were isolated; epidermal cells were placed onto a silicon membrane and allowed to adhere. Dermal cells were placed on top of the epidermal cells, and the silicon membrane was flapped over a full-thickness wound on the dorsal side of a nu/nu mouse. (*A*) A tuft of hair was generated in 3 weeks. (*B*) A magnified view of the newly created hair. (*Courtesy of* Aderans Research Institute Inc, Marietta, GA; with permission.)

incorporated into existing follicles and transformed them into vibrissae follicles. The second mechanism implies a stem cell homing characteristic of follicular-derived dermal cells. Additional evidence of this homing was provided in the work of Bernaskie and colleagues.[46]

DELIVERY OF CELL THERAPY

Various methodologies of delivering cells into the scalp have been successful in producing emerging hair follicles that are cosmetically acceptable. The variations in these methodologies are dependent on the donor cell mechanisms, which initiate the formation of new hair. Superficial placement of donor cells can yield a completely new hair follicle through fusion of the epithelial component of the new follicle with the recipient scalp epidermis, facilitating shaft egress (**Fig. 4**). Alternatively, injection of donor cells into the upper dermis of the scalp, where the vellus follicles reside, can result in integration into existing follicles and initiation of these vellus follicles into terminal hairs (see **Fig. 4**). Through this methodology, the scalp's natural density, orientation, and distribution of resident hair follicles are leveraged to produce cosmetically acceptable hair growth. However, for cases where there is a loss of vellus hairs, as in cicatricial alopecias, this methodology may not be successful.

Recently, Toyoshima and colleagues[47] created a bioengineered hair follicle germ using embryonic skin-derived epithelium and mesenchymal donor cells. The transplanted germ integrated with the host epithelium, producing a fully functional hair follicle demonstrating connection to the host nerves as well as to the piloerection ability. They further demonstrated that through the use of a guide, the interaction between these donor cells and the host epithelium was independent of placement depth. Taken together, these studies demonstrate that cells delivered in the appropriate package are able to integrate with the host tissue to produce a hair follicle. This technique would provide the clinician the ability to control the pattern, density, and orientation of the follicles resulting from this cell-based therapy.

FUTURE DIRECTIONS

Recent developments in the field of regenerative medicine indicate that a cell-based solution for alopecia is coming soon. Multiple groups have produced human hair follicles using cultured cells in a mouse model. Strategies are being developed to expand and maintain trichogenic cells in culture. iPS cells provide an additional strategy to

Native Morphogenetic Pathway

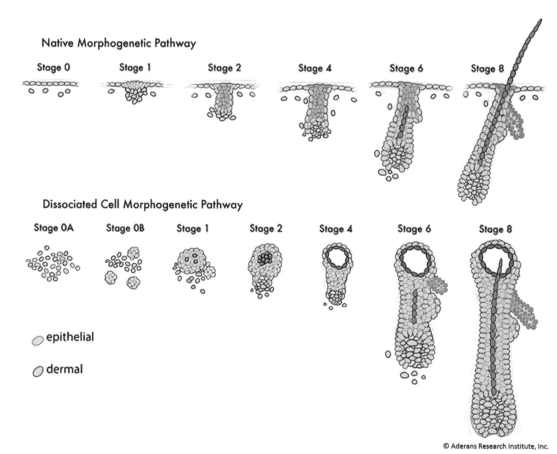

© Aderans Research Institute, Inc.

Fig. 4. Morphogenesis. Follicular morphogenesis is orchestrated by reciprocal signaling between dermal and epidermal cells. The initial morphologic evidence is the formation of the epidermal placode (stage 1). The morphologic events are identical for both the native and dissociated cell morphogenetic pathways. (*Courtesy of* Aderans Research Institute Inc., Marietta, GA; with permission.)

obtain follicular progenitor cells. The challenge is to exploit these methods and determine the most efficient and efficacious method of culture, expansion, and delivery of follicular progenitor cells.

A major hurdle to a cell-based solution to alopecia is the development of a clinically relevant model of the human scalp. Currently there is no laboratory model that allows for the investigation of the delivery of cells into the human scalp and the mode of action in a cell-based therapy. Without a model, it is difficult to determine the appropriate method of delivery, cell types, and cell ratios to achieve therapeutic efficacy.

REFERENCES

1. Orentreich N. Autografts in alopecias and other selected dermatologial conditions. Ann N Y Acad Sci 1959;83:463–79.

2. Ellis JA, Sinclair RD. Male pattern baldness: current treatments, future prospects. Drug Discov Today 2008;13(17–18):791–7.

3. Stenn KS, Paus R. Controls of hair follicle cycling. Physiol Rev 2001;81(1):449–94.

4. Cohen J. The transplantation of individual rat and guineapig whisker papillae. J Embryol Exp Morphol 1961;9:117–27.

5. Horne KA, Jahoda CA. Restoration of hair growth by surgical implantation of follicular dermal sheath. Development 1992;116:563–71.

6. Jahoda CA. Induction of follicle formation and hair growth by vibrissa dermal papillae implanted into rat ear wounds: vibrissa-type fibres are specified. Development 1992;115(4):1103–9.

7. Jahoda CA, Oliver RF, Reynolds AJ, et al. Human hair follicle regeneration following amputation and grafting into the nude mouse. J Invest Dermatol 1996;107(6):804–7.

8. McElwee KJ, Kissling S, Wenzel E, et al. Cultured peribulbar dermal sheath cells can induce hair

follicle development and contribute to the dermal sheath and dermal papilla. J Invest Dermatol 2003; 121(6):1267–75.

9. Oliver RF. Ectopic regeneration of whiskers in the hooded rat from implanted lengths of vibrissa follicle wall. J Embryol Exp Morphol 1967;17:27–34.

10. Oliver RF. The induction of hair follicle formation in the adult hooded rat by vibrissa dermal papillae. J Embryol Exp Morphol 1970;23:219–36.

11. Blanpain C, Lowry WE, Geoghegan A, et al. Self-renewal, multipotency, and the existence of two cell populations within an epithelial stem cell niche. Cell 2004;118(5):635–48.

12. Morris RJ, Liu Y, Marles L, et al. Capturing and profiling adult hair follicle stem cells. Nat Biotechnol 2004;22(4):411–7.

13. Kim JC, Kim MK, Choi YC. Regeneration of the human scalp hair follicle after horizontal sectioning: implications for pluripotent stem cells and melanocyte reservoir. In: Van Neste D, Randall VA, editors. Hair research for the next millennium. Amsterdam: Elsevier; 1996. p. 135–9.

14. Tang L, Madani S, Liu H, et al. Regeneration of a new hair follicle from the upper half of a human hair follicle in a nude mouse. J Invest Dermatol 2002;119(4):983–4.

15. Reynolds AJ, Lawrence C, Cserhalmi-Frideman PB, et al. Trans-gender induction of hair follicles. Nature 1999;402(6757):33–4.

16. Lichti U, Weinberg WC, Goodman L, et al. In vivo regulation of murine hair growth: insights from grafting defined cell populations onto nude mice. J Invest Dermatol 1993;101(Suppl 1):124S–9S.

17. Prouty SM, Lawrence L, Stenn S. Fibroblast-dependent induction of a murine skin lesion with similarity to human common blue nevus. Am J Pathol 1996; 148(6):1871–85.

18. Zheng Y, Du X, Wang W, et al. Organogenesis from dissociated cells: generation of mature cycling hair follicles from skin-derived cells. J Invest Dermatol 2005;124(5):867–76.

19. Gilmour SK, Teti KA, Wu KQ, et al. A simple in vivo system for studying epithelialization, hair follicle formation, and invasion using primary epidermal cells from wild-type and transgenic ornithine decarboxylase-overexpressing mouse skin. J Invest Dermatol 2001; 117(6):1674–6.

20. Kobayashi K, Nishimura E. Ectopic growth of mouse whiskers from implanted lengths of plucked vibrissa follicles. J Invest Dermatol 1989;92(2):278–82.

21. Qiao J, Philips E, Teumer J. A graft model for hair development. Exp Dermatol 2008;17(6):512–8.

22. Lee LF, Jiang TX, Garner W, et al. A simplified procedure to reconstitute hair-producing skin. Tissue Eng Part C Methods 2011;17(4):391–400.

23. Jahoda C, Oliver RF. The growth of vibrissa dermal papilla cells in vitro. Br J Dermatol 1981;105(6):623–7.

24. Messenger AG. The culture of dermal papilla cells from human hair follicles. Br J Dermatol 1984; 110(6):685–9.

25. Horne KA, Jahoda CA, Oliver RF. Whisker growth induced by implantation of cultured vibrissa dermal papilla cells in the adult rat. J Embryol Exp Morphol 1986;97:111–24.

26. Jahoda CA, Horne KA, Oliver RF. Induction of hair growth by implantation of cultured dermal papilla cells. Nature 1984;311(5986):560–2.

27. Jahoda CA, Reynolds AJ, Oliver RF. Induction of hair growth in ear wounds by cultured dermal papilla cells. J Invest Dermatol 1993;101(4):584–90.

28. Botchkarev VA, Paus R. Molecular biology of hair morphogenesis: development and cycling. J Exp Zool B Mol Dev Evol 2003;298(1):164–80.

29. Rendl M, Lewis L, Fuchs E. Molecular dissection of mesenchymal-epithelial interactions in the hair follicle. PLoS Biol 2005;3(11):e331.

30. Kishimoto J, Burgeson RE, Morgan BA. Wnt signaling maintains the hair-inducing activity of the dermal papilla. Genes Dev 2000;14(10):1181–5.

31. Rendl M, Polak L, Fuchs E. BMP signaling in dermal papilla cells is required for their hair follicle-inductive properties. Genes Dev 2008;22(4):543–57.

32. Osada A, Iwabuchi T, Kishimoto J, et al. Long-term culture of mouse vibrissal dermal papilla cells and de novo hair follicle induction. Tissue Eng 2007; 13(5):975–82.

33. Jahoda CA, Oliver RF. Vibrissa dermal papilla cell aggregative behaviour in vivo and in vitro. J Embryol Exp Morphol 1984;79:211–24.

34. Fernandes KJ, McKenzie IA, Mill P, et al. A dermal niche for multipotent adult skin-derived precursor cells. Nat Cell Biol 2004;6(11):1082–93.

35. Shimizu R, Okabe K, Kubota Y, et al. Sphere formation restores and confers hair-inducing capacity in cultured mesenchymal cells. Exp Dermatol 2011; 20(8):679–81.

36. Kang BM, Kwack MH, Kim MK, et al. Sphere formation increases the ability of cultured human dermal papilla cells to induce hair follicles from mouse epidermal cells in a reconstitution assay. J Invest Dermatol 2012;132(1):237–9.

37. Chen D, Jarrell A, Guo C, et al. Dermal β-catenin activity in response to epidermal Wnt ligands is required for fibroblast proliferation and hair follicle initiation. Development 2012;139(8):1522–33.

38. Li S, Thangaparzham RL, Wang JA, et al. Human TSC2-null fibroblast-like cells induce hair follicle neogenesis and hamartoma morphogenesis. Nat Commun 2011;2:235.

39. Higgins C, Jahoda CA, Christiano AM. Human hair follicle neogenesis using dermal papilla cells. J Investig Dermatol Symp Proc 2012;132:S135–48.

40. Takahashi K, Yamanaka S. Induction of pluripotent stem cells from mouse embryonic and adult

fibroblast cultures by defined factors. Cell 2006; 126(4):663–76.

41. Bilousova G, Chen J, Roop DR. Differentiation of mouse induced pluripotent stem cells into a multipotent keratinocyte lineage. J Invest Dermatol 2011; 131(4):857–64.

42. Itoh M, Kiuru M, Cairo MS, et al. Generation of keratinocytes from normal and recessive dystrophic epidermolysis bullosa-induced pluripotent stem cells. Proc Natl Acad Sci U S A 2011;108(21):8797–802.

43. Bonfanti P, Claudinot S, Amici AW, et al. Microenvironmental reprogramming of thymic epithelial cells to skin multipotent stem cells. Nature 2010; 466(7309):978–82.

44. Holbrook KA, Minami SI. Hair follicle embryogenesis in the human. Characterization of events in vivo and in vitro. Ann N Y Acad Sci 1991;642:167–96.

45. Millar SE. Molecular mechanisms regulating hair follicle development. J Invest Dermatol 2002;118(2): 216–25.

46. Biernaskie J, Paris M, Morozova O, et al. SKPs derive from hair follicle precursors and exhibit properties of adult dermal stem cells. Cell Stem Cell 2009;5(6):610–23.

47. Toyoshima KE, Asakawa K, Ishibashi N, et al. Fully functional hair follicle regeneration through the rearrangement of stem cells and their niches. Nat Commun 2012;3:784.

Index

Note: Page numbers of article titles are in **boldface** type.

Facial Plast Surg Clin N Am 21 (2013) 529–549
http://dx.doi.org/10.1016/S1064-7406(13)00113-2

H

Moving?

Make sure your subscription moves with you!

To notify us of your new address, find your **Clinics Account Number** (located on your mailing label above your name), and contact customer service at:

Email: journalscustomerservice-usa@elsevier.com

800-654-2452 (subscribers in the U.S. & Canada)
314-447-8871 (subscribers outside of the U.S. & Canada)

Fax number: 314-447-8029

Elsevier Health Sciences Division
Subscription Customer Service
3251 Riverport Lane
Maryland Heights, MO 63043

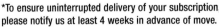

*To ensure uninterrupted delivery of your subscription, please notify us at least 4 weeks in advance of move.

ELSEVIER

Printed and bound by CPI Group (UK) Ltd, Croydon, CR0 4YY

03/10/2024

01040370-0002